# 28 stories of AIDS in africa

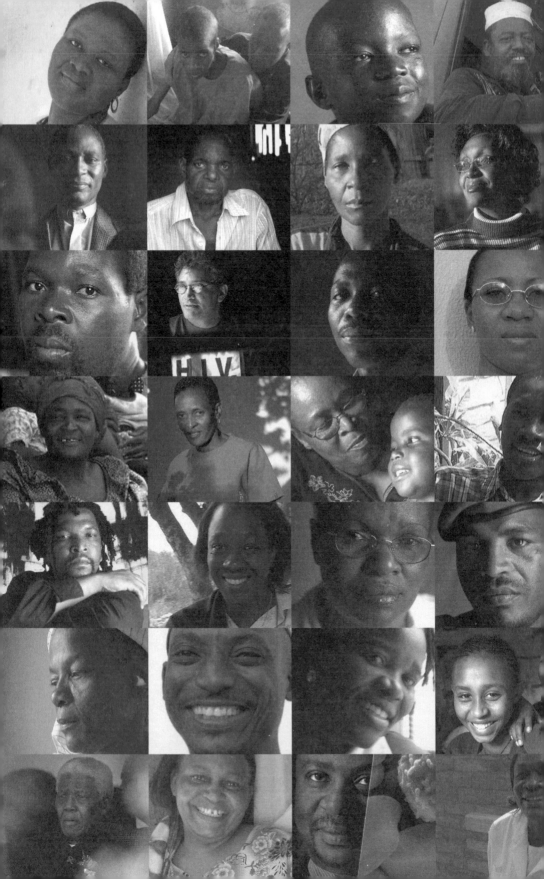

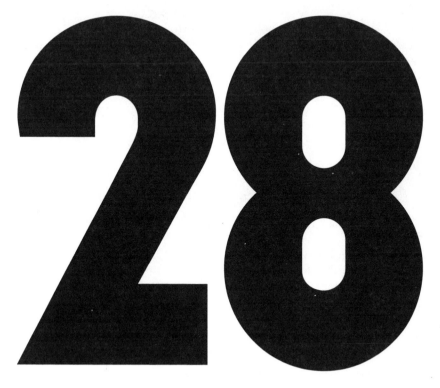

# 28

## stories of AIDS in africa

STEPHANIE NOLEN

*Portobello*
BOOKS

Published by Portobello Books Ltd 2007

Portobello Books Ltd
Eardley House
4 Uxbridge Street
Notting Hill Gate
London W8 7SY, UK

A CIP catalogue record is available from the British Library

9 8 7 6 5 4 3 2 1

ISBN 978 1 84627 037 6

www.portobellobooks.com

Designed by C S Richardson

Printed in Great Britain by MPG Books Ltd, Bodmin, Cornwall

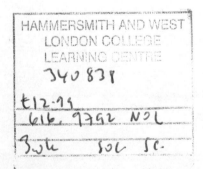

# CONTENTS

# HIV/AIDS PREVALENCE IN SUB-SAHARAN AFRICA

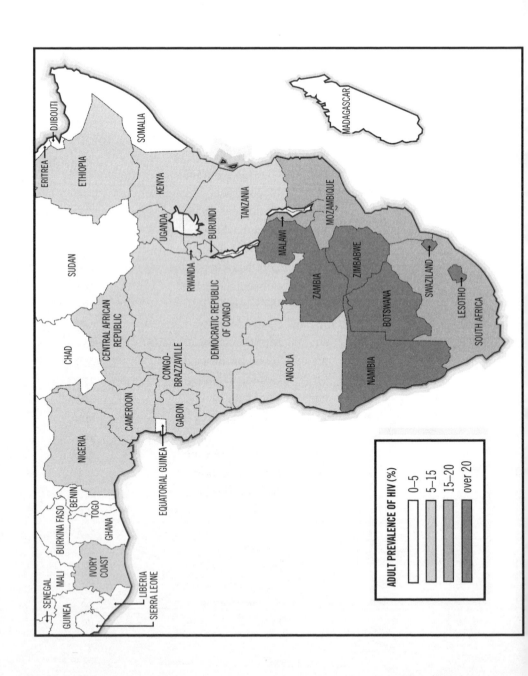

# 28 STORIES ACROSS SUB-SAHARAN AFRICA

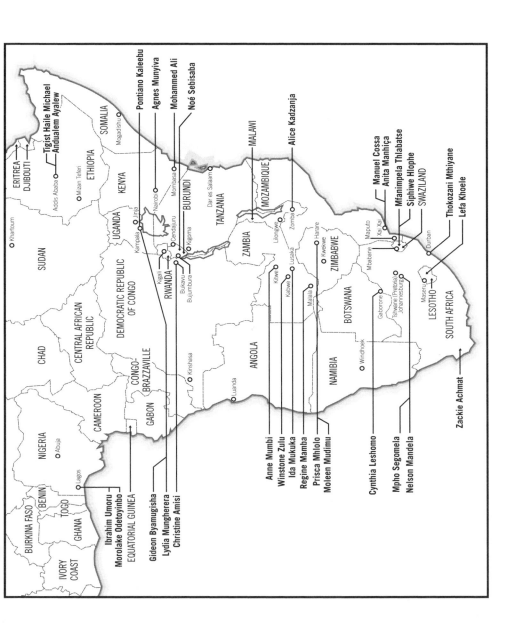

# Why28

I looked at AIDS in Africa for a long time before I understood what I was seeing. That moment came on the shady porch of a small mud-brick house in a village called Nkhotakota in Malawi, early in 2002. The house belonged to Lillian Chandawili. She was thirty-five years old, and I met her through the local AIDS organization. We sat in the softening heat of the late afternoon and she told me how she was raising her five children on her own—her husband was gone. She confided that she was plagued by diarrhea and a racking cough; some days she barely had the strength to lift a hoe, but her little plot of land was the only source of food for her family.

While we talked, Lillian's children ventured up to sit near us, and neighbours and relatives stopped by, polite and eager to greet a visitor. There were a great many children. Lillian explained that in addition to her five she was raising two of her late sister's children and two orphaned cousins. She laid one gentle hand on their heads as they crept in close—"This one has it," she said. "And this one, I think he's infected." When the neighbours moved on, she gestured with a lift of her chin at one or another—"She is infected. He is positive. Her husband is dying. He lost his wife."

And as I listened, I suddenly understood that it wasn't just Lillian and the dozen people in her support group in Nkhotakota who had AIDS. On paper, it was one in six adults in Malawi. But in this village, it was hundreds of people. If they weren't sick themselves, they were caring for the sick. They were sheltering their sisters' orphans, their dead brother's young wife and baby. One way or another, everyone had the disease. And it meant that they earned less, that they grew less food, that fewer children went to school, that no one had any savings.

# I looked at AIDS in Africa
## I understood

Lillian talked of all the people who had "passed," and I had a sense of a community quietly evaporating around me.

A few days later, in the Malawian capital, Lilongwe, I set out early one morning for the main hospital, where the lone doctor in charge had agreed to speak to me about the country's HIV epidemic. When I got to the hospital, however, no one was quite sure where he was, and people suggested I try one ward or another, check this corridor or that office. I wandered the halls in a state of growing horror. I had by that point seen many basic and overcrowded African hospitals, but never anything like this. There were people everywhere: three to a bed, lying head to foot to head; under the beds, lying on grass mats in the stairwells and in the verandas off the wards. They were bone thin and covered in lesions and abscesses. As I stepped gingerly among them, they shifted their heads slightly to look up at me through eyes grown huge in sunken faces. I could not find the doctor; I did find a nurse—perhaps the only nurse—who was stout and slovenly and clearly drunk, her hairpiece of copper curls askew. Looking around the ward, I couldn't blame her: it was barely 8 a.m., but I felt in desperate need of a stiff drink myself.

I had realized, long before that day, that AIDS was a unique and savage phenomenon in Africa. Back in 1998, in a rural hospital in Tanzania, the chief medical officer had led me on a tour of the wards. In one, we passed rows of antique but tidy beds lined up under billowy mosquito nets. Then we came to three men off by themselves, lying in a row on a thin mat on the floor. Their legs were like twigs, and their breathing was audible from the other side of the room. I was puzzled at first, and stopped in front of them. Then realized what this must be.

## for a long time before what I was seeing.

"Do they have AIDS?" I asked.

The doctor and his assistants whipped around. A nurse seized my arm and began to pull me out of the ward.

"*Shh, shh, shh,*" she scolded. "You can't just say that word."

The sight of those men stayed with me. Over the next few years, I kept going back to Africa, drawn to what I began to believe was the biggest story in the world. Not the wars or the refugee crises that occasionally—very occasionally—made the evening news back home, but the slow, almost incalculable devastation that HIV/AIDS was wreaking in country after country I visited.

I know something about what makes news. In the fifteen years I have worked as a journalist, I have reported on some of the biggest stories in the world. I watched Yasser Arafat and the Palestine Liberation Organization move into the West Bank after making peace with Israel in the early 1990s. I saw tentative women venture out of their homes for the first time in five years as the Taliban lost their hold on Afghanistan. I watched Saddam Hussein's army flee Baghdad in the face of an onslaught of U.S. Marines. There is an undeniable thrill that comes with being in the centre of the big story.

But nothing I was sent to cover anywhere in the world compared to what I saw AIDS doing in sub-Saharan Africa. And yet this story never made the news at all.

In 2003, I persuaded my editors at *The Globe and Mail* that we were missing something important. They did not yet share my conviction about the urgency of the story, but they were willing to let me try to tell it. I moved to Johannesburg and began what would turn out to be years of travel through the heart of the epidemic: the Swazi villages, the slums outside Durban, the highlands of Lesotho, the urban hospitals of Botswana. I found hundreds and hundreds of communities like Nkhotakota on the verge of disappearing. I knew people in North America who had been living with HIV for years, taking antiretroviral medication that does not cure AIDS but will keep a person with HIV healthy for decades. But no one in Africa had the drugs. No one was even talking about getting them the drugs. AIDS was a fully preventable illness at home. But in Africa, it was a plague, and people like Lillian Chandawili could do little but sit and watch its inexorable progression. And I began to wonder how this could be happening—how we could be *letting* this happen—almost entirely unremarked.

Over the years, I've learned the way to work in war zones: get in, get the story, write it down, get out without getting hurt. Reporting on AIDS is different. You don't get in and get out on a story like this: you get in, and sit down, and start a very long conversation. AIDS is not an event, or a series of them; it's a mirror held up to the cultures and societies we build. The pandemic, and how we respond to it, forces us to confront the sticky issues of sex and drugs and inequity. The relentless spread of this one virus raises difficult questions about why we do the things we do, why we believe what we believe—about who we are and what we value.

In a Botswana research lab in 2003, I saw the human immunodeficiency virus through an electron-microscope for the first time. And I gasped out loud: HIV *looks* nasty, a sphere bristling with small vicious spikes. One vaccine researcher in South Africa later confessed to me that she always pictures HIV with clawed feet and fangs; another told me he could swear that sometimes, when he is injecting the virus into cell cultures, he hears it give a B-movie villain's ominous chuckle.

The more I learned about the virus, the better I understood these brief episodes of melodrama in otherwise rational people. We know more about HIV than we do about any microbe—any germ, any bacterium or virus—in history. But HIV is both devious and complex in the way it operates, and it has thwarted more than twenty-five years of scientific effort to render it harmless or even slow its march.

HIV belongs to a group of pathogens known as retroviruses, which carry their genetic material not in the familiar double-stranded loop of DNA but on a single piece of RNA. HIV, like all viruses, cannot replicate on its own but needs a host cell; when it enters the body, it goes looking for the kind it likes best. These are a variety of white blood cells called lymphocytes—the ones that normally fight off infection. On their surface, they are studded with molecules with the rather unglamorous names of CCR5 and CD4. For HIV, these act like a piece of Velcro: when the virus finds those molecules, it binds to them, using its own surface as the matching piece of Velcro, and forces its way in. In a move worthy of science fiction, it commandeers the cell's DNA and turns it into a factory, churning out copies of itself. One cell can produce ten thousand new viruses. These burst out of the host cell, destroying it in the process, and make their way through the body, looking for more cells to invade and start the process again. Within days of infection, millions of copies of the virus have burrowed into the lymph nodes, and they can hide out there—resisting the toughest barrage of drugs—only to pop out and start reproducing years later. It takes only ten days for HIV to spread to the brain and other major organs; by then, a single drop of blood from an infected person contains 100 million viruses.

After a couple of weeks of this assault, the body musters a response. It produces new killer T cells; these can drive the virus back, but they can't eliminate it. Instead, a slow war starts between the virus and the immune system. In some people, depending on which of the several different strains of the virus they have, how healthy they were to start and other factors that remain a mystery, this part of the fight can take a couple of years or more than a decade. But eventually, inevitably, the virus wins: the immune system is destroyed, and the person succumbs to one or a series of infectious diseases that someone without the virus might easily fight off. From an evolutionary point of view, it's a brilliant strategy: HIV lets its host live long enough to pass the virus on to plenty of other people.

By the standards of virologists, HIV is only a moderately infectious bug: it's not that easy to catch, unlike tuberculosis or Ebola—you can't get it from being breathed on or shaking hands, and a single exposure does not

# AIDS is not an event, or a
## it's a mirror held up to

guarantee infection. The problem with HIV is that its transmission, in blood and sexual fluids and breast milk, preys on our most intimate moments. It targets the subjects we least like to discuss—the drugs we inject, the sex we have, especially the sex with people we aren't supposed to have sex with—and the interactions least open to honest discussion or to change. HIV grows best in imbalances of power; it has erupted and spread out from the most marginalized groups in human societies, from sex workers and drug users and gay men and migrants. And so we have been correspondingly slow to respond.

The recorded history of AIDS begins in the United States in 1981, when doctors in New York and San Francisco noticed an outbreak of several unusual diseases, including a very rare skin cancer and a severe pneumonia, among gay men. The phenomenon began to be known as GRID—gay-related immune deficiency—and the Centers for Disease Control in Atlanta soon began to suspect that it was sexually transmitted. While the CDC said at first that there was "no apparent danger to non-homosexuals from contagion," cases of the same rare bugs were soon being reported among heterosexual injecting drug users. By July 1982, a total of 452 cases had been reported to the CDC, and the next month, the name of the new disease was changed to acquired immune deficiency syndrome, or AIDS. It began to show up in hemophiliacs—igniting fears that it might be carried in the blood supply—and then in recent immigrants from Haiti. By 1984, teams of French and American researchers had isolated the virus that caused the disease, and designed a test to screen for it; after some debate, they agreed to call it the human immunodeficiency virus, or HIV.

This is the standard story of the "emergence" of AIDS: it erupted overnight in the bathhouses and leather bars of New York and California; a hemophiliac child, Ryan White, was barred from school; and Rock Hudson

series of them;
the cultures and societies
we build.

died. Haitian boat people were interned; ACT UP took to the streets; Diana, the Princess of Wales, had her picture taken embracing infected people; and there was a dawning awareness that more than just gay men were at risk. But not until the mid-1980s, as researchers began to consider the question of where AIDS might have come from, did the scientific establishment in the developed world begin to realize that in fact an epidemic not just isolated incidences of the disease but a plague of terrifying scale— was already well under way on the other side of the world.

Nobody was asking—but if they had, doctors and nurses at rural clinics and mission hospitals in the Rakai district in Uganda could have told them that something momentous had been happening as far back as the mid-1970s. They saw larger and larger numbers of previously healthy young people turning up stick thin with recurrent diarrhea, tuberculosis all through their bodies (not just in the lungs) and oral thrush, none of which responded to treatment. Locally, they had taken to calling the illness Slim, in a macabre understatement. But these hospitals were far away from the surveillance sites and the careful monitoring of the CDC. And one more outbreak of mysterious disease in Africa didn't raise an international eyebrow.

In 1983 doctors in Zambia and what was then Zaire began to suspect a connection between the emergence of a viciously aggressive form of Kaposi's sarcoma, the rare skin cancer, in their patients and the new disease being reported among gay men in North America. That year, two teams of North American and European researchers went looking for HIV in central Africa for the first time, and found several dozen cases of what was clearly AIDS in Kigali and Kinshasa—all of them among heterosexuals. In 1985, Ugandan doctors did a survey of one hundred patients in Rakai, diagnosed twenty-nine with the symptoms of Slim, and used the new test for HIV antibodies to check their blood for the virus. All of them came back HIV-positive. In 1986, Rwanda became the first country in the world to do a national survey of HIV prevalence, covering everyone from babies to the elderly. The results exceeded even the worst nightmares of the government: a staggering 17.8 per cent of people in cities were already infected. Only 1.3 per cent of people in rural areas—the majority of the population—tested positive, but this offered faint consolation. In epidemiological terms, anything above one per cent is considered a "generalized epidemic," indicating that a disease is spreading in the population as a whole and is difficult to control.

Physicians working in East Africa started to reconsider cases they had treated in the late 1970s in Kampala and Dar es Salaam, cases which in hindsight they were sure were AIDS. Starting in the mid-1980s, blood samples collected in central Africa for other studies (such as the presence of malarial parasites) and kept frozen were retested, looking for HIV. The results were astounding: the virus was already present in the former Belgian Congo, Rwanda and Burundi in anywhere up to 3 per cent of the population, in the 1970s. One sample, generally regarded as the oldest confirmed case of HIV, had been taken from a Congolese man in Léopoldville in 1959. Clearly the disease had been in central Africa much longer than it had in North America. (This provides one possible explanation for HIV's early appearance in Haiti. When Congo won independence in 1960, the Belgian colonial rulers decamped en masse, leaving just nine people with college degrees in the country. The UN recruited thousands of Haitian professionals to help build the new country; some may have carried the virus with them when they returned to Haiti a few years later.)

But where did AIDS come from in the first place, and how did it suddenly appear in people in central Africa in the 1950s or '60s? These questions have been the subject of ferocious debate over the past twenty-five years, much of it the result of rigorous scientific investigation and some the product of good old-fashioned conspiracy theory. Gradually, the pieces of the puzzle are falling into place—we know, in broad strokes, how it happened, although plenty of smaller questions remain unanswered. By unravelling the genetic threads of HIV, researchers have found that it is a descendant of SIV, simian immunodeficiency virus. HIV comes in two types. HIV-2, the more rare strain of the virus, descends from a strain of SIV found in the sooty mangabey, which is indigenous to western Africa. HIV-1, the much more common and lethal form of the virus, comes from an SIV found in chimpanzees. Viruses can jump between species, including into humans. This process, called zoonosis, occurs fairly often (think of the global panic caused by bird flu). And a microbe that causes no symptoms, or only mild ones, in its original species can frequently morph into something deadly in its new host.

How did SIV become a human virus? The most widely accepted theory involves the hunting and consumption of monkeys, which was common through most of the last century in much of Africa, although rare now because some primates, such as chimpanzees, are protected species, and because many have been hunted nearly to extinction. This theory posits that a person killing or skinning a monkey or preparing it for the pot cut himself and got monkey blood—including the virus—in his system. The virus survived, to be passed on through blood and other bodily fluids in a new and increasingly lethal form. This has to have happened at least twice, once for HIV-1 and once for HIV-2, in different parts of Africa, and some scientists argue that it has to have happened a dozen times to explain every subtype of the virus.

In mid-2006, Beatrice Hahn and her team of researchers at the University of Alabama, who have traced the genetic relationship between HIV and SIV for more than a decade, analyzed the feces from hundreds of wild chimpanzees in central Africa and, in an astounding piece of detective work, reached the conclusion that HIV-1 jumped to a human from a chimpanzee in southeast Cameroon about seventy years ago. Hahn and her colleagues were able to pinpoint the date because viruses mutate at a fairly constant rate. We know how fast HIV changes, and so comparing the oldest known HIV strain with its progenitor chimpanzee virus, they worked backwards and deduced when the two diverged and one crossed the species barrier.

The puzzle piece that is still missing, and may never be known, is how the virus got from one person in Cameroon down to Kinshasa, a thousand miles away—because the stored blood samples and the infection levels of the late 1970s make clear that the disease first began to spread widely in the urban environment in Congo. While it may seem remarkable that HIV could be present in humans for fifty years before being identified, and reach such a vast number twenty-five years later, in fact this is the classic pattern for the spread of a moderately infectious agent. Some researchers also believe that once HIV had a firm foothold in central Africa, its spread was accelerated by the widespread use of unsterilized needles in mass vaccination campaigns and by rural health clinics. Records of early vaccination efforts in central and East Africa show that many thousands of people were vaccinated over several days using fewer than a half-dozen needles.

The idea that the virus had come from Africa—one more disaster from the Dark Continent—was seized upon in the West in the late 1980s, and many African leaders, sensing the racism that lay behind the enthusiasm for the theory, dug in their heels in response. They denied AIDS was a problem, long past the point that their countries were in grave trouble. Yet there is little doubt about the origin of AIDS: monkeys from Asia and South America have never been found to have viruses related to HIV. And however the jump happened, by the 1960s a virulent strain of HIV was unquestionably circulating in the population of central Africa (and a less vicious one in West Africa, originating out of the Portuguese colony of Guinea-Bissau). Then individuals—well-travelled sailors and flight attendants in particular—took the virus to North America and Europe, and it found fertile ground in the heady days of gay liberation in the United States.

Back in Africa, Slim was being reported in communities of traders, smugglers and prostitutes on the shores of Lake Victoria, near the borders of Tanzania, Rwanda and Uganda, in the early 1970s. As urbanization increased, and people migrated seeking work, the disease began to move into the general population, and by the time AIDS was a recognized global health problem, the pandemic was raging across Africa: nearly one in five adults had the virus in Uganda in 1990; a survey in Francistown, Botswana, in 1993 found that 37 per cent of pregnant women were infected. When I set out to write this book, in 2005, 70 per cent of the burden of disease in the global pandemic was in sub-Saharan Africa. At least twenty million Africans had died.

AIDS has now been reported in every country in the world, and it is present in epidemic levels in many. Some 37 million people around the world are living with the virus. In terms of absolute numbers of people infected, India is the country with the worst epidemic, while the fastest spread of the disease is occurring in Russia and the Ukraine, among injecting drug users and prisoners. China, too, has a looming AIDS crisis, with an estimated 1 million people infected but very limited public knowledge of the disease. But AIDS in Africa is unique. The epidemics in eastern Europe and Asia do not compare to what is happening in sub-Saharan Africa: the disease is spreading quickly in Russia, yes, but the prevalence, the percentage of people with HIV in the population, is barely one per cent. And while India has six million people infected, the country's huge population means the prevalence is still less than one per cent. Consequently, the impact on the economy and on society is marginal. Africa—where some countries have an HIV prevalence greater than 30 per cent—offers a lesson for all of these places, a grim example of what happens when we don't react quickly or with openness to the spread of HIV.

There is always a danger in talking about "Africa"—as if it were one place, one country, one homogeneous story. Africa is fifty-three countries, many of which are themselves made up of hundreds of peoples and cultures. Prosperous South Africa has more in common with France than it does with anarchic Somalia or the deserts of Mali. And there is no one monolithic story of AIDS in Africa. HIV infection rates range from 43 per cent of pregnant women in Swaziland in the southern tip of the continent to less than one per cent in Senegal on the west coast. And yet there are factors common across sub-Saharan African countries, from the legacy of colonialism to the patterns of conflict and migrant labour, that have had a direct influence on how the story of AIDS unfolded in the region.

A great many things made Africa particularly susceptible to AIDS, some of them innate to the communities where the disease flourished, and

# The problem with HIV is in blood and sexual fluids preys on our most

many others imposed from outside. The key factor is poverty. Put simply, millions of Africans are living with a virus from which they might easily have been protected if they had had access to education about it, or to the means of defending themselves. At the same time, their lack of resources led them to do things—to sell sex, to stay with a philandering husband, to leave their families and seek work far away—that they might not otherwise have done; this too spread the disease. And the destitution and weakness of many sub-Saharan states crippled their ability to respond once their populations were infected. Congo didn't have the surveillance systems to detect or track the disease when it first emerged; Kenya didn't have the money to reach its populations with protective measures; Zambia didn't have the nurses or doctors to care for the sick; Lesotho couldn't buy the drugs that would have saved the dying.

That poverty has its roots first in the slave trade, when the Western world's pillaging of Africa began, and in the colonial era, when Africa was viewed as one huge source of raw materials for the European powers, its economies deliberately undeveloped, its peoples kept, often through violent repression, as a sort of indentured workforce. Independence didn't make things much better: hard on the heels of the liberation struggles of the 1960s came the Cold War, and a different sort of meddling. The superpowers used Africa as a board in their global chess game, arming insurgencies such as Mozambique's RENAMO, propping up cooperative tyrants, assassinating elected leaders—as the CIA did Congo's Patrice Lumumba—and warping politics and development all across the region in their ideological battle and quest for control of Africa's rich resources. In the 1980s came a new focus on development and poverty alleviation, but this was little help. The massive international financial institutions, the World Bank and the

## that its transmission, and breast milk, intimate moments.

International Monetary Fund, ordered the most debt-ridden African nations to overhaul their economies or find themselves cut off from assistance. It may have looked like a good idea at the time, but structural adjustment, as it became known, was one more disaster: its ill-conceived user fees denied poor people access to whatever health and education systems existed, while its other interventions failed to produce significant economic growth. Then, in the 1990s, when more than a century of foreign meddling had reduced much of the continent to a corrupt, conflict-torn, impoverished mess, the rich donor countries in North America and Europe refused to send more money to bail out African governments, asking how they could possibly be expected to put funding into such a disaster.

On AIDS in particular, on the pandemic that emerged as an "African problem" at the height of this donor fatigue, there has been a monstrous failure to fund a response anything near commensurate with the scale of the crisis. The United Nations said the global response to AIDS needed $6.6 billion in 1999; donor nations gave $560 million. (These and all other figures are in U.S. dollars.) Eight years later, the funding gap has scarcely narrowed. In 2002, the UN created the Global Fund to Fight AIDS, Tuberculosis and Malaria, intended to target the pandemic and two of its most deadly co-infections with swift and comprehensive programs. The fund struggled, from its first days, to cover its pledges to AIDS-ravaged countries; by mid-2006, it had a billion-dollar shortfall.

That said, some of the blame for the gravity of the AIDS crisis rests on the shoulders of Africans. The continent has been plagued by massive failures of leadership: by corrupt despots who plundered state coffers and exercised brutal repression on movements for democracy, and specifically by heads of state and local government who chose to shun and condemn people with

AIDS rather than mobilizing resources to assist them. People in many parts of the continent still maintain cultural and social practices—such as having multiple concurrent sexual partners and eschewing condoms—in the face of the horrible evidence of what AIDS is doing to their communities.

When I started to write about AIDS, my editors asked a sensible question: Why single out this disease when there is so much "wrong" in Africa? Why is AIDS any different from the famines and the wars and the corruption and the dozens of other terrible diseases, the shortage of schools and clinics and clean water?

The difference is that AIDS underlies all of these things—that it is amplifying the damage even as it undermines the ability to respond. Because it targets the young, productive generation, AIDS robs countries of the people who grow the food and work in the factories and teach in the schools. It makes existing epidemics of tuberculosis and malaria a thousandfold more lethal. It makes countries more vulnerable to political instability and environmental disasters. In country after country, AIDS is stealing away the hard-won gains of the past couple of decades, lowering school enrolments, productivity levels, life expectancies, child survival rates and economic growth.

Many people at home, I know, think of AIDS as one more disaster in Africa, as inevitable and unchanging. And yet over the last nine years—since that day in the Tanzanian hospital, with the dying men on the floor where no one would speak the word *AIDS*—I have seen something change. In most of the places I travel today, people and their governments are deeply engaged in the response to AIDS, in an effort to heal the wounds it leaves. And although the pandemic is still outstripping the response, I have seen AIDS treatment come to Africa. I was familiar with the "Lazarus effect" of antiretrovirals in North America, and had seen friends with AIDS become well again and flourish, but watching it happen in Africa has nevertheless been mesmerizing. I saw African activists put pressure on the pharmaceutical industry until they won access to cheap generic drugs and drove down the prices of brand-name ones. I have seen projects with limited staff and minuscule budgets, working without reliable electricity or in wildly remote areas, get drugs to people in conditions—even in the middle of wars—that the West deemed impossible. I have seen people at the edge of death get suddenly, gloriously well again, just like they do at home.

Something else changed, too: the pandemic started, very slowly, to attract political attention, media coverage and serious funding. This is due to the work of thousands of tireless African activists, and a few high-powered champions of the cause in the West—particularly Irish rock star Bono, former U.S. president Bill Clinton, software billionaire Bill Gates, and Stephen Lewis, a Canadian diplomat who from 2002 to 2007 served as the UN's special envoy on HIV/AIDS in Africa, a role in which he was a dogged and effective advocate for the continent's women and children. This combined pressure produced, first, the Global Fund. Then in 2003 U.S. president George W. Bush announced a five-year, $15-billion program—the President's Emergency Plan for AIDS Relief, or PEPFAR—to fund AIDS prevention and treatment in the developing world, with a focus on Africa. That program was soon mired in controversy (its architects insisted on designating funds for abstinence-based prevention efforts and on buying brand-name drugs made by large U.S. companies instead of cheaper generic medications that could treat more people). But it was the biggest international health intervention ever attempted, and it quickly brought new attention to the African pandemic. In 2006, Bono launched the Red campaign—a marketing effort that soon had people snapping up iPods and T-shirts from the Gap in support of the Global Fund—and suddenly the crisis was trendy.

And yet the response remains muted. Few people outside Africa seem to understand the scale or the epic gravity of what is happening here. When I talk to people at home about the pandemic, I get the sense that they feel a dying African is somehow different from a dying Canadian, American or German—that Africans have lower expectations or place less value on their lives. That to be an orphaned fifteen-year-old thrust into caring for four bewildered siblings, or a teacher thrown out of her house after she tells her husband she is infected—that somehow this would be less terrifying or strange for a person in Zambia or Mozambique than it would be for some-one in the United States or Britain.

And so I wanted to tell their stories—to tell how they want to go to high school, or build up a small taxi business, or meet their grandchildren. When people in Tanzania or Botswana find themselves fighting govern-ments—their own and those in the West—and multinational pharmaceutical companies and their own families and the neighbours who isolate and fear them, that is every bit as bizarre and daunting for them as it would be for you and me. I have met the beauty queens and the soldiers and the young lovers and the scientists who live with AIDS in Africa, and I know that the only way that they are different from me is that they have the misfortune to live in countries that are economically and politically marginal—that they are black and they are, quite often, poor, and so their lives can slip away unremarked.

I can't tell every story. I decided to tell twenty-eight—one for each million people infected in Africa. Their stories explain how the disease works, how it spreads and how it kills. They explain how AIDS is horribly, inextricably tied to conflict and to famine and to the collapse of states. They explain how treatment works, when people can get it, and how the people who can't get it fight to stay alive with virtually no help and no support.

Let me say, here, a word about numbers. This book could equally plau-sibly be called *26*—or *30*. The data collection on the number of people living with HIV/AIDS in sub-Saharan Africa is extremely weak. Many countries draw their statistics only from HIV tests at prenatal clinics, because that's the one time adults reliably come into contact with the health system. But those numbers can be artificially high compared to the overall population, because by definition pregnant women have had unprotected sex. A few countries have done door-to-door surveys, and these data are more reliable, but people who know or suspect they are infected are much more likely to decline to be tested by the surveyor who knocks at the door, even when promised anonymity. So that pushes the numbers in those surveys down. Many nations lack the skilled people to accurately process and maintain these kinds of statistics, and in those countries, the UN agency responsible, UNAIDS, is guessing too. Still, today, only an estimated 10 per cent of those who have the virus in Africa have actually been tested for it. Meanwhile, national governments have played down their infection rates—not wanting to scare off tourists or foreign investors—at the same time that international agencies have sometimes inflated them, out of a desire to attract more attention and more funding. In recent years UNAIDS has revised its infection numbers for most African countries downwards (while a few shot up); part of that decline is the result of people dying, and part of it of more reliable statistics.

The latest epidemiological survey for the continent gives a range of twenty-five to thirty million people with the virus. My own feeling, after nine years of watching the African pandemic unfold, is that the figure twenty-eight million in Africa is conservative. Again and again, I travel to areas where the estimated prevalence is 15 per cent, but it seems obvious from looking around that the rate of infection is higher; or I speak to doctors and government health officials who have just done new surveys and found much higher numbers than they expected. I suspect that when accurate survey methods finally reach into rural areas and all segments of the population, the figure will be still higher.

This is, of course, on some level immaterial. The African pandemic is as much of a crisis with twenty-eight million people infected as it is with twenty-three or thirty-three million. The inaction of the previous two decades is ample proof that numbers alone, no matter how high, are not enough to motivate us to respond in any adequate way to the crisis.

Some of the people in this book I have come to know well, and come to call friends, and I have followed their stories for years. Others I met only once, over a day or two in their shattered villages, and so I can tell their stories only as a snapshot as their lives unravelled. Some of these stories show us what success in fighting AIDS looks like, and others tell us how desperately far we have to go.

Some make for painful reading. Many of the people I meet wage a daily struggle to stay alive. All of them have suffered a level of loss of which I can barely conceive. They have been betrayed by their lovers and their families and their neighbours and their governments. AIDS has robbed them of much more than health.

And yet each day in my travels in these worst-affected countries, I meet people caring for their sick families and their neighbours, fighting drug companies and their governments for treatment, sheltering their orphaned siblings, overcoming shame and fear with breathtaking bravery. Along with all the pain and all the needless loss, theirs are stories of triumph and resilience, and they give cause for hope in the most unlikely circumstances.

People ask me all the time why I do this job, when "it must be so depressing." Here are twenty-eight of the reasons why.

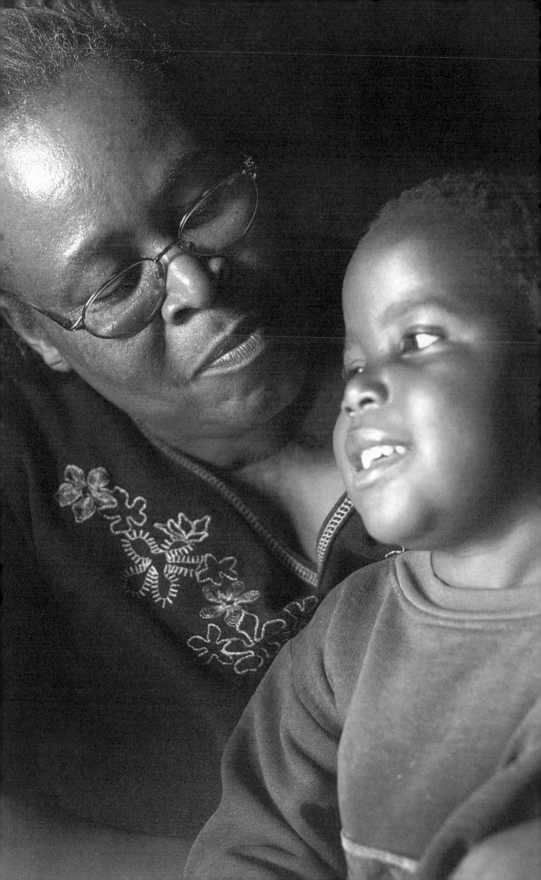

# ONE

# SiphiweHlophe

**W**hen I hug her, she feels like rock. She is solid, Siphiwe is—solid courage and grit and determination. She has more strength and more forbearance than I can get the measure of. There seems no end to what she has to give—or to what is asked of her.

Siphiwe (pronounced *Spee*-way) comes from Lundzi, a village in the north of Swaziland—well, she tells me, it's really too small to be called a village. "What's smaller than a village?" I ask. She laughs. "Mmm. A community?" Lundzi is a collection of scattered homesteads, of low, round thatch houses surrounded by fields. When Siphiwe was a girl, her father was a truck mechanic who earned a weekly wage of 10 emalangeni, then worth $2, enough to support three wives and a great many children. The first wife had twelve, and then came Siphiwe's mother, who had seven more, of whom Siphiwe, born in 1960, was second; the last wife had six of her own. Of those twenty-five children, eighteen were girls, and her father imagined he would be a rich man in his old age, with all the cattle he would collect in *lobola,* the traditional bride price. It didn't work out that way: only five girls married. There were changes coming in Swaziland that Siphiwe's father could not fathom.

Her parents quarrelled a great deal, and when Siphiwe was five, her mother went back across the border to family in South Africa. (The tight-knit

Swazi community inhabits both sides of the arbitrary colonial line that separates tiny Swaziland from its huge and powerful neighbour.) Siphiwe and her siblings went into the care of the first wife, but she died when Siphiwe was twelve, and so the third wife inherited them all. "Life was not good—there we didn't get the love of a mother," Siphiwe recalled. "We were made to work from morning until sunset. In the morning before school my sisters and I did the cooking for all the children. After school we collected firewood and then we had to cook or water the garden. We would get to sleep very late. Sometimes we didn't get soap for bathing. She would tell us that she is not the one who sent out our mother—it's our father—so why should she provide for us? It was a very hard life for us."

Her father beat and terrorized them, but he paid for them to be educated—although when she went off to secondary school, Siphiwe was the only student without shoes, an offence for which the headmaster could have dismissed her. She hated this visible sign of her poverty, and after a few weeks of school, she walked to town, to the office of the aid agency Save the Children, in through the door and right up to the director. She delights in telling this story. "I said, 'You know I'm poor, and I need to continue my education.' That man, he is retired, but still when I see him now he says, 'I remember when you came into my office in your gym dress and bare feet.'" Impressed by her spunk, the director found a family in Finland to pay for shoes and the cost of boarding school, so she could get out of Lundzi. The Finnish family continued to sponsor her until she graduated from university in 1984. Back then she thought, "Maybe when I grow up I will take care of some orphans to pay back what they have done for me." She told me this with an amused little snort—funny how *that* worked out.

She thought at the time that she might like to be a nurse. But then she went before the scholarship committee. "They said, 'Eh! Siphiwe Dlamini! You will do agriculture!' without even looking at the report card. They just tell you. I said, 'I want to be a nurse.' They said, 'No.'" It was authoritarian and absurd—and it worked out well. "I'm happy that they chose a career I really liked, rather than nursing . . . In agriculture you work with older people and you have to recognize the experiences of older people and make sure they take the decisions—not you. It expands my knowledge to work with these people."

Siphiwe grew up to be an indomitable, independent woman—in a place that doesn't encourage that sort of thing. The first time I went to Swaziland, in 2003, women had recently been forbidden by royal decree from wearing trousers. The king, the last absolute monarch in Africa, makes a habit of plucking a new teenage bride from among the bare-breasted virgins who carry reeds and dance in the annual *umhlanga* ceremony. There is much to admire in the way Swaziland has kept its distinct culture strong, even as it sits on the border of imperialist South Africa, and the reed dance is a beautiful rite. But it is centred, as so much of Swazi culture seems to be, on men's control of women's sexuality. Women have the same legal status as children in Swaziland; until a new constitution was adopted in 2006, women were not allowed to own property, no matter how successful they were in business.

Siphiwe is a marvellous story teller, and her stories—long, meandering tales punctuated with her huge laugh—give a vivid picture of life for Swazi women. She got pregnant the first time in 1979—by Frank Hlophe, a handsome fellow five years her senior—when she was in high school. That wasn't a tremendous scandal; in Swazi culture, a girl who has proved her fertility goes up in value. Frank's mother looked after the baby while Siphiwe finished school. Three years later, she and Frank had a second baby, and then a third in 1984 as she struggled to finish her degree. Her mother-in-law told her, "Go to the clinic like these other women and do something so you don't have all these babies." Siphiwe had never heard of condoms then, and they weren't sold publicly in Swaziland. She went to the clinic, but the doctor there told her she could not gain access to contraception without a letter from her husband. But she didn't have a husband—Frank was stalling. "I was thinking, 'Who will marry me now, with all these children?'" One child was a helpful selling feature—but three, that was a burden. Her father began to mutter that she was unmarriageable. Finally Frank made good on his promises and paid *lobola* for her, plus a five-cow penalty for having impregnated her out of wedlock.

# Her mother-in-law told these other women so you don't have

They married in 1985, and at last Siphiwe could get the all-important letter for the clinic, where she had an intrauterine device inserted. But five years later it began to trouble her and she had it removed; she found herself pregnant for a fourth time just a month later. That, she thought, is quite enough. She wanted a tubal ligation. She went back to the clinic. This time the doctor said she needed her mother-in-law's consent. Her mother-in-law said only her father-in-law could assent to such a thing. He roared, "How many cows did we pay for you and you want to stop at four children?" Only the ancestors could approve such an idea, he said. Siphiwe knew she wasn't going to get a permission letter from the ancestors, no matter what kind of ritual she performed. "So I thought, I must be a bit smart." She disguised her emerging fourth pregnancy and went to a different doctor. "I said I had eight children and my husband was dead. He said, 'Is your mother alive? No? Well, get your older sister.'" When Siphiwe, who was then thirty years old, brought her sister to the clinic to sign the papers, she was finally given permission to have the procedure. There was still Frank to negotiate—but Siphiwe tacked the operation on after the birth of the baby, and had her sister tell him that she needed to stay on in hospital because of some vague "complications." This story made her chuckle, a bit ruefully, when she told it.

After college Siphiwe was hired as an outreach worker for the Ministry of Agriculture, teaching better farming techniques to the subsistence farmers who are the bulk of the Swazi population. She was good at her work, and revelled in it—and led her colleagues in a union drive that won them higher wages. When an angry boss told her she should be behaving "like my wife"—that is, docile and obedient—she took a complaint to the highest level of the ministry. Soon, she said, managers decided to stay out of her way. In 1996, she left the children with Frank and his mother and spent two years in Lusaka, earning a degree in agriculture at the University of Zambia.

The next year, Siphiwe won a scholarship to study for a master's degree at the University of Bradford, in England. It was a rare and wonderful opportunity for a Swazi woman, and her whole family buzzed with pride. "Mama is going to England," the children boasted to their friends, and Siphiwe hummed the words to herself: "I'm going abroad, I'm going abroad." The scholarship required a medical report, and so Siphiwe went to her family doctor carrying the sheaf of papers he was required to fill out. She was completely healthy and not the slightest bit worried. But when she went back to get the papers a few days later, the doctor pushed them at her roughly and said, "You won't be going to the U.K."

Unbeknown to Siphiwe, one of the tests required was for HIV—and she had tested positive. The scholarship was automatically rescinded; the committee was not going to invest its resources in someone who would imminently die. She went home in a daze. She told Frank why she wouldn't be leaving for England after all, and he was enraged. He accused her of having had lovers when she was studying in Zambia, of having all manner of illicit sex when she was visiting farm sites around the country, alone and unsupervised in her ministry pickup truck. He moved out of their home, saying, "I can't live with a prostitute."

The news raced through their extended families. Siphiwe had never had sex with anyone but Frank—but she knew that he had had many other partners. "Men cannot hide when they are in love," she said with a sigh. "Sometimes he would not come home. Now, a person who does not drink, who comes at 2 a.m., where is he coming from?" He had girlfriends almost from the time they were married, she said. But no one in the family wanted to hear about Frank's infidelity—only to gossip about Siphiwe's shame. The aunties shook their heads: they had always said she was too independent.

Her test result was not the first Siphiwe knew of AIDS. Five years earlier, her sister Gciniphi had fallen ill, and Siphiwe helped nurse her in the hospital. In the corridors she heard people talking about a virus that made people terribly sick, with symptoms that sounded much like those troubling her sister. The doctors had tested Gciniphi, and told Siphiwe she did indeed have this new virus. They wouldn't, however, tell the sick woman that news, and Siphiwe kept it from her, too. She was afraid to touch her sister, wondering if the rumours were true, if she could catch this disease by bathing or feeding her. Three days after the test, her sister died. "If only I'd had information about HIV, maybe she'd be alive," Siphiwe said. But it would be years before she learned any more. "The page of HIV was closed to me until I discovered my own status."

But even then, five years later, people didn't know any better. "Disclosing your status made you an outcast—it was the leprosy of that time." Beyond the shame of her diagnosis, she was full of fear, remembering her sister's painful, lonely death. By then Swaziland had an HIV infection rate above 20 per cent of the population, but Siphiwe had never heard anyone say publicly that they were infected. There was one group, the Swaziland AIDS Support Organization, and she made her way to one of their meetings. For the first time, she met people who were openly HIV-positive. But it wasn't much comfort. They were young people, activists—"even street kids," she said. Nobody like her, an educated civil servant and a married mother of four. "I thought, 'I can't join that group.'"

Word of her infection had spread quickly—Swaziland, where everyone comes from one of five big clans, often feels more like an extra-large village than a country. Now as she taught workshops and supervised projects in rural areas, many people shifted away, avoided meeting her eyes. But a few women sought her out. They were her age, and their experiences were much like hers: they had unexpectedly found out they had HIV after medical tests, and had been cast out by their husbands, shunned by their communities—told they could not use the village well, must not touch other women's children.

In 2001, Siphiwe and four of these women formed Swaziland Positive Living—Swapol, for short—as upbeat a name as they could think of. At first, they met to talk and to encourage each other. Then they started trying to organize help for the increasing numbers of orphans in every community, and homecare for the sick. Soon they had a small office in Manzini, the bustling commercial capital, and every day or two, another stout woman in a cardigan and a sober serge skirt would tentatively edge in the door and say she needed help.

Two years later, they had five hundred members, and Siphiwe's boss at the Ministry of Agriculture kindly suggested that perhaps AIDS had become her job. She was seconded to the National Emergency Response Committee on HIV/AIDS, the government body trying to coordinate prevention and care projects, most of which were piecemeal community efforts like Siphiwe's. Soon she was back to travelling the country in a pickup truck, this one with a big red ribbon painted on the door. She might be dying, but in the meantime, she had a great deal to do.

I first met Siphiwe in Mbabane, the other of Swaziland's two cities. I was reporting on the government's response to AIDS and I dropped in on a meeting of people living with HIV who were petitioning the UN for help. There were many hot-headed and angry young people in the room, but when they were finished throwing around their denunciations, Siphiwe rose. She is just over five feet tall, round with a generous bosom, stout arms and smudges of grey in her short hair. She began to speak, in a voice deceptively soft, painting a picture of a nation overwhelmed and of a floundering government with little idea how to respond to a crisis of this magnitude. She spoke with crisp precision, and in just a few minutes she had laid out the whole complicated web of ways that AIDS was destroying Swaziland: no parents for the children, no women to work the fields, no nurses to staff the hospitals. After the meeting, I arranged to travel on her rounds with her, and it was the first of many journeys I would take with Siphiwe as she helped me understand what AIDS is doing to her country.

A few years later, in November 2005, we were driving down a valley road about an hour outside of Manzini, when she gestured with one plump arm out the window, over the hills dotted with thatch rondavels and the occasional splash of fuchsia bougainvillea. "I was driving on that road," she said, pointing across the valley. "And they saw my car—the AIDS car, they call it—and they sent one woman running, running across the whole valley to meet me. She was waving, waving, and when I drove up to her she started to cry. I stopped and said, 'What, is someone dying? Is someone sick?' And she told me they sent her because they needed to talk to me—she said, 'You must come up here.'" So Siphiwe drove her truck as far as it would go down the stony track and walked the rest of the way. In a village of three hundred people, she found fifty-one orphans. Some people came out to meet her, but she went door to door, wanting to know who couldn't rise to greet a guest. How many people lay dying on grass mats in the houses?

Siphiwe made a plan. She organized the twenty-two people in the village who knew they were HIV-positive and, drawing on what she does best, she helped them plant a huge garden near a stream running out of the mountains. She arranged the money for seedlings, fertilizer, a fence to keep the cows out and hosepipes for irrigation. Everyone in the village who was well enough contributed labour; soon there were fresh vegetables to feed the sick, food parcels for the houses where the orphans lived alone, and a surplus of leafy spinach and beets to sell in town. Villagers decided together how to use the proceeds: mostly for medicine and funerals.

Siphiwe stopped off to show me the garden—it was clearly a source of pride as well as vital income for the village. But still, things were grim. Lindiwe Shabangu, thirty-four and gaunt, told me that the nearest clinic for AIDS patients was Mbabane, two hours away, and she couldn't afford the 20 emalangeni, or $4, each way to pay for a seat in a shared taxi. A wide-eyed four-year-old, also named Lindiwe, followed me as I toured the garden; she had abscesses on her scalp and the clubbed fingertips that mark a child with chronic respiratory trouble. When her mother lifted up her dress, I saw that she was covered in scabs and rash. I raised an eyebrow at Siphiwe, who nodded once and looked away. "She's been tested. But there is no money to take her to the city for treatment."

We drove back down through the mountains, past tiny towns built around a crossroads, each with a general store and a church. Siphiwe had an urgent visit to make, to a home where three orphans had been living together since their parents died three years before. The household consisted of five small mud-brick buildings—bedrooms, storage, one for cooking. Now only one was occupied, the three children sharing a twin bed. Tengethile Tshabalala, thirteen, was doing her best with her four- and six-year-old siblings; each morning they got up and dressed in their school uniforms, even though they had no money to pay to go to class since their parents died. Instead they sat in the shade and watched the other children in the village walk past on the way to school.

Swapol was keeping the children in food and AA batteries for the ancient transistor radio that is Tengethile's lone joy in life, and Siphiwe was trying to find a sponsor for their school fees. Our mission that day was to drop off an emergency ration of sanitary napkins for her: Siphiwe was worried that to buy them, Tengethile would resort to having sex with a man down at the trading centre, who might pay her $2. "We bring them food and clothes every month because we are afraid of men abusing them. These orphans say, 'We can have sex in exchange for food.'"

We spent an hour or so with the children, Siphiwe coaxing words out of them. The littlest one spent our whole visit in her lap, delighted by the novelty of a broad adult bosom to snuggle into. Tengethile tugged at the skirt of her too-small uniform, trying to keep it over her knees. Her bravery left me on the edge of tears, and as we drove away I wondered, as I had a hundred times before, how Siphiwe could keep going, when every single day brought another visit like this.

The scenes like this were being repeated all over the country. In May 2004, Swaziland, with its population of 1.1 million people, won the grim title of the nation with the highest rate of HIV/AIDS infection in the world—38.6 per cent of adults, based on figures from prenatal clinics, the best data available. The national AIDS agency swore to redouble its efforts, and aid groups pledged more money. Even the king said the issue was a crisis (although it did not stop him from selecting a twelfth teenage bride at the *umhlanga*). Then, a year later, the Swazi government did another national survey. The results were a horror.

Not only had the infection failed to decline in the face of the renewed prevention efforts—it had risen. To 42.6 per cent. What becomes of a country—of a small, poor, isolated country—when nearly half of its adults have HIV? What does that even look like?

It looks like Siphiwe's family. Of her twenty-four siblings, six are still alive. One died in a car accident; the other seventeen died of AIDS. Her brothers, she told me angrily, got sick but refused to go for the dreaded HIV test. Instead they ordered their still-healthy wives to go. Siphiwe put a stop to that: "You have infected her and now you are using her to test!" It was no mystery to Siphiwe why the infection rate was still climbing. "In our culture a man is stronger, he has more integrity if he has more wives and girlfriends, and that has continued even in the time of HIV/AIDS. More partners is more prestige—they're not seeing that it's killing us and killing them and killing our children." Women, legally subservient and dependent on husbands or fathers for food and shelter, could do little to protect themselves from exposure to infection.

As we drove along, I asked Siphiwe, "What would you say to the king if you could get to see him?" Despite the enormous influence he wields over Swazis, King Mswati has made only trifling efforts to fight AIDS. I had interviewed him briefly the year before, and thought he resembled a fraternity boy in a splendid traditional outfit. I added, "Would you kneel?" (In Swazi tradition, a woman must kneel in the presence of the king and come before him shuffling on her knees.) "If I was not on my knees, I would be talking to a statue, he would not even see me there," she replied. So she would kneel—"And I would tell him this issue of HIV/AIDS is killing the nation. He must change his attitude and be a role model and not take another wife. He goes to the people and says 'Be faithful'—and then takes another wife. He needs to talk to people about multiple partners. What he does has an effect. People will listen to him."

In the meantime, he isn't helping the country to get the assistance it needs. "Donors say, 'Why should we bother about Swaziland when half the population is HIV-positive? We'd be wasting our resources.' But we are human beings and have a right to all the matters they also have—to life and health. Or they say our governments are corrupt and if they give us help it will just be stolen by the government." Although Swaziland has staggered under the twin burdens of AIDS and drought in recent years, the country alienated international donor agencies when the king used state funds to build lavish palaces for all his wives, then added to his luxury car collection. He was only narrowly dissuaded from buying a personal jet. "Yes, we cannot say they are not corrupt. But we are dying because of that corrupt government. They"—the king, his courtiers, the parliament he appoints—"have private hospitals or fly to America, but we don't have even one cent to move. So give your money to NGOs and be confident where it will go. HIV is like the Asian tsunami: they don't say, 'There is a tsunami but you are not democratic so we are not rescuing you.' AIDS is an emergency just like that."

Those days of making rounds in the truck leave Siphiwe fuming. She hates the hospitals, where people lie three to a bed, and she hates that so many people never make it to the hospital at all, and that the waiting lists for drugs are full of the names of twenty-five-year-olds who die long before they get to the top. She hates the bureaucracy that keeps the government from getting medication out beyond the cities, and she hates that Lindiwe Shabangu will die because she can't manage $8 for taxi fare once a month. Unnecessary deaths, she calls them. They enrage her.

And yet she remains convinced that the country can recover. She talks about Uganda, Africa's great AIDS success story, which drove its infection rate down from nearly 20 per cent in the 1990s to under 7 per cent today. Uganda is a much larger country, and better off, but Siphiwe retains a stubborn faith in Swaziland, convinced her country can do it, too.

In 2004, her estranged husband sought out Siphiwe and apologized. "I know I am the one who infected you and I'm sorry about that," Frank told her. It was an admirable gesture, although Siphiwe sardonically questioned his motives—he had recently been laid off from his accounting job and knew she was comparatively well paid for her work with Swapol. In addition, his health was then erratic, and one of his long-time girlfriends had recently died of what appeared to be an AIDS-related illness.

Frank wanted to live with her again, and, over the protests of her children, Siphiwe took him back. There is no divorce in Swaziland, she reminded me: a woman remains the property of her husband all her life. Frank, she pointed out, had title to her house—but there was more to it than that. Despite all that has happened, she loves him, and she wanted him to come home. Frank moved back in with her, their two youngest children, and three AIDS orphans she had taken under her wing.

When we talked in late 2006, Siphiwe was battling a flu she couldn't shake, and she speculated frankly about whether this was the onset of AIDS. The thought of death didn't seem to trouble her nearly as much as all she had left to do. "If I die now, I won't be happy—these women I'm working with in rural communities are so ignorant of HIV/AIDS. My heart becomes heavy when I see these women die like this. I just think, 'Now is not the time for me to go.'"

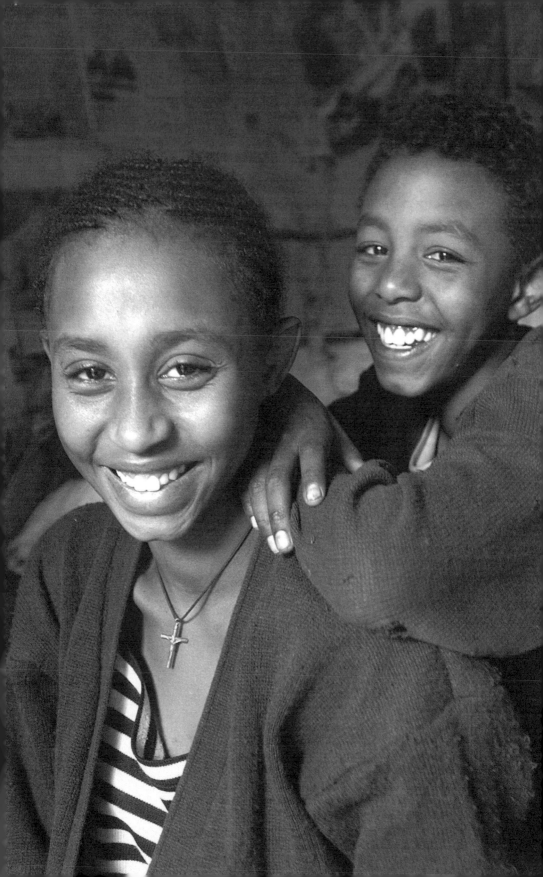

# TWO

# TigistHaileMichael

S ometimes she forgets for hours at a time. On the weekends, she sits with her friends from school. They braid each other's hair in fancy spiral patterns, and look at Bollywood film stars in scavenged magazines, and paint each other's toenails (delphinium blue is all the rage). Then Tigist feels like a kid, like all the other kids.

But when it's coming on dusk, and she walks back home, when she takes the jerry can to the standpipe around the corner to buy water, puts a few pats of cow dung to burn in the brazier and boils a small pot of lentils—when she calls her brother, Yohannes, in from the street and chides him about his homework—then the illusion crumbles. After Yohannes falls asleep sprawled on their one narrow bed, and she has nudged him over to make room for her own long arms and legs, then she lies in the dark and runs through the list. Is there money for their rent. Is there money for their fees at school. Is there money for more lentils, more dung, more water. And just where, exactly, is she going to find the money for another sweater for Yohannes, because his wrists now dangle four inches below the cuffs of the one he has.

"I shouldn't be worried about this," Tigist said to me. She spoke without bitterness or rancour—simply to make clear that she knew what she had lost. "It should be for others to worry."

"I shouldn't be worried
me. She spoke without
simply to make clear that

Those nights when she lies awake in the dark, she thinks about her mother, Buzunesh, who died in 2002, when Tigist was ten and Yohannes just six. He has little memory of a time when it wasn't up to them—when there was anyone but Tigist to scold him for staying too late in the streets playing soccer, anyone but Tigist to answer his questions and tell him what to do. But Tigist is old enough to remember when Buzunesh bought the food, made the meals, supervised the lessons—and did the worrying.

"Now there is no one for me to ask for advice. I think about my mother when I'm worrying about what to do to provide for my brother. If my mother were around I wouldn't have the responsibility of my brother and we'd have her love and we could focus just on our education."

Tigist's father died when she was very young, and she doesn't remember him at all. "I just have stories about him from my mother." Then Buzunesh met the man who would become Yohannes's father; he moved in with them, and Tigist remembers him a bit better. He grew thin, was sick for a long time, and then he too died, before she was six. So it was just the three of them living in a small room in Kazachis, a crowded Addis Ababa slum full of bars and flophouses where rent was cheap. Buzunesh baked injera, the flat, sour bread that is the Ethiopian staple food, to sell in the streets, and she took in washing. She didn't make much money, Tigist said, but it was enough to pay their fees at school and sometimes to buy them little treats—small toys or shiny new pencils.

But then Buzunesh fell sick, too. She couldn't work, was confined to her bed off and on for two years, Tigist said. At the public clinic, they gave her treatment for tuberculosis—a six-month course, twice—but it didn't work. She got weaker. The neighbours helped a bit with nursing; Tigist brought her mother water and tried to make the meals the way she directed.

about this," Tigist said to
bitterness or rancour—
she knew what she had lost.

She reckoned Buzunesh was about twenty-eight when she died, although she has no documents—no birth or death certificate, no identity papers. "She was quite young, that's what I know."

That left Tigist and Yohannes together to fend for themselves in one of Africa's largest cities. They sit with their limbs tangled up together; they walk arm in arm in the road; they keep their eyes on each other all the time. "I'm lucky, because he doesn't cause me many problems," Tigist told me, trying to stifle a smile. "We don't fight, because he does what I tell him." Her brother rolled his eyes at this. The child is still visible in Yohannes, with his tangle of curly hair—he would rather run than walk, he likes to tease, and he can't quite muster embarrassment when he confesses that he sometimes gets strapped for cheekiness at school. Tigist, though, has an air of timeless patience, other-worldly in a child of fourteen. Only the sparkly blue toenails give her away.

Ten or fifteen years ago, it wouldn't have been up to Tigist: someone would have stepped forward to take care of an orphaned ten- and six-year-old when their mother died. It would have been as unthinkable in Addis Ababa as it would be in Toronto or Dallas or Birmingham for two small children to set up house on their own. But in the age of AIDS, the net of family and community that once caught and cared for children such as these has frayed and worn and finally unravelled altogether.

As Ethiopia's HIV prevalence neared five per cent in the 1990s, it had a devastating impact on families. First came the "serial orphans": parents died and their children were taken in by an aunt or uncle. But then the aunts and uncles sickened or died. The children went to other aunts, then to grandparents. The grandparents died, and the children went to neighbours. Each move unsettled already traumatized children—and eventually, there was nowhere left for them to go. Most African cultures have no tradition of orphanages or adoption in the Western sense of taking in unknown children. But fostering—caring for a late sister's or neighbour's children—was standard practice in communities where it was not uncommon for adults to die young, even before HIV began to spread. The sheer scale of AIDS, however, changed that dynamic: each family can take in only so many children, and the dead, of course, can take none at all. The fostering system has long since been exhausted.

Inevitably, serial orphans became something else: little "families" of children living on their own because there was no one left to take them. In the bland language of AIDS, they are called child-headed households, a term that does nothing to convey the surreal quality of a nine-year-old gathering firewood, cooking, washing and telling bedtime stories to the seven-, five-, three- and one-year-old left, by default, in her charge.

Even as HIV infection rates have flattened in response to prevention campaigns, and more people have gained access to treatment, one massive problem has remained largely unaddressed. An estimated fourteen million children across Africa have been left without parents because of AIDS. These children can't go to school if no one pays their fees, and many end up either struggling to grow food on land they have never been taught to farm, or living wild on city streets. Aid agencies express fears about the cost to countries of a generation growing up without education or even socialization, and alarmed political leaders talk about orphans as a threat to national stability. And while some of the steps to fight AIDS are simple enough if the money is there—put condoms in the truckers' bars; put drugs in the clinics—what these children need is parents, and no cash infusion, no matter how great, permits a country such as Ethiopia to buy parents for 700,000 AIDS orphans.

Ethiopia's HIV prevalence was 4.4 per cent in 2006—moderate by the standards of sub-Saharan Africa. But with a total population of seventy-eight million, that means one and a half million infected people, in a nation singularly ill equipped to respond. Ethiopians take enormous pride in being the only African country to have successfully resisted European colonization (save for a brief occupation by the Italians from 1936 to 1941), but its own leaders have done a fine job of ravaging the nation without external help. Emperor Haile Selassie lived a life of obscene luxury while keeping 90 per cent of the population as peasants in a feudal system. The Marxist guerrillas who ousted the emperor in 1974 replaced the monarchy with an equally brutal junta known as the Derg. A million people died in the famines of the 1980s even as the dictator Mengistu Haile Mariam insisted there was no food shortage. He and the Derg, in turn, were ousted by a coalition of rebel groups in 1991, after a brutal seventeen-year civil war—just as HIV sank its teeth into the country.

The new government held elections, made primary education free, and tried to reform the agricultural sector on which virtually the entire population depended. It built roads and clinics and schools. But it also began an absurd and vicious border war with Eritrea that left an estimated hundred thousand people dead by 2000. Then the government began to fear that democratic elections might cost it power, and in 2005 launched a campaign of political repression that evoked memories of the dictatorship it had usurped. The foreign donors on whom Ethiopia is entirely dependent began to freeze and withdraw their funding.

All of this exacerbated an incipient AIDS crisis. The virus had killed an estimated 900,000 Ethiopians in the fifteen years since the first cases were recorded, in 1986. The government started mustering resources to combat the disease, but the challenges were enormous. The country was desperately poor, with an annual per capita income of just $100. Half the population had no access to any medical care, and there was scarcely capacity or infrastructure to educate about AIDS, let alone treat it.

Tigist's mother was a casualty of that underfunded system. Although Buzunesh received treatment for tuberculosis, the TB drugs were useless in the face of untreated HIV. "I was surprised my mother died," Tigist said softly. "She was on medicine—we had the hope she would get better. No one was suggesting she would die."

Buzunesh had left her home village, Addis Alem, more than a decade earlier; she was one of hundreds of thousands of young people fleeing Ethiopia's benighted countryside, where population pressure, persistent drought and an archaic land tenure system has made survival from agriculture increasingly difficult. As a teenager, she travelled the eighty kilometres by dirt road into Addis Ababa, looking for work. Over the years, she returned home to visit only once, and she lost touch with the village. But when Buzunesh sensed she might die of her illness, she went back to her family, taking Tigist and Yohannes with her. Village life came as a shock to children used to the crowds of the capital city: it was so quiet and so slow. There was so little colour. Their young cousins spent most of their days working—plowing or herding cows, walking kilometres to collect water and firewood. They weren't much interested in school.

Buzunesh died not long after they arrived in the village, and Tigist's aunts suggested that she and her brother could stay on and live with the family—they would be welcome, and cared for. But the idea alarmed the children. They didn't know any of these people. Even the way they talked was different. "And we wondered if we would get to go to school," Yohannes told me. "I might have to plow." Tigist, crinkling her snub nose, added that she is more of a city girl. "We decided it was not in our interest to stay there—there is more education and more prospects in the city." And so they politely declined the offer. Neighbours from Addis Ababa had come out to the village for the funeral, and Tigist asked to go back with them. Her aunts and uncles, already struggling to feed the mouths they had, wished the children well and let them go.

Back in the city, Tigist and Yohannes stayed on in their mother's rented room. Tigist washed their uniforms and they went back to school. The neighbours helped a bit with food. Then some nice ladies from the *iddir*, the burial society, came to call. The societies are a fixture of life in Ethiopia. There, and in many other African countries, great value is placed on funerals at which the family of the dead person provides food and hospitality for the whole community. But the expense can be crippling. Members of the burial society pay a small monthly premium (between 50 cents and $1), and when they die, the *iddir* pays for food, coffins and gravediggers. *Iddir* are present in nearly every community, have elected directors and are trusted by the people they serve, and so in 2004, the international aid agency CARE began to approach the burial societies about responding to HIV/AIDS. The *iddir* leadership resisted initially, saying they cared for the dead, not the living. But CARE saw them as uniquely well placed to pick up some of the burden for Ethiopia's desperately poor government. Meanwhile the *iddir* leaders realized that they were going bankrupt as AIDS killed so many of their members; doing HIV support work might help slow the pace of death. So the societies began to supervise orphans and care for the sick, helping to distribute small grants from CARE through their vast network.

When the *iddir* in their neighbourhood heard that Tigist and Yohannes were living on their own, the directors came calling. The society began to pay the children's rent and their school fees. Just as important, the motherly older ladies took to dropping in from time to time to see how the children were doing. It was one of these ladies who first took me to meet the children, and who explained that their mother, and likely both of their fathers, had died of AIDS, although no one says the word in front of Tigist and Yohannes.

As Tigist got older, and prettier, a problem was brewing: men from other families living in their compound began to pay her more and more attention. When the *iddir* ladies prompted her to tell me about it, Tigist looked at her feet and whispered that they said she would have to have sex with them if she and Yohannes were to continue renting there. The men grew more persistent, and Tigist more afraid. "There were nights I couldn't sleep in the old house—I feared someone would break in and do harm to me," she said. Finally she confided in the *iddir* ladies, and they quickly began to look for somewhere else for the pair to live.

They found a one-and-a-half-square-metre shack made of bits of salvaged tin, in a neighbourhood still poor but less known for bars and sex work, and the society rented it for 70 birr, or $8, a month. The shack sits in a cramped courtyard above a polluted river that runs through the city. Tigist papered the walls with old newspapers and decorated them with a couple of film-star pictures torn from magazines. There is room in the house for their thin straw-mattress bed, for the wobbly bamboo bench and trunk their mother left, for a small cabinet to hold their handful of dishes—and then just enough space to turn around. An electrical wire that runs from the main house in the courtyard powers a single yellow bulb in the ceiling, although Yohannes noted sadly that it doesn't cast enough light for them to read their school books at night. In the yard is a *mitad*—a flat iron plate over coals where each day Tigist and the other women in the compound bake injera. Cut into the hillside, seven stones lead down to a hole over the river that serves as a latrine. The compound is owned by a strict middle-aged matriarch, and Tigist feels safer here: "Now this room, we lock it and I don't worry." And indeed there is a stout bolt and a padlock on the door—although the walls are so precariously pieced together they could easily be pushed in.

Even a heavy bolt cannot ease her larger worries. "The thing I fear the most is housing. Right now I pay 70 birr—tomorrow it might be 90 or 100." As the *iddir* struggles to care for more and more orphans, it has less money to give to Tigist. She worries that the next time she approaches them, for school fees or help with food, there will be nothing left. "We will have to live on the street. We would have no other option. That's what I worry about all the time. Just in a room, let alone in the streets, it's quite risky—I understand it's very dangerous on the street." Tigist and Yohannes pass street kids on their way to school—there are thousands of such children in Addis, swarming car windows at stoplights, filthy and haggard and begging for food—and Tigist knows that very little stands between her and that life.

And yet, in the years since her mother died, she has kept herself and Yohannes clean and fed and in school. In 2006, she stood nineteenth of fifty-two students in her Grade 8 class; Yohannes is sixteenth of twenty-nine in Grade 4. Education in Ethiopia is ostensibly free until Grade 10, but the children must pay 360 birr a year in "development fees" and 140 birr each for a uniform (a total of about $75). CARE helps, and Yohannes sometimes earns a few birr shining shoes—although more than once he has been robbed by older boys who steal his money and the brushes and polishes for which he saved for months. Tigist earns a bit, too: she's good with hair, and the neighbours will give her three or four birr (40 cents) for an afternoon of braiding.

On weekday mornings Tigist makes tea in a battered aluminum pot over a pan of hot coals, and they breakfast on bread dipped into small cups. They put on their uniforms, and at eight o'clock they set out on the kilometre-long walk to school along a congested main road where fleets of honking taxis compete with herds of sheep for pavement space. The school is big, with two thousand students and a hundred teachers; two-storey cement buildings house classrooms lined with sturdy wood benches and desks. Tigist loves school, the safety it provides. If she can find the money to keep going, she would like to be a teacher herself. One of her favourite classes is English, although she was much too shy to speak it with me, ducking her head every time I tried to coax out a few words. Her notebook is filled with romantic pictures cut from magazines; she practises writing "I love you" with all her coloured pencils.

After school, Yohannes plays football with other boys from the slum, and Tigist shops at a stand that sells single tomatoes and tiny twists of salt or sugar—groceries in quantities for the very poor. If they have saved a little extra money from shining shoes or braiding hair, they add cabbage to the lentil stew, and once a month, usually on a religious feast day, they splurge on a small piece of beef to add as well.

When they walk down the main road on the way home from school, the children look in all the shop windows. Yohannes tries to catch a few minutes of movies playing on the TV screens, while Tigist likes to look at the clothes and the books. If they had more money, she said practically, she would spend it finding them better housing, and newer clothes, and proper cooking pans. When I put the question to Yohannes, he answered instantly that he would pay for them both to go to the best school in the city. And then he would buy trays and glasses, the things they need in the house. And perhaps, if there were *lots* of money, a television. When his sister was out of earshot, he confided, "I'd use it to take care of her."

And when Yohannes had gone back out to run with his friends in the street, Tigist watched him from the doorway, her head against one slim-fingered hand, and she said it too. "If we had more, I would try to take better care of him. I have to take care of him."

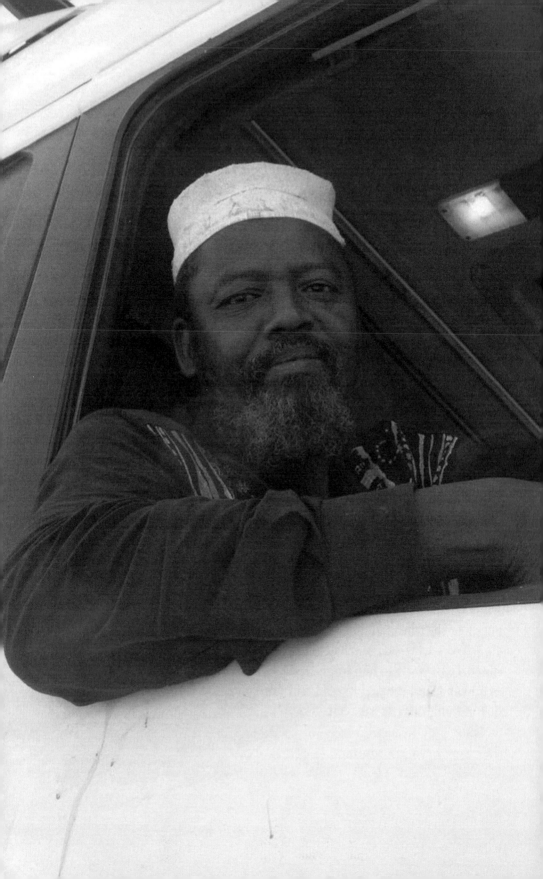

# THREE

# MohammedAli

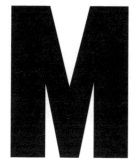ohammed Ali stroked his little tuft of greying beard, caressed the steering wheel and thought about it for some time. Eventually, his voice barely audible over the crashing of the gears and the rumbling of the engine, he told me his conclusion. "One hundred thousand," he said.

I bounced in the passenger seat and endeavoured to keep the disbelief out of my voice as I asked if he was sure.

"I think so," he replied with a nod. "One hundred thousand, more or less."

In a lifetime of driving the pitted highways of East Africa, Mohammed reckoned he had had sex with 100,000 women. For the next few kilometres we rumbled along an outrageously bad Kenyan road, and I tried to do the quick calculation on whether that was even possible. He was forty-eight. He had started driving at eighteen. Could a person have sex with 100,000 women in thirty years? And still have time to work? Or eat? I concluded that his math might be a bit off, or that pride had perhaps caused him to inflate the numbers—but it didn't matter much in the end. Mohammed's point was that he had had sex with so many women in so many roadside brothels over the years that they were beyond counting.

I met Mohammed at a truck stop outside Nairobi in mid-2005. I had long been interested in Africa's long-haul truckers, the tens of thousands of men who move most of the goods on the continent. Their transient lives have made them key players in the spread of HIV, and I was hanging around in the dust, looking for a trucker who might let me ride with him for a while and get a sense of his life. Mohammed, an affable and generous fellow, double-checked that I knew what I was asking—I wanted to come with him on the highway to Uganda? If I was sure, then he was willing to take me, and he would try to help me understand just how it is that a man ends up with 100,000 lovers. Give or take.

The day before I clambered gracelessly into the cabin of his eighteen-wheeler, Mohammed had loaded it with cement in the Kenyan port of Mombasa, where he and his wife, Maryam, live with their eight children. The truck was filled quickly, but Mohammed had spent the rest of the day in the maintenance yard and hit the highway only after nightfall. This trip to Jinja in Uganda would take just a week, if he didn't sleep much and he found the right customs officials to bribe at the border. He was to pick up another load in Jinja, and if he was lucky, he would be hauling it back to Mombasa, although sometimes these consignments—industrial parts or generators or vehicles—take him as far as Lubumbashi in the Democratic Republic of Congo, or Bujumbura in Burundi. A trip like that can keep him on the road for a month or more.

By late afternoon the next day Mohammed had arrived at the edge of Nairobi, a transport hub called Mlolongo where I was loitering in the diesel fumes. He had stopped to pray, in a small bare room off a sheet-metal tea shop with prayer rugs tacked on the wall. When he had heard my request, and agreed to take me with him, we sat down for hot sweet Somali tea served by the light of smoky kerosene lanterns; the other patrons, all drivers, stared unabashed at the strange pair we made. Tea drunk, we climbed into the truck as the sun set, and headed into the nightmare traffic of Nairobi. It took hours to traverse the city, and it was close to midnight when we made it to the edge of the escarpment and started down the twisting turns into the Great Rift Valley. Another hour on a cratered highway and we arrived in Maimaiu—one of the last trucks to pull off the road to look for a berth in the wide dirt lot that banks the highway in all the truck-stop towns.

Most everything in Africa moves on trucks like Mohammed's: air freight is too costly for the kind of cheap consumer goods or bulky building parts that are bought and sold, and long-haul trucking carries virtually all the fuel as well as the products of industry and agriculture. Goods enter and leave Africa through a handful of major ports—Lagos and Dakar in West Africa, Durban and Maputo in the south, Mombasa and Dar es Salaam in the east. From there, it's all by road, snaking from the edges into the heart of the continent. In the landlocked nations in the centre of Africa—Uganda, Rwanda, Zambia, Zimbabwe, Malawi, Burundi, Botswana—everything moves by truck. AIDS is no exception.

Mohammed got us the last two rooms in the Toa Jam hotel (the name is Kiswahili for the optimistic "get rid of the traffic jam"). For 200 shillings ($2.50), we each had a room of one and a half square metres, a bed with a wood frame, a simple chair, and a nail in the wall on which to hang our clothes. The walls didn't reach the ceiling, so the activity in the adjacent bar, and rooms, was clearly audible; the sheets were a topographic map of several days' transactions. The toilet was a rough hole cut in a cement floor across the courtyard. The proprietor brought us plates of greasy lamb chunks and cold chapattis. Mohammed ate quickly, washed his face in water dribbling from a small tin cistern into a filthy bucket and headed for his room.

We did not sleep for long: the proprietor pounded on my door at five o'clock, when the moon was still a bright crescent in a sky full of stars. One by one the trucks in the lot added their roar to a noise that sounded like lions. Mohammed prayed before stepping out into the clouds of dust, then swung himself up behind the wheel, somehow keeping his black jeans and black cotton shirt clear of the dirt. The road deteriorated badly from that point on, and all day long he wrestled with the wheel, coaxing the truck through craters that could swallow one huge tire. We drove through savannah where zebras grazed and baboons paced at the side of the road, and through crowded dusty towns, but we rarely managed to travel at a speed above thirty kilometres an hour. There were police check-points every fifty kilometres or so, where Mohammed had to hand over the obligatory 50-shilling bribe. Those, and the "fees" at weighbridges, all come out of his 4,000 shilling ($54) travel allowance from the trucking company. He complained about his salary, 15,000 shillings a month ($210)—not a fortune, but a decent wage in Kenya, which has 40 per cent unemployment. When we slowed at the weighbridges, he bought snacks—peanuts, bananas, small bags of fresh water—from vendors who clambered up the steps of the cab and thrust baskets through the window. A couple of times we had engine trouble that required tinkering; the rest of the time, the truck shuddered and shook so hard it made our teeth snap together.

And so the respites, when they came, at the Sweet Banana Bar and Hotel or the Silver Star Butchery, Bar and Lodging were wondrous relief. Cold beer. Soccer on the television. The latest hit from Congo thumping on the stereo. And clean, warm women with wide smiles and quick wit.

At sundown, Mohammed parked at Salgaa, where three hundred trucks stop every night. We watched the drivers streaming into the bars, where women waited on plastic stools. Younger women moved between the rows of parked trucks, looking up, working to catch the eyes of the drivers. The negotiations were remarkably brief—a driver would nod, and the woman would either climb up into the cab or tell him which bar to meet her in once he was done tending his truck.

"There's not much conversation—these are prostitutes, they don't want much conversation," Mohammed explained. "You do the finances first. I say, I will give you 200, okay? Okay. Then sex. Then I pay." For an extra fee, the pair might spend the night together in one of the small hotels. "Different people do different things, some say they must do it every day, some every two-three days, some go once a month, some must sleep where women are every night. Some have a push-and-go for 50 shillings, and some stay together in the lodge for 150. The important thing is to have sex."

Truck drivers are vilified all over the continent for spreading HIV—and there is some truth in the accusation. Truckers were what are called vec-tors in the early years of the African epidemic. In the 1970s, once the virus had a firm foothold in communities in the Great Lakes region, it spread outward on the transport and trade routes, from border points, cities, ports and bustling transport centres back to rural villages. No one else in Africa travels like the truckers do: public transport is limited in most countries, and only those seeking work in the towns have reason to need it. Save for disaster and displacement, the majority of people spend most of their lives in one small patch of the world. Truckers and the handful of other migrants—soldiers, traders and miners—are the exception, and they have played a correspondingly key role in the evolution of the epidemic.

Job Bwayo, a researcher in immunology at the University of Nairobi, noticed in the late 1980s that he was seeing more and more of this new disease, AIDS, among sex workers. Groups of prostitutes he screened tested as high as 80 per cent for HIV, and he wondered about their clients. He started testing truck drivers for the virus in 1989: 36 per cent of the Ugandan drivers were infected, 19 per cent of the Kenyans, 51 per cent of the Rwandans. And while sex workers are a relatively static population, the truck drivers who patronize the prostitutes often have families to whom they return at the end of a journey.

These days, long-haul truckers such as Mohammed have an HIV infection rate that is roughly twice that of the general population. And they remain a key group for the transmission of the disease: because they have what is, by regional standards, a good income; because they spend most of their lives in environments where sex is bought and sold and little social stigma is attached to the transaction; and because many truckers, like millions of others on the continent, have refused to modify their sexual behaviour in the face of frightening evidence of the risks involved.

Some efforts have been made to get drivers to change. The U.S. aid organization Population Services International, for example, has a project called Corridors of Hope that targets drivers at border points across Africa, with condoms, education and health care provided at the truck stops. And yet everywhere I have travelled, and everything I hear from people in the field, makes clear that the trucking culture remains remarkably unchanged from what it was twenty-five years ago, in the era before AIDS. A couple

## "These women are in marketing. They show you are ready to serve it, so buying it. You look at her doing the calculation,

of years earlier, at Chirundu on the border between Zambia and Zimbabwe, where trucks were parked in lines kilometres long waiting for customs clearance, I had watched women—teenagers, most of them— climb in and out of the truck cabs, spending fifteen or twenty minutes in each and then on to the next. Along the highway through the sun-bleached centre of Tanzania, drivers had explained to me that a man has to have sex every day—the impact on his health, if he didn't, could be crippling. At the Maputo port in Mozambique, drivers waiting for freight to come off ships had told me they would never wear a condom when they had sex—it would be undignified, messy, beneath them. All the men I spoke with knew about AIDS, knew of other drivers they thought had likely died of the disease, but they didn't believe it was a risk for them, or at least not the biggest risk. Not a risk outweighed by the benefits.

"Drivers see other people playing with fire and getting burned and then they go to play with the same fire," Ahmed Omar, deputy chair of the Kenya Long Distance Truck Drivers' Welfare Association, told me. We were sitting in a truckers' café in Salgaa, and Omar waved one despairing hand at the women waiting outside on stools, and the men milling around them. "They don't value their lives."

But it's not as simple as that, as Mohammed wanted me to under- stand. When he was growing up in Mombasa, his father was a snack-shop chef and his mother sold chapattis in the road, and they had only enough money for him to go to school for four years—"just enough to read a little

## business—they know
## a piece of cake and they
## there is no problem
## and immediately you start
## How can I get her?"

and speak a little English—we didn't see the importance of school at that time." That limited his options; he apprenticed as a mechanic and got a lucky chance to drive a truck. He liked the independence, liked the physical work of navigating the highways, and yet as he saw it, the hardships of the job—the time away from home and the delays at the borders and the bandits and the bribery—made it almost inevitable that he would come to grief, one way or another.

"Many truck drivers end up having AIDS because they have so many problems," he explained. "The state of the roads, police corruption, low wages—all these problems affect the driver psychologically, so he finds a place to have entertainment and get relief." Working in such conditions, a man could be weak in the face of temptation. "There are so many women on the road and they are tempting, the way they dress is very alluring and I'm very tempted by them." Uganda, in particular, where we were bound with the load of cement, is a hotbed of Mohammed's particular type of temptation. "Uganda has the best women, they are very welcoming, very kind," he said seriously. "Very entertaining. And a good body—middle size, not fat but with a big backside and a small waist, and not very big breasts. That's what Ugandan women are all about." Some men like the very tall, very thin Kenyan women, and some like the delicate Tutsi girls in Rwanda and Burundi, but Mohammed is a Ugandan fancier himself. And then there are the clothes the women wear—not wildly provocative by the standards of a Las Vegas strip bar, but racy for here: miniskirts and scoop-neck tops or halters, outfits that reveal the belly. "Their clothes show parts that are not normally exposed—their hips or backsides or breasts," he said. "In Africa it's not normal to see even the upper part of the knee. Once you see that and you are away from your family for a long time it's hard to resist. And these women are in business—they know marketing. They show you a piece of cake and they are ready to serve it, so there is no problem buying it. You look at her and immediately you start doing the calculation, How can I get her?"

The women are as much a part of this life as the police roadblocks or the border delays. When Mohammed began his life as a driver, working for a big Mombasa transport firm, he bought the company of a woman every night. When, at twenty-three, he married Maryam, he cut back to just once a week or so. There are no condoms in the bars or lodges, and Mohammed said he has never seen them available anywhere on the routes he drives. Until a few years ago, he had no idea that Africans even used them; he thought they were strictly a foreign phenomenon.

The lack of condoms reflects the tension between the conservative cultural and political environment and the reality of the pandemic. Sex with prostitutes causes an estimated 40 per cent of HIV infections in Kenya. Yet here and elsewhere in sub-Saharan Africa, sex workers are rarely included in national AIDS plans: buying sex is illegal, and while authorities tend to turn a blind eye to prostitutes, policy-makers won't include them in government strategies. Donor countries don't like dealing with the business either; the United States AIDS funding agency, PEPFAR, which is the largest donor to AIDS groups in Africa, specifically requires the groups it funds to sign a pledge condemning sex work. So no one is rushing to put condoms into the Sweet Banana—not, Mohammed said, that it would likely make much difference if they did. "The use of condoms among truck drivers, if I can be very frank, is not very common—they don't get enough enjoyment using condoms," he said, hunting for words to explain it delicately. "You don't get the feeling. You're getting the pleasure from a third party—it's going from the woman to the condom and then to you. So truck drivers don't use them."

Some of the women might initially suggest using one, but a few more shillings will usually persuade them otherwise. Anyway, he said, they don't insist for a married man. Single men are one thing, but married men buying sex are perceived to be much safer. And many of the drivers have long-standing relationships with women in each truck-stop town—women they call on once or twice a month, each time they come through. A driver may help with school fees for the woman's children, or buy her a cellphone. And he would no more think of using a condom with her than he would with his wife. "This is the driver's way of thinking."

Mohammed understands this, and yet he also has a new and vivid sense of the risk involved. In September 2003, the truckers' welfare association opened up an outreach centre in an old shipping container parked at the Mlolongo truck stop where we met outside Nairobi, offering drivers counselling and HIV testing. Mohammed said he had heard about the disease— ukimwi, something that makes you thin, in Kiswahili—over the past decade, and knew that it was transmitted by sex. He had seen other drivers die, perhaps from that disease, although one never knew for certain. He had been feeling flu-like symptoms for some time, and he had taken malarial cures with no improvement. Nevertheless, when he went for a test in November, he said, his sole motivation was to "set a good example," to give this new truckers' service some business.

"What did the test say?" I asked. Mohammed raised his eyebrows all the way up to the edge of his frayed white prayer cap. "Positive?" I asked. He nodded. "It was a very big shock," he acknowledged. "But I took it very easily because I'm a truck driver and I could die any time." It was a sentiment I had heard many times before, from soldiers and miners, too: there was little point in worrying about a tiny germ, given all the other dangers. And no sense denying oneself comforts, either.

Mohammed wasn't sure when he had been infected—obviously, there was no shortage of opportunity. "I'm sure not many of the women are infected, but by chance or by luck I ended up with one who was positive. It was just bad luck." He felt well enough, and so he had declined the counsellor's referral to a clinic, saying he preferred to manage his health

# "My wife doesn't know I had all these partners."

on his own. "After that, I decided to stay away from cigarettes, from drinking—I was drinking a lot, and having a lot of outside entertainment. I thought I should rather concentrate on my family and eat a balanced diet. Up to now I feel very strong and very healthy and I think something that creates better health with HIV/AIDS is your own mind—if you think all the time about AIDS, it will kill you very fast. But my positive status doesn't trouble me and that's why I think I'm very healthy."

His positive status does, however, trouble his wife, Maryam, whom he told of the diagnosis, although they have not told their children or anyone else. "But she has to accept my state," Mohammed said with a shrug. "My wife doesn't know I had all these partners"—well, not specifically— "but she knows about drivers and she takes me to be the same." Maryam went for an HIV test after he told her of his results, and she tested negative. Since then, he said, they don't have sex, and he has given up sex on the road as well. That made me arch an eyebrow of my own. What were the odds that I would be picked up by that rare creature, a celibate trucker, when I was taking a trip to learn about AIDS? But Mohammed was so honest about his sexual history that I had little reason to doubt him, and he talked with great sincerity about his return to Islam.

In our long conversations on the rutted highways, Mohammed gave voice to a range of contradictory views. In one breath he would tell me how essential it was for a driver to have sex every few days; in the next, he would talk about the shame of having sex outside marriage, how wrong that is "in African culture." His religion didn't trouble him through all the years he bought sex, he said: "In the Muslim community you have drunkards and other people doing evil, Muslims in name only." He and many others had found a place to live between the official prescriptions of religion and conservative culture and a reality that was much more permissive. "I wasn't devout then—but I'm very sorry about it. I wish I could go back and do it over."

At noon on his third day of this journey, Mohammed reached the Ugandan border and submitted his paperwork at the customs office. The engine had to be oiled and tuned; when that was done, he unrolled a mat beneath the high bed of the truck and lay down in the shade. Men were streaming past, on their way to the bars. Mohammed stayed put.

"Do you worry about getting sick?" I asked him.

"Yes," he said. "But everybody dies one day."

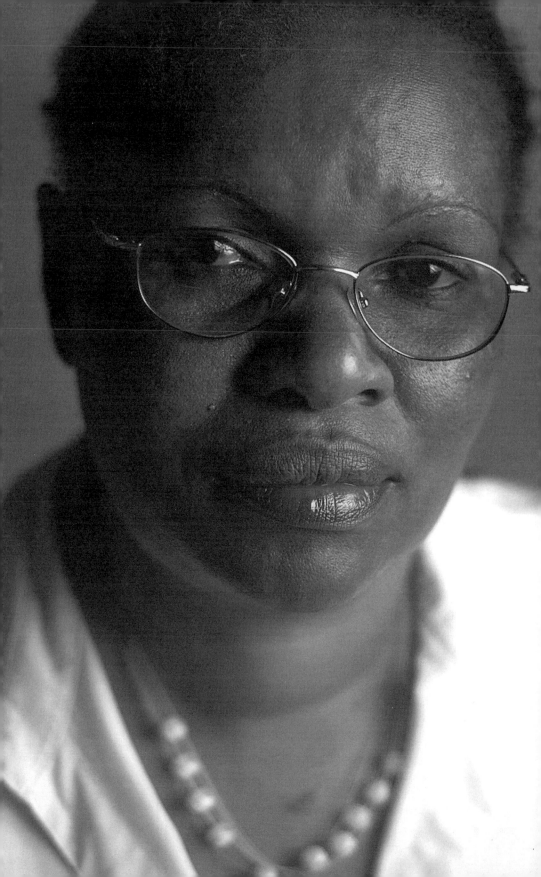

# FOUR

# PriscaMhlolo

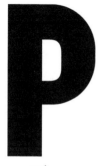risca Mhlolo took an inventory of all the fear and shame and hurt.

The scar on her forehead, that's where her sister hit her with a bottle. "This here," she said, running her fingers over a scar at the back of her head, "this was a bench, my brother hit me with a bench." Next was a raised keloid scar on her chest. "I had a big cut there. I don't even know what hit me. That was my other brother."

What prompted it? "The word *AIDS*. That word was enough."

In 1997, Prisca decided that ten years of keeping her secret was plenty, and she confided to her closest family members that she was living with HIV. "It didn't go well," she said dryly as we settled on the lumpy couch in her house in Harare in early 2006. I had known Prisca for years, as an outspoken counsellor and advocate for people with HIV in Zimbabwe, and I knew she had had a hard go of it: she has a flinty fearlessness that comes with losing a great deal. So one day I asked her to tell me the whole story—it took her that day and well into the warm night, until even the neighbourhood dogs had ceased to bark, to chronicle the cost HIV has exacted from her.

It began with a sick baby. In 1987, Prisca and her husband, Bruce, both twenty-seven, were living in a small house in Mabvuku, a low-income neighbourhood on the outskirts of Harare, the capital. It was an era of new prosperity in a country independent for just seven years. Bruce was an army medic, earning a decent monthly wage, and Prisca was as much in love with her soldier husband as the day she first laid eyes on him, as a schoolgirl of eighteen. They had married at 23, against the wishes of his family, because she is from the Shona ethnic group, while Bruce was Ndebele. But no matter: they had found a house they could afford in the city. They had friendly neighbours. They had two bright and healthy children, Bianca and Richard.

In 1987 came a third child, Agnes. By her first birthday, it was clear something was grievously wrong with her. "She was always in and out of hospital with swollen eyes, with diarrhea, you name any disease," Prisca said. "Of course, we didn't think—we didn't know what it was. Each time we would take my daughter to the hospital, they would say a lot of things: 'It could be liver, do you have asthma in the family, do you have cancer?' But there was nothing of that sort in the family." Finally one doctor took Prisca aside. "He said, 'Look here, we need to do some tests.' He never said what tests, and it was okay with me. They were going to find the problem."

The doctor drew a vial of Agnes's blood to test her for HIV, the first cases of which had been reported in Zimbabwe six years earlier. "The thing I knew about AIDS was that AIDS was for sex workers, prostitutes, not married women, not baby girls. If you were a promiscuous person, automatically you could get AIDS. But there I was, a married person. I had slept only with Bruce."

Two weeks after the doctor took blood, Prisca carried her daughter back to the clinic to collect the results. The doctor himself didn't turn up. And the nurse, although she knew Prisca well after all her visits, spoke to her coldly, without any of the formal greetings that would normally begin such a meeting in Zimbabwe. "She was just looking at me, she didn't want to talk to me, she didn't want to play with my daughter," Prisca recalled. "Then she took a letter and threw it at me. I said, 'What is this now? I came here because I want to see the doctor, I want to get the results.' She said, 'Those are your results, Prisca. Your daughter has AIDS and she is going to die. Don't waste your time.'"

All the anger, shock and pain of that moment were clear in Prisca's face twenty years later. "The way she said it was something else: AIDS! Where did the AIDS come from? I looked down at my daughter in my lap and she was not a child any more, she was something—she was now AIDS to me. I didn't want anything to do with that child. I took her and threw her—she hit the corner of the desk and got a big cut. She collapsed. And I ran from that hospital into the street screaming. Doctors were coming and they wanted to get hold of me but they couldn't because I was running. In Mazoe Street, just by the entrance, I collapsed. The next thing I knew, I woke up and it was two weeks later."

When she awoke in a hospital bed with her husband standing next to her, she turned to him in anguish. "I said, 'Bruce, we are dying, we are already dead.' He said, 'Why?' I told him about Agnes. I told him, 'Because of AIDS. I'm a moving grave as you see me.' That's what I told him.

"He laughed. Up till now, I can hear him laugh.

"He said, 'Prisca, look here. There is nothing like AIDS, there is nothing of that sort. AIDS is a white man's disease. There's been a mistake in this hospital. The results given to our child were a white child's results. You don't have to worry. I still love you, I still love Agnes. We can go home and rejoice. These doctors don't know what they are doing.'"

His words didn't entirely make sense, but Prisca was comforted regardless. "When it's coming from your husband, who is learned, whom you trust, the one you don't suspect has other partners—I was okay for that moment. Though it was a lie, it helped me. It made me feel better."

Nonetheless, a full month passed before she was strong enough to be discharged. She ached with guilt each time she looked at the scar on Agnes's forehead. Before they left the hospital, she made a request of her husband: just to be sure, she wanted the two of them also to be tested for this AIDS business.

"He didn't refuse. He was a cool guy. He said it was okay with him." He was, she said, gambling.

Their results came back positive. Prisca said she knew as she read them that it was true, there was no laboratory mix-up. How else could Agnes have got the disease? "I said, 'Okay, I have AIDS.' I asked the doctor, 'How long will we live?' He said, 'You will not survive.' He gave Agnes two weeks, he gave me three months."

# "So if you dare talk about HIV/AIDS to anyone, I am going to kill you."

Her sole experience of the virus came from a neighbour who had gone away to work in South Africa, died there of AIDS and been shipped home in a biohazard bag in a sealed coffin. "At that time it was said that if you looked at someone with AIDS you will get the virus." Now Prisca could picture her own imminent death. "I'm going to die, I'm going to be put in black plastic and my coffin will be sealed. What about the church people, what are they going to say? What about my parents, what of my neighbours?"

She was discharged from hospital, and carried Agnes home to her house in Mabvuku, where the other children were anxious to have her back. But her joy at the homecoming barely lasted until they were through the door. "When we came, something funny happened. That loving and caring husband changed into a monster." She had climbed straight into bed, and now Bruce stood over her. "He said, 'Prisca, look here. Your AIDS, we left it at the hospital. In this house I am in charge, I am in charge of you—don't forget I paid *lobola*. I am also in charge of the children. So if you dare talk about HIV/AIDS to anyone, I am going to kill you.'"

Prisca understood that this was no idle threat. "He was a soldier who used to bring a pistol or even rifles home. Even up to now, soldiers can do anything." Men from the army regularly beat and sometimes murdered their wives, and there was never an investigation. Prisca knew she could easily die the same way—at the hands of this grim stranger, her husband.

Looking back, she has little doubt that Bruce knew his HIV status long before she took Agnes to the hospital for the test. She reckons he had tested positive some time before, in a military screening, and he either hoped that somehow the hospital test would be negative—in the mid-1980s, HIV testing was a more imprecise science—or that doctors would not tell Prisca the truth. Now he told his wife about a close friend, a fellow soldier, who had tested positive a year earlier "for this AIDS"—a man who was still strong and healthy. Whatever the doctors said about the days or weeks they had to live, Bruce said, it was all garbage: his colleague was fine.

Prisca began to take Agnes from clinic to clinic across Harare, searching for someone who would give her a new diagnosis. "My life was packed with lies—because I knew what was wrong with my daughter and I was also in denial, saying, 'No, it can't be, not my daughter, not me.'" But the doctor's prediction haunted her, and she sensed her days running out. She gave away her clothes, offering no explanation to the startled friends in whose arms she heaped skirts and blouses.

"Then it was two months, then three months, then ten months, a year, and we are still alive. But in this home there was no happiness. It had stopped. We couldn't talk the way we used to because of this AIDS thing." If she put on nice clothes to go out, Bruce would call her a whore. He was critical of any plan she made, fearing that she might confide their secret to someone outside the home. "Even church—I stopped going to church." Instead, she sat at home and wondered what she could possibly have done to bring AIDS upon her family.

They all remained alive through the next four years, although Agnes was always frail and fighting one ailment or another. Prisca did not take Bianca or Richard to be tested. "I was confident the other children were healthy—but really, I didn't want to know. To think of looking after another child who had AIDS, that was too much."

From the outside, they looked like a normal family. They had relatives nearby, Bruce's colleagues from the military and friends from the Anglican Church. But her secret made Prisca feel horribly isolated. "I was with my problems alone."

And then one day in 1992 she heard on the radio about a support group for women with AIDS. She wrote down the address and set off right away, without telling Bruce where she was going. With Agnes in her arms, she walked into a room where a dozen women were gathered, and felt instant, immediate relief at the sight of these others—some black, some white—all of them also infected with HIV. They told Prisca about Lynde

# "If people know about me won't want anything

Francis, a tough white Zimbabwean woman who ran a building company and who had been living openly with HIV for an almost unheard-of eight years. That afternoon, Prisca carried Agnes to Lynde's graceful old house and told her the child had the disease. Lynde took Agnes and put her in the bathtub (Agnes had constant diarrhea) and then gently explained to Prisca about HIV—the virus she had—and AIDS, the disease to which Agnes had clearly progressed.

Prisca joined the group of women who met regularly at Lynde's house. They called themselves Tariro, or "hope" in the Shona language. "Everyone who was there had hope: we will live with the virus." Yet hope notwithstanding, they lost members regularly. "Death was surrounding us. At every meeting you would hear, 'So-and-so who was here last week is here no more, is dead, and So-and-so is very ill.'"

And by 1995, it was Agnes: she was skeletally thin. Prisca was awed that her child had lived even that long. "She was strong. And she got all the love, from me—and from Bruce. Each time Bruce went out to Tanzania or Mozambique he would bring something for Agnes, a new dress, a pair of shoes or a toy. He loved that child—maybe because he knew he was the one who had caused all the problems."

Prisca took her daughter to stay in a palliative care hospice full of AIDS patients. Eight-year-old Agnes had a lesion on the side of her face that would not heal, and at the hospice, they diagnosed the skin cancer Kaposi's sarcoma. It was easier to care for her there, with professional help, but the atmosphere was horrible. "When I got there, I started crying. I saw a lot of people who were sick. I never thought that in this world I would see people who were sick like that." And Prisca was afraid—that people would know, because Agnes was in the hospice, that she had AIDS. "I was afraid of Bruce and his threat, that's one thing. But also for myself: if people know about me and my AIDS status they won't want anything to do with me." By then nearly 20 per cent of Zimbabwean adults were living with HIV, yet as Prisca remembers it, the fear and stigma remained almost totally unchanged from the day of her diagnosis.

She knew that Agnes, lying in bed, could overhear voices from the corridors, heard when people died in the rooms on either side, or when everyone gathered to pray for a person in the last moments of life. "It's harder than your own diagnosis, looking after a dying child with AIDS," Prisca said. "The pain was there written all over her face. She would cry and say, 'I think I'm also going to die, because the pain is too much. My whole body is painful.'" Finally, sensing Agnes had only a few days left, Prisca took her home again.

On November 20, 1995, Bruce had a day off and decided to go into Harare. Agnes first pleaded with her father not to go, saying he might find her dead when he returned. Then she asked him to bring her favourite treat, chicken and chips from the city. But soon after he left, she asked for the pastor, saying she wanted to be prayed for. As the pastor finished his prayers, she died. Bruce came home several hours later to a house and yard overflowing with people. Toting the chicken in a paper sack, he rushed to the bedroom and found the neighbours washing his daughter's wasted body.

At her funeral a few days later, he became completely hysterical. "Some people thought he was drunk," Prisca said. "He even wanted to throw himself in the grave." The drama was just starting. While still at the cemetery, Bruce developed diarrhea. "He was pouring profusely. He didn't even see the end of the funeral, he had to be ferried back to the house. And that was the beginning of a new era."

Her husband, the strapping soldier, never walked again. "He was so depressed. He started talking in tongues. He had dementia." At times he would weep and apologize to Prisca for having killed their daughter. Another time he confessed to infidelities while posted in Mozambique. "Because of Agnes's death it came into his mind that this is real and he is going to die."

Prisca believes the shock and stress caused him to progress rapidly to full-blown AIDS. But still, from his bed, he tugged at her skirt and pleaded with her not to tell. "I kept the promise." No one had suspected AIDS when the child was ill, because her parents were still so healthy. And now, although Bruce was clearly desperately ill, Prisca looked fine. "I was surprised they never thought of AIDS, but I was happy for that. I was safe."

Except that, instead of AIDS, Bruce's family began to suspect his wife of having cursed him. "One day his parents brought a traditional healer who waved a wand and pointed at me, saying, 'This is the witch. If you leave your son here, he is going to die. You must take him away.'" Many people in Zimbabwe and elsewhere in Africa invest great faith in traditional healers, who heal the sick with natural medicine and use visions and divination, like healers in aboriginal cultures around the world, to try to explain events, good and bad, that befall their followers. But along with legitimate healers, there are charlatans who invoke the spirit world to justify actions like those of Bruce's parents, who now accused Prisca of having first killed Agnes and now attempting to kill Bruce, in order to get his money. They picked her husband up by his shoulders and legs and carted him out to the car. Even as he was carried out of the house, he pleaded with her not to tell the truth about his illness.

Prisca was still standing in the doorway, stunned, when a truck pulled up a few minutes later. Supervised by a few of Bruce's relatives, workers packed up the family belongings. "They took everything, even the utensils, even my clothes, even the children's clothes." The neighbours looked on in astonishment. That night she and the children slept on the floor of their empty house, on a thin blanket loaned by friends.

A few days later, she travelled the two hundred kilometres out to Kwekwe, where Bruce's family had taken him. But at the door of the house, she was turned away. Perhaps, she said, her in-laws really believed it was witchcraft. Or maybe they had an inkling of what might be wrong, but the idea that Bruce had this mysterious disease that struck down healthy young people when they behaved immorally was too awful, too shameful, to contemplate. If the workings of sorcery were hard to understand, AIDS was worse. Everybody knew about greedy wives who cursed their husbands; few understood viruses. Prisca turned away and made the long journey back to Harare without catching sight of her husband. She feared his family might unwittingly contract HIV as they nursed him—at her support group she had learned of the risk of infection in blood or diarrhea—but she could think of no way to warn them without giving away his secret.

Bruce died a few weeks later, but the family did not notify Prisca. She learned the news only two weeks after his death when a good Samaritan travelling from Kwekwe slipped an unsigned note under her door. "I remember screaming. I screamed so that all the neighbours came." She went back to Kwekwe, and the family begrudgingly let her visit the grave, but she could not stay long enough to perform any of the rituals that a Zimbabwean wife is supposed to offer at her husband's grave.

And then it was Prisca's turn: the shock of her husband's death and her sudden impoverishment caused her own health to collapse. "I wanted to tell my mother but I didn't know how to start. I was so sick. I got a terrible headache, I got a terrible rash. My hair fell out, there was nothing left. My lips became red with sores everywhere. I couldn't stand on my own, I couldn't sit, I couldn't even feed myself. But because my family members didn't know what was happening, they took care of me at that time. I was dying. I was on my way to heaven."

In the meantime, she had a very earthly problem. Until he was hopelessly ill in the last weeks of his life, Bruce had insisted they have sex—"naked sex," as they call it in Harare, sex without a condom. "He would say, 'Prisca, I married you, not a condom, and we are not going to use one.'" Their house was sandwiched in between the neighbours', with just screens in the windows, and she couldn't bear for the neighbourhood to hear their arguments. "That would make me a no-good woman, because if you are married in our culture, you have to abide by your husband's rules." So she acquiesced.

A few weeks before Bruce died, Prisca had gone to the hospital to try to enrol in a drug trial she had heard about at the support group. The trials, run by big North American and European pharmaceutical companies, were then the only way of getting access to AIDS medication in Zimbabwe. A physical exam, including a pregnancy test, was part of the trial screening—and now the doctors told her she was six months pregnant. She was stunned. In the drama of Bruce's death, it had never occurred to her that she might be pregnant again. "It wasn't good news. I started thinking of Agnes . . ." She could not bear the thought of nursing another dying child. But the doctors told her she was too far into the pregnancy to end it. She was hysterical. "I told the doctor, 'If you don't abort me, I will kill myself at your home.'" Her threats persuaded them, and although she was not well, her health stabilized.

Now, however, she was penniless, with two children to raise and no idea how to make money. Prisca talks about many of the most difficult episodes in her life with poise and calm, but when she told me this part of the story she broke off and wept. A friend told her she could make money by having sex with men from the pub. She could think of no other way. She refused to go and work in the bars, but the friend brought men to her house late at night. She felt filthy, she said, full of guilt and shame and nearly crushed with the weight of her secret, with the knowledge she might be passing HIV to these men. But she saw no other way to take care of her children. "There was no food and I wanted to pay for school so much."

And then, when she felt trapped and panicky and nearly mad, came rescue. Her support group received donor funding to send two members on a year-long college course to train as HIV counsellors. Prisca was chosen, and immediately excelled. "It was like I was born into it. I was doing the course with nurses and doctors and here I was, a nobody just with my O-levels, but I did well." She earned, in fact, a 95 per cent in her first semester. Lynde Francis had in the meantime turned her support group into an organization she called The Centre. It provided testing, counselling and HIV education built on a philosophy of "positive living"— Lynde told people that with good nutrition and a good attitude, they could live healthily with the virus for years, as she had. Lynde offered Prisca a job as a counsellor. "It answered all the prayers that I was praying all the time. I stopped the dirty work and started a new life."

But before she had even finished the counselling course, Prisca received more dreadful news. Richard, her second child, who was in high school in Mutare, had taken his own life by drinking pesticide. As he explained in the letter he left for her, written on notebook paper in his messy schoolboy's hand, he had been sexually abused by a teacher and he was certain that he had been infected with AIDS. "He knew his sister and his father died of AIDS, although he didn't know about me. He wrote me, 'I don't want to die like Daddy and my sister, that's why I'm killing myself. I don't want to die of AIDS, that's why I'm taking my own life.'"

At the funeral in Mutare, Prisca made a decision. "Something in me just said, 'Enough, enough. It is high time.'" First she read Richard's letter out to the family, revealing that Bruce and Agnes had had AIDS. Bruce's father had snuck away from his own family to attend his grandson's funeral, and Prisca felt relief that now he would know the truth, and could tell the others what had really killed her husband. Then she told them she was also infected. After a moment of stunned silence, her siblings launched themselves at her with the bottles and the bench. "I was beaten like a thief."

Prisca got away from them and ran out of the house, and a friend took her to a clinic. She needed dozens of stitches. Her spectacles were smashed, her clothes so drenched in blood they could not be salvaged. Friends urged her to return to Harare immediately, but Prisca felt she could not leave without visiting her son's grave the next day. She slept that night in a hotel, her wounds throbbing.

The next day, when she arrived at the cemetery, her family was already there, and there was another scene. "Prisca, do you see your mother here?" her older sister Mercy asked nastily. Their mother was not there: Prisca's siblings told her she was in the hospital with perilously high blood pressure, "because of your AIDS." Prisca performed the rituals at the grave and left quickly, heading for the hospital. But when she approached her mother's bed, her mother thrust her arms out. "She said, 'Prisca, don't come near me, you with your AIDS. Don't ever, ever come. I don't want to see you.'" Prisca dropped the fruit basket she was carrying, sending oranges and bananas scattering across the floor; she moaned and sank to her knees, and nurses came running. Her mother insisted she get out. Prisca collected Bianca and headed back to Harare.

"AIDS, it brings a lot of problems and hatred," she said to me, still wistful.

But she had crossed a line and she was not going back, regardless of how her family behaved. Days after Richard's funeral, she was asked to do a national television interview on HIV testing and counselling. "The presenter asked how I felt dealing with people with AIDS. I said, 'It's okay with me, because I am also HIV-positive. I have the virus.'"

Her colleagues were shocked at her bold disclosure, but congratulated her on her courage. Prisca's siblings, however, were also watching. "That night my sister Mercy came. She gave me good, good, good, good claps"—blows to the head. "I didn't fight back because I respected her—she's older. She said, 'You have shamed the whole clan,' that our family was now dirty because of me." (That, as Prisca would soon learn, was a most ironic statement.)

She quickly discovered that others beyond her family were not impressed with her public stance either. "Things had been going better for me. I was gaining weight, I was okay, I was respected in the community, I was a professional, working, earning good money. But coming out on television was a big blunder. It didn't go well with my neighbours. If I was seen talking to a male neighbour they would say, 'Ah, our man, he will get AIDS from this AIDS victim.'"

Yet while she was publicly shunned, there were many evenings when she would hear a soft tap on the window frame after dark—people too embarrassed to come to her house in daylight came at night to seek advice. "They would say, 'I have developed this rash, does it mean I have AIDS?' or, 'My husband is ill, can you come?'" By this time, a quarter of Zimbabwean adults were living with HIV, and scarcely a single family was untouched, but still only a handful of people had the courage to go public. It made Prisca a magnet for those seeking help.

The next few years went well, except for the pain of the estrangement from her family. "But I was okay with that. I was surrounded by people who were like family." Then, early in 2004, her brother Lovemore died—of AIDS. Months later, her sister Mercy died of AIDS, and two days later, her younger brother died of meningitis, a common HIV-related infection. Finally her last surviving sister, Violet, fell ill.

Now Prisca found herself back in favour with her mother, who came asking for money for seed and fertilizer to put in the next year's crop. She couldn't resist asking her mother if she was sure she wanted to accept cash from a person with AIDS, but she gave her the money. "Even though these are the ones who made me to suffer and no one ever asked for forgiveness or said they were sorry for what they did." Family is family.

Through more than twenty years of living with HIV, Prisca has had a lot of time to think about the fear and disgrace that dog this disease even though so many people have it themselves, or have partners and children and sisters and cousins who are infected. "In the early days, when it first came, it was a disease for prostitutes. There were posters with a guy and a bottle of beer and a lady in a miniskirt. Those were the ones who were supposed to get HIV—not married people," she said. "Now people know better." Yet the stigma remains, as does the belief that bad things don't just *happen* but rather are earned, or engineered through witchcraft.

The policy of confidential HIV testing, imported from the West where AIDS began as a gay disease, hasn't helped either, she said. "This confidentiality is killing a lot of people. Let's look at the woman's side: the husband goes and he is tested, but he doesn't come home and disclose his status. What does that mean? The wife is going to be infected. Because he doesn't have guts, she is going to die." Or women are tested, in prenatal visits, but won't tell their husbands if they are positive for fear of being accused "as the one who brought it."

Coming to the end of her story, she sighed and slumped back on the couch. "In our culture, you don't tell. We don't talk, and that is killing the nation."

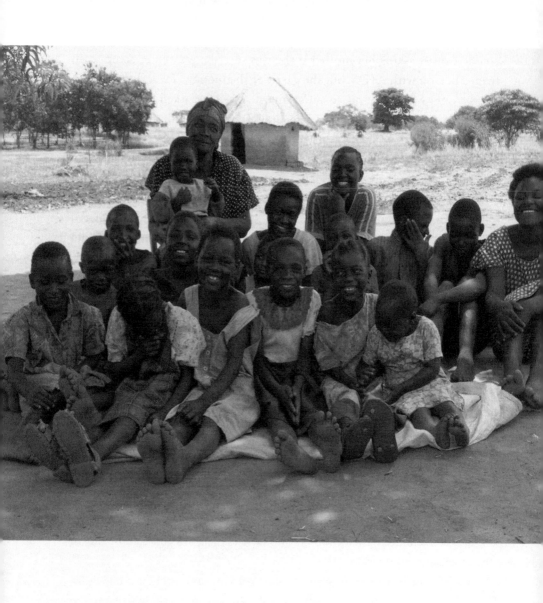

# FIVE

# RegineMamba

n the natural order of things, these would be quiet days for Regine Mamba. She would sit in the shade of the large neem tree in her swept dirt yard in Malala in southern Zambia. She might sift through a basket of beans in her lap, picking out the stones and twigs, and she might keep an eye on a pudgy baby just learning to totter. They should be peaceful, these days at the end of her life.

Instead, Regine works. She is up before the sun to start a fire for the maize porridge the children eat, and still up well after the sun has set, trying to comfort them with a story or a hymn when they sit by the embers of that fire. And although she is exhausted, she often lies awake long after the children have fallen asleep all crammed together in two round mud houses—there is much to occupy her mind. Instead of the quiet twilight of old age that should be hers, Regine has work and worries and children.

A huge number of children: so many that when I arrived at her house, on a walk through Malala, I thought at first that it was a primary school. There were children peeping around the doors of the houses and children sitting in the shade of the thatch-roof overhang, children tussling by the kindling pile and children beneath the tree.

"These children, their mothers and fathers died," Regine said by way of introduction.

We sat beneath that tree and Regine told me about the past few years, how it came to be that they are all her children now. As a young woman, she had given birth to seven who survived, most of whom went off to the capital, Lusaka, to work as teachers and clerks and maids. There they got married and had children of their own. In the usual way of things in a place like Malala, those children would have come home every few months, bringing their own families—they might time their visit to help with the planting, and bring a sweater or a fluffy new Chinese-made blanket as a gift. Regine would have sat on a rough wood chair and listened to the stories from the city. Her children would have stayed for a couple of days, and then they would have gone home again, taking their own children with them.

It didn't work out that way. In 1998, one of her daughters died in Lusaka, and she took a rickety shared taxi into the city. "I went and assessed the situation. Their father did not have much life left in him. According to our tradition, as the grandmother you are responsible. You cannot just disregard your grand-children." So she brought those children home to Malala. Then a second daughter and son-in-law died, and their children were sent to Regine. Then her third daughter, Lovegirl, lost her husband and came home, bringing her one surviving child and two orphans from another daughter. Before long there were more than a dozen children, in city clothes rapidly starting to fray, and at the age of seventy-four, Regine's days of sitting in the shade were over.

In Zambia today, basic demographics are horribly skewed. One in three children is an orphan. One in five people has HIV/AIDS. In a country of eleven million, at least 600,000 people have already died, almost all of them young adults. They have left behind a good part of a generation of children without parents. And in so many cases those children have wound up, after a few detours to aunts or neighbours, with their grandmothers.

Nearly two-thirds of orphans in southern and eastern Africa are in the care of grandparents. One in three heads of household in Zambia is over fifty

# twilight of old age that has work and worries and children.

years of age; two-thirds of them are female. In other words, grandmothers. It is the grannies, more than any other group, who carry this burden. Regine was already widowed and long past the days of sexual activity when the virus took hold in Zambia—women her age have largely escaped it. They remain healthy as their children waste away by the age of thirty. When I met her in 2003, Regine had lived to twice a Zambian woman's life expectancy, by then reduced to just thirty-seven years because of AIDS.

Regine and her family live at the end of a winding dirt track on a low hill. There is one big rondavel, about two metres across with smooth mud-plastered walls, where she sleeps with the little ones; one rough rondavel where they cook and keep their small store of maize; a third, small rondavel where the older children sleep, and one last round hut. Regine led me inside this one and introduced her youngest daughter, Jacqueline, who was then exactly my age, thirty-two. She was lying on the floor on a fresh grass mat, and dying. Every hour or two her toddler daughter crept up to the door and peered around it to where her mother lay. Sometimes Jacqueline gave her a little wave.

Regine has a constant struggle to care for this brood, ranging from one lanky fifteen-year-old boy to several grubby babies. Lovegirl, the only other adult in the family, is fifty-one, has grandchildren of her own and could also reasonably expect to be retiring. Instead she had moved back home to help her mother.

"It's trying, it's difficult—the only way I manage is that what little I get, I give them," Regine said. "Even if it's not very nice food—as long as it helps them to live. The biggest problem is that I have to till the land, and I have no animals to help me plant a big maize field." Her back aches, and it pains her to hoe and plow, but she has no cash to hire labourers from the village and must rely on the work of the older children. Her worries have given her high blood pressure; after she slowly lowered herself to the ground, to sit and rest for a minute or two, she rubbed her swollen calves with gnarled hands.

The children were dust-smeared and grimy, wearing short trousers made out of feed sacks. It is a source of some shame for Regine, who knows that her grandchildren are less well off than her own children were. The newest child in the house that day was an infant a few weeks old, born to a fourteen-year-old granddaughter. Regine said, looking pained and embarrassed, that she was surprised by the pregnancy, but then, it isn't uncommon for orphaned village girls to have sex with older men for cash or food.

She wants the children to go to school, but in Zambia it costs 8,850 kwacha per year per child, or about $2.50—a huge burden. On the holidays and between terms, the oldest children go out to hoe the fields of better-off farmers near town to earn a few kwacha; thus far, it had been enough to keep them all enrolled for another term. Sometimes there is a bit left over for a new shirt or a pair of shoes, shoes that are worn only to school and church and otherwise kept stored away.

Regine's situation, the sheer quantity of children she has inherited, should be extraordinary. And yet in Malala, this story—of the young people dying and their wide-eyed children turning up back in the village—has become the norm. In 1999, the old women decided to organize, to pool their resources. They made a registry, and came up with 376 orphans, out of a total population of four thousand in Malala and two villages nearby. In other words, nearly one of every ten people in these villages is a child whose parents have died of AIDS. The grandmothers made a plan: committee members set out to visit each family with orphans, to see how they were coping. That chance to talk is important, Regine said—it gives the guardians an opportunity to share their worries, and the children time to air their grievances. The local branch of the Salvation Army said it would help, with blankets, food parcels and pens and notebooks. But there wasn't enough money for the one thing every grandmother wanted: money to pay the fees and keep all the children in school.

As I sat with Regine that day, several of her neighbours, elderly ladies dressed, as she was, in a print wrap and blouse, scarves knotted round their heads, walked slowly up over the hill. They joined us in the shade of the neem tree, stretching out callused bare feet. The grannies said they could cope with the young orphans, but the pain of their parents' deaths makes the older ones a handful. "There's a problem with teenagers," one neighbour confided, while Regine slowly nodded in agreement. "With younger children you can manage, but teenagers say, 'You are not my mother or father.' Like any teenager, they go out and we are afraid they will be infected themselves, by the older men in the drinking places." Regine glanced toward her teenage granddaughters, one with the new baby on her back.

Regine was keeping the children fed and clothed—in itself something of a miracle—but she worried a great deal about their spirits. "I try by all means to make the children happy, because if I look sad they will worry and wonder what is happening, so I must tell them jokes. In the evenings when we sit around the cooking fire, I tell them stories, I sing them songs. I wish them happiness."

She and the other grandmothers listed off the people who were sick in Malala; they could name almost two dozen children who would lose their parents in the coming year. What, I asked, would happen to those children? Someone will take them in, the women said. We will continue to take care of them until all of us are dead.

But that, of course, was Regine's predominant worry. She was acutely conscious of her age. What will happen if she dies? If Lovegirl gets sick or can't manage? She told me that her great fear is that if the children are orphaned again, they will be separated, each one parcelled out to a different family; no one, she knows, could be expected to take all thirteen. "I worry. I think the children will suffer . . . I am old now, but we thank God that I can still manage."

She was sitting with her back against the tree trunk, and one by one the smaller children had crept forward to listen to the visitors. First one, then a second, jostled for space in her lap; she moved her legs so that a couple more could cuddle up beside her. An impish girl of about four wanted to drape around her granny's neck, and Regine made room for her too.

"I never imagined it this way," she said.

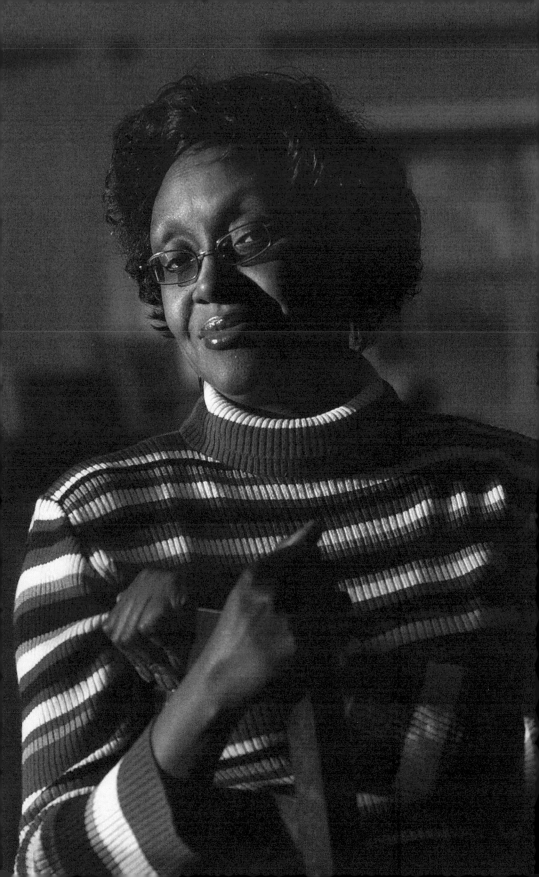

# LydiaMungherera

**D**r. Lydia Mungherera runs briskly through the list of symptoms: tuberculosis, candidiasis, pneumonia, skin lesions, advanced dementia. Not a single organ or bodily system left unaffected. Total immune collapse. Death just hours away. Beyond grim: hopeless.

The broad-shouldered Ugandan physician pauses, counts off the maladies on her long fingers, taps a chic-booted toe impatiently. Is she missing one? "The only thing I *didn't* have was cryptococcal meningitis," she says.

This is not a patient's file. This is her own list: this is what she had in June 1997, when AIDS very nearly killed her.

In a healthy person, the CD4 count—a measure of the number of CD4 cells, or helper T cells, in the blood—would be about 1,000 per cubic millimetre. On that June day, Lydia had rather fewer. "It was one. Just one. Imagine." Lydia chuckles about it sometimes—and it seems preposterous when I see her now, when she strides through an airport, a leather handbag fat with files swinging at her side, or when she addresses another audience from a lectern, the light glinting on her impeccable accessories.

I had heard about her for years, this doctor who came back from a CD4 count of one to be a key figure in the fight for AIDS treatment. I had seen her speak at conferences and meetings around the continent and abroad. But it was not until 2005, when a leg injury had Lydia laid up for a few days, that I got her to sit still long enough to tell me her story.

Once, years ago, it mortified her, the idea that she, a doctor, could get HIV and end up at the very edge of death from AIDS. But it's been a long while since Lydia has had time to worry about that sort of judgment, from herself or anyone else.

She is, by Ugandan standards, a person of considerable privilege. She was born in 1959 in Jinja, a good-sized city to the east, where the Nile flows out of Lake Victoria. Her father worked for the British colonial government as a community development officer. Her mother was a social worker and teacher who for forty years ran the Young Women's Christian Association in Uganda. Lydia's family put a great premium on education: of the six children, four are doctors, one a journalist and one a lawyer. Lydia, a middle child, always felt medicine was a natural choice for her, a field where her forthright personality would allow her "to talk to people directly." She enrolled at the medical college of Makerere University in the capital, Kampala; despite the civil war that had raged in Uganda for years, it was still the premiere university in East Africa. When the brutal despot Idi Amin was overthrown by rebels in 1979 there was sporadic fighting all around the school, but it stayed open for all but a week or two.

In her fourth year of medical school, Lydia was drawn to a fellow student named David Mwere, an affable, thoughtful member of her gang of pals. "For a long time we were just good friends—good relationships are based on that." They married when they finished school in 1985. They were each given jobs at Mulago Hospital, the big public facility on a hill above Kampala. But there was no staff housing, and they had to live crammed into a tiny apartment in town. (There is only limited commercial housing in most African cities, so accommodation is often a benefit offered with public service posts.) Uganda lay in ruins after the years of war, the economy was a shambles, and Lydia said they didn't see much future there. So they began applying for jobs outside the country and were soon offered posts working together in Zimbabwe, where the government was pouring money into the health system. In 1986, they headed for

Masvingo, Zimbabwe's third-largest town. "It was just after independence and Zimbabwe was wonderful," Lydia recalled with a sigh. Their first child, Diana, was born there; they had a big house with a lush garden and plenty of household help.

But they weren't in Zimbabwe long before they realized that even better opportunities were to be had next door in South Africa. In 1988, David and Lydia landed jobs in a hospital in a "homeland," one of the remote regions the apartheid government declared independent nations for the black population. The politics of it were dubious—Lydia said hostile black South Africans often asked them why they were working for the white-rule state—but she reasoned that people had to have health care, and the government was not going to send white doctors to work in the homelands. Besides, she and David needed the comparatively well-paid jobs to send money home to family in Uganda. "With what you earned, you could buy a car in a week." As foreigners, they were largely insulated from the brutality of apartheid. "We loved South Africa. All the hospitals were manned by foreign doctors, Ghanaian, Kenyan, Ugandan, we were all one big family. And it was good medical experience—you did everything."

They both liked their work, they were building up savings, they had a second child and named him for his father—life was good. Then in 1990, David developed fevers and severe chest pain. Eventually he was diagnosed with disseminated tuberculosis: the bacteria had spread from his lungs to his other organs. After a long hospital stay in Durban, he started to get well, and the family made their first trip back to Uganda to visit. But the TB treatment involved swallowing handfuls of tablets every day, and even though David, as a doctor, knew that the drugs had to be taken for at least six months to eliminate the disease, Lydia said he stopped taking them after a couple of months when he felt better.

Both Lydia and David had begun to suspect, because of TB and other infections he caught, that he might have HIV. They were just starting to see the first cases in the hospitals where they worked in South Africa, which had been isolated by apartheid. But Uganda had one of the earliest

# They stuffed her full of Valium so that she would die quietly.

epidemics; they had heard both about the ravages of the disease back home, and about President Yoweri Museveni's ground-breaking public-education campaign on safer sex. They discussed whether David should be tested—but then a Ghanaian colleague warned them of the apartheid government's hard-line policies on the disease: "If they find you with HIV they will send you away." So David didn't test. Instead he left for a post-doctoral course in psychiatry in Pretoria.

A few months later, Lydia travelled up to see him, and found him frighteningly unwell. "He was very, very sick but so determined to live," she said. "I told him to stop working and let me bring him home, but he refused—he had so many plans for the future." Reluctantly, she returned to work in the south without him.

Four months later the phone call came: David had died. Lydia made arrangements to send his body home to Uganda, hardly able to believe that her kind and vital husband was dead. She considered having an HIV test herself. "But I saw myself as healthy, so I put it out of my mind. I knew I might have it, but I just *couldn't* have it!"

For a few years, things were all right. She had the support of friends, she had plenty of work in South Africa. But by 1996, when she was trying to obtain additional qualifications of her own, in ophthalmology, she started to feel weak and perpetually tired. "My body just started to break down—I had thrush, then boils, and then I started really going downhill." She blamed the stress she was under—trying to raise two children on her own, working long hours including many night shifts. She thought about HIV. But there was still no cure, still no treatment, and still huge fear of the disease. And so even though she was a doctor who could clearly recognize the symptoms, she refused to consider that she might have the virus.

LYDIA MUNGHERERA

But when she checked into a nursing home to convalesce, the staff, without consulting her, tested her for HIV. She was positive.

Before Lydia could take any further steps, she became gravely ill. She developed AIDS-related dementia, as the virus attacked cells in her central nervous system. She did not recognize her children, didn't know where she was. The maid she had brought from Uganda struggled to care for her; the children, then four and nine, were terrified. In June, she was admitted to hospital in the small coastal city of East London. There the nurses told her, "Go home to Uganda and take the disease with you." They would not feed or bathe her; they stuffed her full of Valium so that she would die quietly and not distract them from their work. "They were waiting for me to die as soon as possible," Lydia said. "People with HIV in South Africa were rubbish. In 1996, the country was where Uganda was in 1982."

Her sister Margaret, the youngest doctor in the family, flew down to South Africa and made preparations to bring her home, arranging intravenous drugs and support for the flight. Yet by the time Margaret got her to the airport hotel, Lydia—skeletal and totally addled by the dementia— was so ill that the family began instead to make arrangements to transport her body.

Lydia remembers none of this, but she survived to make the flight. Her horrified parents met the plane at Entebbe, armed with more medical supplies. She had no idea who they were. It was the start of a concerted family effort to which, Lydia said, she owes her life.

In those next few weeks in Kampala, Lydia got very, very lucky. Margaret had attended the International AIDS Conference in Vancouver the previous year, and she had heard an American researcher, Dr. David Ho, make a stunning announcement. In the West, people with HIV had been treated for nearly a decade with a type of drugs called antiretrovirals, or ARVs, which disrupt HIV's ability to replicate itself. The first such drug, commonly known as AZT, was approved in 1987, and it and others that followed slowed the progression from HIV infection to AIDS, extending the life of people with the virus by two or three years. But Ho said he had found that by using three or more different ARVs together, combined in a kind of "cocktail," he could suppress the virus almost entirely in his patients. It wasn't a cure—but if they took the pills every day, they would stay healthy for a long time. After Ho's announcement, patients seized on the combination ARV therapy, taking a regimen of a dozen daily pills, and by the time Lydia landed in Uganda, people with HIV in the West were managing their HIV infection like a chronic illness such as diabetes.

But the drugs cost tens of thousands of dollars, and no one was talking about offering them to people with AIDS in poor countries. In fact, there was only one place in all of East Africa to get the treatment: the Joint Clinical Research Centre, a few miles away from Lydia's home in Kampala. People with HIV were coming from as far away as Kenya and Zambia to buy the tablets there. The centre was selling "recycled" drugs—leftover pills donated when patients in rich countries switched medications—at a relatively low cost, using the proceeds to bring in more drugs. Still, the fee was $1,500 a month, a fortune in Uganda.

Staff at JCRC told Lydia's family that there was little point in them buying the drugs: a person simply could not recover from all that ailed Lydia. But her mother, Joyce, quickly sold her land to buy the first few months' worth of medication, and then sold many of their household furnishings; other relatives lent money. Joyce and Margaret stayed by Lydia's bed every moment, desperate to see the drugs have some effect. It took months, but just as they were about to give up, Lydia began to recognize them, to make sense, to want to sit up and eat. By August she remembered that she had children. Soon she was out of hospital, learning to walk and talk again. Her father would sit and count out her regimen of tablets and watch the clock, making sure she took each one at the correct time.

By January, she said, she was well. "My CD4 count was 196, still low—but I was my old self in mind and my body had healed." She decided to return to South Africa, thinking she would resume her old job. In East London, she dropped in on the hospital where she had been left to die. "A nurse looked at me and said, 'Funny, you look so much like a Ugandan doctor who died.'" Lydia took immense pleasure in explaining that in fact she was the same doctor, and that AIDS treatment had done this for her. The nurse gaped, uncomprehending. (It would be six more years before public hospitals in South Africa had any treatment to offer.)

Not long after returning to South Africa, Lydia had a dream. "People were calling me, 'Help, help,' people were reaching to me. They looked like familiar faces, although I couldn't name them. But they were not South Africans. I thought, 'I should go home to people who need me.'" So she returned to Kampala, hoping to work there. Not long after she arrived, her father mentioned to her that an old friend, a retired army major, had started a national network of people living with AIDS. With some trepidation, Lydia went to her first meeting. She left a few hours later filled with a new euphoria. Even though so many people were sick or dead from the disease, few were public about having HIV—but the network was made up of vibrant people who were comfortable with their HIV status. Lydia was eager to throw herself into their kind of advocacy. But there was a problem: activism didn't pay, and she was broke. All her savings were going to pay for her drugs.

Then she got lucky once more: there was an opening for a doctor at the outpatient clinic at The AIDS Support Organization. TASO, as it is called, was the first such group in Africa—founded in 1987, when many countries were still denying that there was any HIV within their borders at all. It had begun with members meeting informally in each other's homes to share their stories, and quickly expanded into offering formal counselling and home-based care for the sick. TASO championed the rights of people with the virus and popularized the idea of "positive living." Here, Lydia could confidently go public. "At first I was scared. What are people going to think of me as a doctor?" she recalled. "But all the educated people were hiding. I thought, 'Someone has to break the stigma and it's going to be me.'" So she told everyone who came to TASO that she herself was HIV-positive, and found that her patients would relax and talk to her more freely when they knew.

In the early years, the work was frustrating: the price of drugs put the ARV treatment that had saved her out of reach of all but one or two of her patients. So there was a limited amount she could do for them—"A patient this week has candidiasis, next week has cryptococcal, next week has died"—

and soon she was consumed in the effort to bring public treatment to Africa. Her expertise was sought by government, business and community groups both within and outside Uganda. The World Health Organization wanted her to consult on treatment guidelines for poor countries; UNAIDS wanted her help with planning. Lydia offered a rare combination: the first-hand experience of a person living with HIV; a forceful, articulate, powerful personality; and her medical and managerial expertise.

When, years later, TASO received a grant from the United States and was able to start offering ARV treatment, she herself was the most compelling advertisement for the drugs. It is now Ugandan legend that Dr. Lydia had a CD4 count of one before she began the treatment. "I could go and say, 'This is what the drugs can do—I know because I'm taking them since 1997.' So people realize it's not just them, it's me too. They say, 'You're lying.' I say, 'I *do* have the virus and I'm taking the drugs.'"

Treatment is today available to all her patients, but still, the fear of the disease keeps people from seeking the help they need—and that, of course, Lydia can well understand. "Because it means death. Nobody wants to talk about a disease that means death. The whole aura of death is stigmatizing—the idea that a person is going to die and that person has a contagious disease." But Lydia also sees it as a class issue. She remains one of the few professionals in Uganda open about her status, yet a quarter of her classmates from Makere medical school have died of HIV. "So many of my colleagues are dying silently," she said with a sigh. "It has always been seen as a disease of low class and poor people. And it's sexually transmitted. So no prominent people admit to it."

Today Lydia is part of the small band of African AIDS professionals. She sits on the board of the Global Fund, advises the WHO and travels

# drugs can do.. 'You're lying.'"

constantly, to a meeting in Geneva today, a conference in Cape Town tomorrow. She lives on email—five hundred messages a day, sometimes, she told me. At once imperious, demanding and charming, she engages instantly with people; she multitasks so continuously that she's like a child with an attention deficit. She jokes that she is a "terrible mother" but quietly frets that she does not see her children, who are in boarding school, often enough. She sends them frequent cellphone text messages from the road.

Lydia knows that a combination of good fortune, geography and her indomitable will saved her. She was lucky in her loving family, who never blinked at the word *AIDS,* and in their affluence, which got her the drugs when almost no one else in Africa had them. She was lucky to be in Uganda, where the president showed rare leadership and launched an early fight against the disease, creating a different climate from that of so many other countries, including South Africa, where she lay doped in a hospital waiting for death. And she has an acute sense of just how close it came.

"The first reason I survived was the support from my family and friends, the second was that Uganda was open. Drugs are the third. But love and support—those were first."

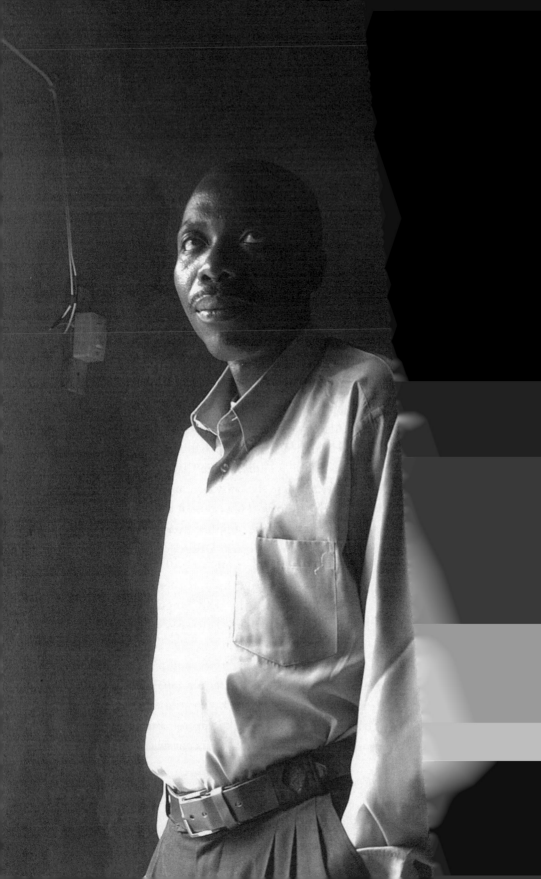

# SEVEN

# NoéSebisaba

oé Sebisaba's mistake was moderation. He was a gentle and judicious man in a harsh, fanatical time, and it cost him badly.

He can laugh about it now, a little bit. Really, he told me gently, you have to laugh when you have had a life like his, or you would weep all the time. He can laugh, and take comfort in the unexpected achievements he has built from his ordeal. But he does not forget what he has lost.

Noé is the second-last of nine children, born in October 1968 to peasant farmers in Cendajuru, a *commune,* or district, in eastern Burundi, a small country of lush and misty hills in the conflict-plagued Great Lakes region of East Africa. Noé was the only one of his siblings to study past elementary school. In fact, only three of them made it that far. But Noé loved books, and philosophy, and language. Teachers encouraged him, and his somewhat bewildered parents did too, selling their only cow to cover the cost of sending him to high school. He was the sixth person in the *commune* of thirty-five thousand people to graduate. "Can you imagine?" he asked me. "Six people, out of thirty-five thousand. It was such a poor place." He went on to study for four years at the École d'administration publique in the capital, Bujumbura. At just twenty-four, he was made administrator of his *commune.*

Burundi shares some of neighbouring Rwanda's dark history: here, too, the Belgian colonial government used a divide-and-rule tactic and elevated the minority Tutsi ethnic group to positions of power. But while the Hutu majority seized control in Rwanda and persecuted the Tutsis, matters played out differently in Burundi, where the Tutsi minority kept power, dominating the government and the armed forces. The country suffered through a succession of coups and waves of violence, most of them massacres of Hutu civilians by Tutsi soldiers and mobs. There was a brief period of hope in 1992, when Burundi adopted a new constitution and a multi-party system; a Hutu named Melchior Ndadaye was elected president in 1993. But he was assassinated just three months into his term. Hutu extremists blamed the Tutsi elite for the murder, and launched attacks; the Tutsi-dominated army led the reprisals. Within days a convulsion of bloodshed shook the country.

When the killing started, Noé was away at meetings in another *commune;* he saw the army arrive there and begin a frenzy of rape and indiscriminate killing, and he escaped to his own village. But the situation was no better there. "The army burned houses, killed people. In just two days they razed a whole path." And so he joined the tens of thousand of Hutus fleeing across the border to Tanzania. Peaceful since its independence in 1961 but extremely poor, Tanzania nevertheless has an extraordinary record of generosity in sheltering refugees from forty years of vicious conflicts around the Great Lakes—more than a million Burundians, Rwandans and Congolese have sought shelter there.

In those first days in 1993, a great tide of Burundians poured across the Tanzanian border to take shelter in camps that sprang up, sprawls of tightly packed mud-and-twig huts on the vast flat plains of yellow scrub. Noé found an epidemic of dysentery in the camp where he arrived, and a shortage of food and shelter. He could not imagine how he would live there. And so, when the worst of the fighting seemed to have died down two weeks later, he went home again. Many of the houses in the village had been burned or looted. Many people were dead.

"I went to see the governor. She said, 'Thank God, you're back—now I ask your help to stabilize the *commune.*'" Resuming his post as administrator, Noé travelled between villages. "I advised people to look long term: 'Can you live here if there is all this fighting? You have to live together.' People were panicked. They were hiding at night in the bush or the swamp, and in the daytime they would come to their houses. The first thing was to inspire confidence. I said, 'Go home. Try to contact those you can—tell them to come home, life is restarting.'" He spread a calming message, but he too was unnerved by the uncertainty that hung in the air. "There was a point where I also refused to live in the town, I was hiding at night."

Noé reckoned it was essential to keep the soldiers away for a while, because the sight of patrols inspired new panic. He persuaded the army that he could do a better job of keeping the peace without them, and that it was in their interest to have him restore order. "I said, 'Leave me with this population, let me calm them.'" And gradually, although thousands of people were dead and thousands more stayed on in the camps in Tanzania, some semblance of normal life did resume. Over the next months, there were more coups, and more spasms of killing around the country, but Noé worked on rebuilding markets and wells, on smoothing relations between Hutu and Tutsi neighbours.

In August 1995, he married a smart and charming high-school teacher named Agrippine from a neighbouring village. They talked of starting a family. But the calm didn't last. A Hutu rebel group from the south was gaining in power and starting to draw more and more supporters. Noé found himself presented with a stark choice: "It was 'Either you work with the Tutsi government to control the rebellion, or you work with the Hutu rebels to overthrow the government.' If I worked with the rebels, the army would target me. And if I worked with the army, the rebels would target me. I was between the nail and the hammer."

To compound the problem, the Tutsi authorities mistrusted him. Even though he worked for the government, he was a Hutu, and every Hutu, especially those in positions of local power, came under great suspicion. After Noé organized an informal collection among friends at the pub to help a pal with some bad debts, he found himself detained and interrogated. The army accused him of raising money to buy weapons for the rebels. The charge was preposterous—but also a sign that his family was no longer safe in this charged atmosphere. "I understood that I was working with people who at any moment could turn against me." Local officials began to meet every few weeks to discuss the military success of the rebels, and to debate how they could safeguard their power. Noé, being practical, suggested the government would have to negotiate with the rebels—and that made everyone suspicious. "I was totally neutral. But I always said what I thought—I wasn't very experienced." He laughed at his own naiveté, a big chuckle that revealed every one of his straight white teeth. "I thought it was part of the job to be honest." Now the bargain he had struck with the army came under new scrutiny: commanders accused him of keeping the troops out of his district, not to restore order but to create a haven for the rebels. "I thought, 'I'm at risk of losing my skin. I have to go.'"

And yet he remembered those two weeks he had spent in the camp in Tanzania in 1993, and he dreaded the idea of taking Agrippine there. Plus, he had so many plans for the *commune*. All the signs said they should go, but they stood to lose so much as refugees.

In the end, the decision was made for them.

"There was one other thing that happened—worse than all the rest," Noé said. Ten years later, telling me this story, his voice cracked with the pain of it. Tears began to roll down the edges of his thin face. He pulled out a burgundy handkerchief, unfolded the square and held it over his eyes for a minute or two, then straightened his shoulders and resumed.

"My wife was raped by soldiers. I was away, I had gone to Bujumbura, and they came then and raped her."

Agrippine was five months pregnant at the time.

"Afterwards, we discussed what to do, whether to make a complaint—but complain to whom?" The memory of his helplessness evoked a rare flash of anger. "It was the army who administered justice!"

They knew they had to flee, but Agrippine was still recovering, and they felt they could not make the long journey until she delivered the baby. They suffered through the next four months, trying to behave normally under the stifling tension in the *commune*. Every time he saw a soldier, Noé wondered whether this was one who had attacked his wife. Agrippine gave birth to a girl they christened Sanctiana, and two weeks later, they fled.

They left separately, because Noé still felt a sense of responsibility to the community and he feared people would panic at the sight of the administrator running away. He left one day as if he was going on government business again, but outside town he met up with a nephew who showed him the way to the border. He walked all that day and into the night, until at 3 a.m. he arrived at the edge of a camp called Kanembwa, home to twenty thousand people. Agrippine came the next day, after heading out in the morning as if she was going to till their plot as usual.

Noé had carried with him only one suitcase from Burundi. It held a change of clothes, their small stash of money, their few photos and his favourite book: *Les Misérables.* In the camp, people from the *commune* greeted them with joy—and trepidation, knowing what it must mean about conditions at home if even the administrator had fled. And indeed, when they realized in the *commune* that Noé was not coming back, a wave of people followed him to the camp.

At Kanembwa, Noé accepted the small parcel of goods that all refugees received, a jerry can and a plastic basin for washing, plus a piece of plastic sheeting to roof the mud-and-grass houses the refugees were expected to build themselves. But Agrippine had arrived exhausted, carrying their two-week-old baby, and he needed somewhere for them to sleep right away. "I looked for a house—well, 'a house.' If you could see what I'm describing as a house . . ." He found a young man who had been in the camp for a few years and had built a comparatively solid mud room, and Noé gave him much of their savings so that he could install Agrippine there. A few nights later, there was a torrential rain, and water streamed through the roof; the only way they could keep the baby dry was by lying over her together.

Refugees were not permitted to leave the camps to seek paid work in the Tanzanian host communities. Instead they were given a ration of maize, beans and oil, but it wasn't enough to live on. Within three months, Noé had spent the last of their savings supplementing the ration. A kind camp administrator gave him work on a ditch-digging project, but Noé the scholar was inept with a pick and shovel, and he berated himself that he could not manage this one opportunity to feed his family. The indignity of it all was paralyzing. "I lost my country, my rights as a citizen, my identity, my personality, even my way of thinking. I was given food without having worked for it and without having decided what I needed. I was dressed without choosing clothes that fit me. I went one day to get a pair of trousers, and they gave me a dress instead—and I couldn't say anything, because I had no other options."

Noé had no illusions about temporary exile. "In the beginning we could see that it was going to take years. I never believed we'd be going back in a matter of weeks or months." It was a huge relief when Agrippine was hired to teach in the camp secondary school, which used the Burundian curriculum and operated in French. Soon after, Noé was hired there, too, as a history teacher. "It didn't pay much, but at least we could buy clothes for the child. It helped a little bit."

They decided to seek third-country asylum, and applied by post to the Canadian embassy in Dar es Salaam. "We knew nothing of Canada except what they taught us in geography class—but people said it was welcoming." Their application wended its way through the tortuous bureaucracy, and in the meantime, life in Kanembwa started to seem, if not normal, at least familiar.

One day when Noé had been in the camp for nearly two years, he was passing the health clinic when a good friend, a nurse, called out to him. A patient needed a transfusion, but the clinic had no blood supply. Noé quickly volunteered: he had type O, the universal donor. "They said, 'We have to do a test on your blood—can you wait thirty minutes?' I said, 'Sure.' They took the sample and left. Thirty minutes went by, then forty minutes, fifty minutes. I was getting worried. I said, 'Hey, tell me, why aren't you taking blood for the transfusion?' The nurse said, 'We've found that your blood doesn't match. You can go.' I said, 'Look, I know I'm an O—it's universal.' I could tell from the way he was talking that something was up, I could see it in his face. I insisted. I said, 'You're a friend, you can tell me anything, I have no problem.'" So his friend broke the news: the rapid blood screening had found HIV in Noé's sample.

He had first heard of the virus in secondary school in 1985, when the principal told students that a deadly new illness had been discovered in the United States. "I didn't know French very well at that time so I didn't understand clearly, and for me, speaking of America—well, I was in Africa. Plus they said it was transmitted by sexual relations. At that time, I was such an innocent virgin. So this was for other people—not me!"

Noé calmly thanked his friend for the information and walked out of the clinic.

"But I can I tell you I was staggered. *Vraiment, vraiment.* I can hardly describe it to you: I felt without life. When I left the clinic, I don't even know how I got to the house." He walked the kilometre back home, slipped silently past his wife in the doorway and lay down on the bed. He turned on the radio, and a cheery pop tune blared out. He turned it off again.

"That night I went to the bar, and the nurse was there. I took him aside and asked, 'This test that you did, can it be wrong?' He said, 'Look, Noé, it can be wrong. You should go and do it somewhere else. It was probably wrong.'" So Noé went home that night, determined to act as though everything was normal. But he was racking his brain to think how he might have been infected. "The first thing was that before I met my wife I had girlfriends with whom I—we had unprotected sex. Is it maybe because of that? And then my wife, she had had boyfriends before we married. Maybe it's that. And then my head was filled with the idea that maybe it was the rape—the soldiers." Many militias in East Africa have deliberately used rape as an effort to spread HIV: it was, for example, a specific strategy of the *interahamwe,* the Hutu killing squads in Rwanda's genocide.

# "My life was broken—going to live. How could I had dreams,

Noé told this part of the story with a bitter laugh. "I blamed everybody, I even blamed my parents for giving birth to me. I blamed God for having created me." But it didn't change a thing. "My life was broken—I didn't know how I was going to live. How could God let me get HIV? I had dreams, dreams for my life. I wanted three things: a family to love, with at least three children; to do things for my *commune*—because I was one of the first educated people; and to build a house, simple but strong. And now none of that was possible. I'd had to flee my country, I had lost our land and our savings, and now my family was totally destroyed. Because in the beginning, I thought HIV was total destruction. I could picture it: I saw my wife dead, my child dead."

A few years before the war, Noé had volunteered as a friendly visitor at a Bujumbura hospital and had seen "very sick people." He realized, from their skeletal frames and what he overheard in the corridors, that this was AIDS, the American disease. "So I knew it existed, but I never thought it could have anything to do with me. I felt healthy, my wife and daughter were healthy. I couldn't integrate this reality. It was a disease for prostitutes."

After three days, he knew he had to tell Agrippine. "I thought, 'How am I going to tell my wife so she doesn't think I'm accusing her, so she can understand, so I can understand her? How can I save my family, save my marriage?'" Noé led her outside, to sit in the shade of a tree beside their tiny house. "I said, 'My wife, I'm going to tell you something very dangerous and very bad. I don't know how you will cope with it.' She said, 'Tell me.' I said, 'When you married me, were you a virgin? She said, 'No—like you.'" Agrippine leaned back and squinted at her husband, wondering where on earth the conversation was going. "And I said, '*Alors,* my family is infected

I didn't know how I was
God let me get HIV?
dreams for my life."

with HIV.'" Agrippine could hardly fathom what he was saying. Why, she asked her husband, did you get an HIV test? "I said, 'I didn't want to get tested, I wanted to donate blood.' I told her what had happened. And I said, 'I don't blame you. Maybe it's me who brings it, I knew women before you. Maybe it's you. Maybe it's what happened before—the rape. We don't know. We can't throw stones.'"

Months passed before Noé worked up the courage to have himself retested. There was no comfort to be had in the results. Agrippine could not bring herself to get tested for an entire year, and when she did, her results were also positive. But they never again discussed how they might have become infected, Noé said: "What purpose would that serve?"

Their application for asylum in Canada was advancing through the process, but now Agrippine overheard people say that European and North American countries required negative HIV tests before they approved immigrants. So they withdrew their application. "If they demanded the test and we refused to do it and dropped the application, people would deduce why and we would be exposed to discrimination," Agrippine fretted. Instead, they claimed patriotism, a duty "to go home and do something for the country. But in fact it was something else."

The next year, Agrippine became pregnant again. "She refused absolutely for us to use condoms. She thought we could not have only one child. She really, really wanted more children, even with the risk." A woman with HIV has a 50 per cent chance of passing the virus on to her baby, and while pregnant women in the developed world were receiving drugs and other interventions that lower that risk, none were available in the camp. Agrippine gave birth to a baby girl they named Lina. By the time she was seven months old, it was clear she was not developing normally. She had a lesion behind her ear that didn't heal, and rather than gaining, she lost weight. "We knew."

A new crisis unfolded. "My mother-in-law, who was also in the camp, wanted to know what was wrong with this baby. Africans don't like to believe that death just comes—they want to believe in fetish or witch-craft. She went to the witchdoctor. He said, 'It's your neighbour who wants a child and she can't have one until another child dies. She made a poison with chameleon skin and secretly fed it to your child.'" Noé's mother spread the witchdoctor's diagnosis, and the childless neighbour was shunned. "Agrippine and I knew the reality—but my wife refused to tell anyone so we wouldn't be stigmatized. Yet here's my neighbour being ostracized. I felt guilty."

Meanwhile, Noé was worried about his students. "I saw them—especially the girls who were living in this very difficult situation where they couldn't buy a pair of shoes, even flip-flops—selling themselves to the NGO workers who had a little money—this happens in the camps. *Et ça m'a touché au coeur*—that touched my heart. I thought, 'If these children knew what I know . . .' So I said to my wife, 'Couldn't we say it openly?' She refused. She said, 'I'm afraid. How would I act in front of my students, my colleagues?' And so I could not say anything either, not without exposing her."

But Agrippine agreed he must do something for his students. So he began to set aside five minutes at the end of each lesson and shared with the class the information he had gleaned about HIV/AIDS—what it is, how they might be exposed to it. In the months after he learned he was infected, Noé looked around the congested camp and thought about how everything in the life of refugees puts them at risk of the disease. They start off in situations of great violence, including rape. In the camps, they may have only sex to trade for food and shelter. They live through harrowing experiences, unsure if they will see another day, "and life becomes cheap."

After a couple of weeks of talking about this in class, four of Noé's students approached him. "They said, 'What you say at the end of the lesson interests us. What can we do? Can we start a small club?' So we started Stop SIDA." (SIDA is the French acronym for AIDS.) He knew his family could not be the only one infected in the vast chain of refugee camps in western Tanzania. "I knew people were ignorant like I used to be—and that AIDS would reach everyone if nothing was done."

AIDS reached his own house a few months later. Their daughter Lina died at fourteen months, and her illness, Noé said in retrospect, was the beginning of Agrippine's as well. Nursing the child had exhausted her. She got very thin, developed lesions and was plagued by the same series of infections that Lina had had. On July 10, 2001, Noé's smart, sparkly wife died, too, at thirty-three.

Once more, people started asking questions. Blame fell again on the childless neighbour, and relations became heated, with his in-laws threatening to kill the "criminal" and wanting to know why Noé was not seeking revenge. Broken-hearted over the loss of his wife and daughter, he could not bear the lie any more. "At the funeral I said, 'Listen, I'm worn out, but I have to tell you something: people must not kill one another thinking one person or another is causing the problems in my family. I know the truth. And I need to rest but I'll tell you in time.'"

A month after Agrippine's death, he mustered his strength and called together the chiefs and the influential people in the camp. "I told them, 'Look, here's the truth: I'm HIV-positive. My wife died of AIDS. My daughter died of AIDS.'"

Just as Agrippine had feared, the news was not well received. In church, a pastor used the sermon to speak directly to Noé: AIDS, he said, was God's judgment against the sinful. Many of his friends stopped coming around; a few confessed sheepishly that they could not be seen with him lest people think they too were infected. Noé's brother's children had been living with him, because he had extra room in his little house after Agrippine and Lina died, but now the brother rushed to collect the children. "He was afraid the utensils would contaminate them." Noé worried about his surviving daughter, Sanctiana. If he died, she would be called an

"AIDS orphan" and perhaps be abandoned. "I regretted speaking out, but it was impossible to retract."

There were 850,000 people in the five huge Burundian camps in Tanzania at that point—and Noé was the only one to have declared publicly that he had HIV.

Word spread, and soon local Tanzanians were confronting the refugees, accusing Burundians of bringing HIV into the country. Refugees who had been doing food-for-work labour projects were harassed; they blamed Noé. (Research by the United Nations High Commissioner for Refugees shows that most refugees in Africa are displaced from areas of lower HIV prevalence into areas of higher infection, but they are nonetheless almost invariably accused by host communities of bringing the disease.)

There was one place where Noé found support: his students. "I said, 'Remember what I was telling you at the end of your lessons? About being careful? You're still meeting people who say HIV doesn't exist, but it does. I have it and my wife died of it and probably you know others who died of it.' And they were sympathetic—they understood I really cared about them." Rather than avoiding him, his students wanted to know what they could do to help.

They had no money or resources, but they wanted to spread the message Noé had given them. They decided to organize a concert. "We had to present it as a festival. Nobody would attend if we said, 'Come and talk about AIDS,'" Noé explained. So the students sang and danced, and then Noé gave a short talk. He said, "I am HIV positive, my child has died, my wife also, but I am still strong, as you are." He said he wanted them to learn from his experience. He spoke about the importance of abstinence ("I couldn't talk about condoms because people would have said that was encouraging children to have sex"), about the responsibility of parents to educate their children and of the whole community to care for the sick.

Despite the fear that had greeted his initial disclosure, he did not hesitate to tell the crowd he had the virus. "I say, 'Yes.' We must have openness. And so when anybody asks, I say, 'Yes. Yes, yes, yes, yes.' That's my attitude to being HIV-positive."

Noé's courage was infectious. Instead of the hostility he had anticipated, he was astonished to see some young people stand up to sing him a traditional song reserved for heroes in Burundi. A flood of parents wanted to know if their children could join his club. The group grew quickly; they organized plays and took their message to sporting events. Now a few other people joined Noé to say publicly that they were living with HIV. Stop SIDA added messages about how to live positively with the virus, and offered care and support to those who were sick (although there were no drugs). People began to confide that their spouses or children had died of HIV, and parents started having frank talks with their teenagers about sex.

But not everyone appreciated his success. Refugees, Noé said in his quiet, thoughtful way, are often seen only as desperate recipients of charity and not as people with skills or even stories of their own. "You see lines of people with bundles of their possessions on their heads who need food or tents or donations—you don't think, That is a doctor, that is a teacher, that's a *commune* administrator. In the camps, the officials and the UN workers say, 'You are a refugee. Don't talk about your education, the posts you held before—you're here at our protection.'" And so when he began to do HIV/AIDS education, he met with a frosty reception from agencies such as UNAIDS, especially when they saw that enormous crowds turned out for his Stop SIDA rallies. But, Noé said, it only made sense. "People respected me, despite my refugee status. I wasn't respected because I held power—my authority came from my experiences, my life. I was speaking in their language, of their culture, of the reality they were living. A refugee is a person living in one country with his thoughts in another, so any program you do that reaches him must take that into account."

Some of the international NGOs tried to hire him, but he preferred to keep his little initiative independent—although he said he would gladly accept any financial support they wanted to provide. Now

"You see lines of people
possessions on their heads
or donations—you don't
that is a teacher, that's a

Noé found himself caught up in the petty politics of the aid world, where bickering over territory (and the funding that comes with it) took precedence over the urgent need to address the spread of HIV. On a continent where emergency and development efforts are a key source of jobs and cash, this phenomenon is depressingly common. "The NGOs complained I wasn't a specialist or qualified," Noé said. They used this pretext to persuade the camp administrators to stop the group's activities, and it took a delegation of Burundian elders to convince them otherwise.

After a couple of years, Stop SIDA had grown from only Noé and his small group of supporters to an organization with thirteen hundred registered members, eighty-five of whom were openly HIV-positive. I heard about it, and sought Noé out, intrigued by this refugee story so different from those I usually heard in the camps. "I ask myself, sometimes, how we did it—starting out as just three or four people," Noé told me, shrugging his thin shoulders modestly.

In 2003, several years of intermittent efforts at peace talks between the government and Burundi's many rebel groups finally produced a deal. Some refugees began to pack up from the camp. Two years later, when Burundi held peaceful national elections, the tide of repatriations picked up, and Noé began to think about going home. He left his daughter with relatives in the camp and made a quick trip, first to his *commune* and then down to Bujumbura, to try to get a real sense of how safe it was. He found the country vastly changed. "Many houses were burned, the gardens were overgrown and not cultivated." The small cement house he and Agrippine

with bundles of their
who need food or tents
think, That is a doctor,
commune administrator."

had been building before he fled had been razed to the foundation. "But in the town people were living together, with no problem. When I fled Burundi, there were areas where, as a Hutu, I would not have dared to walk. I would have been detained or killed. So when I came home that spring, the first thing I did was to walk around in the neighbourhoods that had been dangerous for me." In the congested central market, and along the grassy lakeshore, he walked past Tutsis, and other Hutus; no one paid the slightest attention.

That was a marvellous change, but the overall climate was less than welcoming. "And I understand that—it's because of hunger, and problems related to land. When I arrived, people hoped I would have something to give them, but I was in the same position: I was a person with nothing. They wanted help, but I needed help." Yet he was confident enough in the prospects for Burundi's future that he decided to come home. And that raised the question of what would become of his AIDS work, which had grown from a small after-school club to, he said, "a vocation."

"We had a meeting to talk about what would happen with Stop SIDA, and to the widows, the orphans and people with AIDS—when these people go home, what will their reintegration be like? Will the community accept them? Maybe they have been accepted here because of our work, but they won't be accepted at home." He suspected there would be little awareness of HIV in Burundi, just emerging from war. His first goal was to take the education program home, but he also saw a chance to give refugees a valuable message—"that they have something to bring back."

He signed up for the formal UNHCR repatriation process, in which the UN refugee commission provides transport and a small ration of food to returnees to help them start over at home. "I left the camp very proud"—residents threw a party to thank him for his advocacy and wish him well. He left his daughter with friends to finish the school year in the camp, and he boarded a big UN truck, packed with ebullient refugees and their small piles of possessions, with great anticipation— and one aching regret. "I had to leave their graves in Tanzania," he said of the small plots where he had buried his wife and daughter. "One day a few years from now all the refugees will have gone home and the bush will reclaim the land. Their graves will be there alone in a forest."

Back home, Noé went first to the authorities and formally registered Stop SIDA. The UN refugee agency had made a short film about the group in the camp, called *Love in the Time of AIDS,* which had played several times on national television in Burundi, and he had also done a series of interviews on the radio, the main media in the country. Soon, people were approaching him on the bus or in the street to say, "You're that fellow with HIV who worked in the camps—I've heard about you."

He decided to stay on in Bujumbura rather than return to his *commune,* to try to get Stop SIDA up and running. He rented a small house—one in a row of concrete rooms on a courtyard choked with laundry and children—in a war-scarred neighbourhood on the edge of the sleepy capital. There was reason to be hopeful about the future of the country: the government made primary education and health care for children free, and quickly integrated Hutus and Tutsis into the civil service and the military. Yet there was little money to fund a national development program, or to house the refugees still streaming home, and the accord among the former rebel groups was fragile.

And as Noé had suspected, knowledge of HIV was much lower in Burundi than it had been in the camps. In fact, he said, by the time he left, the refugee population knew more about HIV than Tanzanians, and the camps had more condoms, more funds for educational campaigns and more centrally located clinics for tests. HIV prevalence in Burundi, which stood at 6.6 per cent in 2005, was poised to increase along with the population movement and economic activity in peacetime, and Noé was anxious to use mobile theatres and films to spread AIDS-prevention messages in the poorest parts of Burundi.

He found the government encouraging, but there was no money to fund the group—or to pay him. A friend helped him get work through a local church teaching life skills to young people, earning just enough to pay the rent. "Otherwise I am at risk of having to go back to the camp."

Noé knew his own health was precarious—by then he had likely been living with HIV for at least a decade, but the fledgling government was struggling to provide treatment and only a few thousand people in all Burundi had access to ARVs. Even to get on the waiting list, Noé would have needed tests that cost a couple of hundred dollars, money he did not have. So he began work on a memoir for his daughter, fearing that he might not live long enough to tell her the family story at an age when she could remember the details. "Your mother, your little sister and I loved you very much," it begins. "And we were sorry to leave you."

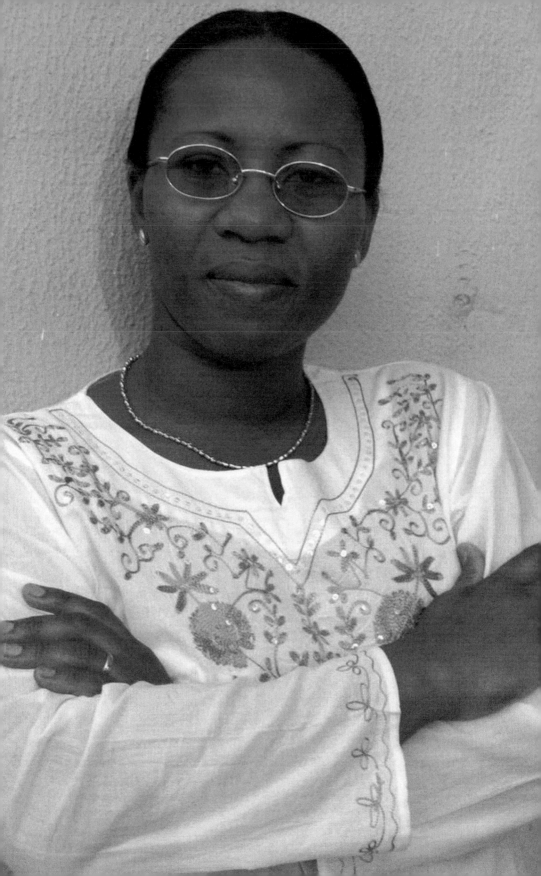

# EIGHT

# ChristineAmisi

**T**hey survived the first four days. Christine Amisi lay on the floor of her apartment with her husband and their three small sons through the days and the long, long nights, listening to gunshots and yelling from the street below. When a rebel militia fought its way into the hilly city of Bukavu in the eastern Democratic Republic of Congo in May 2004, the front line in the fighting was just a few hundred metres from her house. The glass in all her windows shattered from the force of the artillery blasts, the electricity and water cut out, but for the first four days her family was safe.

Then, on the fourth day, when Tina, as she is known, peered cautiously from the corner of the gaping window frame, she saw rebel soldiers scaling the wall around the yard. They began to pound at the main door to her apartment building. Her husband, Fefe Matula, worked frantically to jerry-rig a couple of old batteries and a wire into something that would power her cellphone. He got a charge, and Tina snatched up the phone and dialled the number of her boss, Konrad Putz, a Norwegian who ran the Doctors Without Borders clinic where Tina worked as a doctor. In the first hours of the raid, Putz and the handful of other staff had fled across the border to the relative safety of Rwanda, but only expatriates had been evacuated: Tina and her family had had to hunker down at home.

At first, they thought they could wait it out—Congo had been at war so often in Tina's thirty-one years that she had a certain resignation about events like this. But this time, with the rebels spilling into the yard below, she was sure they would die. The cellphone network was still operating, and Putz answered. She whispered to him that the rebels were breaking into her building. "I don't know if we will live through this," she choked out. She said later that she didn't imagine the team in Rwanda could do anything to help. But she wanted someone to know how they had died.

Putz, however, got on the long-wave radio and made a connection with the United Nations peacekeeping mission in Bukavu. Minutes later, as the rebels reached Tina's apartment door, a UN armoured vehicle pulled into the yard, its horn blaring. The rebels backed off, and Tina and Fefe sprinted out to the truck, carrying their sons. As they drove through the ravaged city, Tina tried to keep her hands over the boys' eyes so they would not see the bloated corpses lying in the roads.

At a compound run by the Mission des Nations Unies en République Démocratique du Congo, or MONUC, they took shelter behind barbed wire, cement blocks and mounted artillery. But the tiny UN mission, chronically underfunded, could do little to protect the rest of the civilians in Bukavu, which was seized that day by Rwandan-backed rebels who had rejected a 2003 peace deal meant to end six years of horrific civil war. The conflict had left an estimated 3.3 million people dead in one of Africa's largest and potentially richest nations. And here in the east of the country, the jungle remained full of heavily armed militias. Bukavu, a verdant city of 600,000 on vast Lake Kivu near the borders with Rwanda and Burundi, had been peaceful for a couple of years, but the calm was over now.

In the UN compound, Tina and her family were safe: there were blankets and food and a sense of order. Yet Tina no sooner had her boys installed than she announced that she was going back into the city. "I had to get to the clinic," she told me few years later, as if this had been a perfectly logical move, "because of my patients. What would happen to them?"

I met Tina, a slight, shy woman with gold-framed glasses and a girlish giggle, in her clinic on a hill above Bukavu. I thought of it as something of a "miracle clinic," where six hundred people with AIDS were on lifesaving treatment in the midst of the chaos. That was no small thing in itself. But the ramifications of what Tina, her colleagues and her patients have achieved has, I would learn, had reverberations far beyond Bukavu.

Doctors Without Borders, better known by the acronym MSF, for Médecins Sans Frontières, has had the reputation of a maverick organization since it was founded in 1971 by a team of French doctors. They were treating victims of the Biafran war, the savage civil conflict that erupted when a southern region tried to secede from Nigeria, and they were disgusted by the deference of traditional aid groups such as the Red Cross, who claimed neutrality and would not criticize military attacks on civilians. The doctors behind MSF vowed they would do things differently: they would provide medical aid more quickly, without getting sidetracked by politics or state sovereignty; they would speak out about violations of human rights by all sides; and they would refuse to seek government or rebel permission to operate in crisis zones. Twenty years later, when MSF staff got involved in AIDS in Africa, they acted much the same way: they were out to save lives, of course, but they also had something to prove.

From the moment in 1996 that David Ho announced his success in treating AIDS, people with HIV in North America and Europe rushed to get the drug cocktail. But five years later, fewer than eight thousand people in all of Africa were on antiretrovirals. Those who did have the drugs were, like Lydia Mungherera, members of the wealthy elite—people who could afford to purchase the medicine privately. And the dominant thinking in the developed world was that AIDS treatment was a luxury that simply could not be provided in poor countries. These incredibly sophisticated medications, the argument went, could be administered only in top-class medical facilities with the most modern diagnostic and laboratory equipment. AIDS treatment needed medical specialists and molecular biology laboratories capable of measuring the amount of virus in a patient's blood. In 2001, Andrew Natsios, then head of the United States Agency for International Development, or USAID, infamously said that Africans would not be capable of managing the pill regimen with the precision needed to avoid drug resistance. "People do not know what watches and clocks are," Natsios told the U.S. Congress, arguing against providing more money for AIDS treatment. "They do not use Western means for telling time. They use the sun." His words came as a surprise to the millions of Africans who wear watches, of course, but more ominous was the implication that AIDS could be treated like a chronic illness in San Francisco or Toronto or Paris, but it would have to go on being fatal in Africa.

MSF was having none of that. The organization had begun to treat people with AIDS in a project in Thailand in 2000. But since the great majority of people with HIV are in Africa, this was the logical location to try to make a point. The next year, Eric Goemaere, an unflappable Belgian with weathered features and sandy hair, a veteran of MSF missions to crises around the world, set up a small treatment project in Khayelitsha—a poor and violent township outside Cape Town in South Africa where 40 per cent of adults were infected with HIV. Goemaere thought it was the ideal place to provide a tangible example. "You have to just start treating people," he told me. "You have to show it's feasible and show that you can do it."

He admits now that he was terrified it wouldn't work—that the naysayers would be proved right, that without any public health system to speak of, treatment would fail. But within weeks of his arrival in Khayelitsha, his patients were showing the same miracle transformation seen in any European clinic. Other projects followed quickly, in Cameroon, in Kenya, in Malawi, in Zambia, and each had the same success. In September 2003, MSF went to Nairobi, to the pan-African AIDS conference that is held every two years, and called a press conference. Exuberant MSF staff in bright red and yellow T-shirts reading "AIDS Treatment

Now!" thumped an extraordinary document down in front of delegates and reporters: the collected results from MSF treatment programs running for at least a year in ten African countries. The data showed patients had survival rates on the drugs and adherence rates (correctly following the daily pill regimen) that were as high, and in many cases higher, than people in North America. So much for the Natsios theory.

MSF presented a ream of data that showed the group was successfully treating AIDS in rural and slum settings across the continent, with a minimum of lab equipment and without the teams of specialists used in AIDS projects in the West. To do it, they had made a couple of key modifications. In the rich world, the progression of AIDS is monitored through two key tests, the CD4 count, which measures the functioning of the immune system, and the viral load count, which measures the amount of virus in the blood. But these required costly infrastructure and were expensive to do; instead, MSF diagnosed stage 3 or 4 AIDS—the point at which a person is completely immuno-compromised and must start ARVs—based on either basic lab tests or simply the presence of a group of clinical symptoms such as severe wasting, tuberculosis, persistent pneumonia and oral thrush. When all of these opportunistic infections are present together in a previously healthy person who is twenty or thirty years old, they almost invariably indicate AIDS.

MSF was treating these patients for a cost of just a few hundred dollars per patient per year in medication (drug costs make up about a third of the total cost of treatment, which also includes tests, staff and infrastructure). The group was using generic drugs from India—because Indian patent law protected a manufacturing process but not a product itself, so Indian drug firms could "reverse engineer" the ARVs to produce drugs that were protected by patents abroad, and then sell them at a fraction the price of brand-name medicines from the multinational pharmaceutical companies such as Merck and Pfizer. In fact, the Indian firm Cipla struck a deal with MSF to sell the group ARVs for less than $1 per patient per day—$350 a year, compared to more than $10,000 for the patented versions of the same drugs. Cipla packaged three ARVs together in one tablet called

Triomune. Patients took only two combination tablets a day, rather than the six or ten individual brand-name drugs in David Ho's original cocktail, and the simpler pill regimen boosted drug adherence. MSF was using medicines that didn't require refrigeration (to which virtually none of their African patients had access) and ones that caused visible side effects such as skin rashes rather than those that are more difficult to diagnose, such as anemia, so that patient management could be done by a nurse or clinical officer rather than a doctor. They were all obvious steps, in many ways, but the medical establishment in both the developed world and Africa was too bound up in protocols, policies and profit margins to see that treatment could be done this way.

Working in the poorest places, MSF designed innovative strategies to get around the problems. Drug adherence was critical in an environment with limited capacity to manage problems, so patients had to prove they could take the pills reliably and accurately before they started ARVs. But MSF taught adherence without a fancy classroom or educational DVDs. Instead, counsellors gave every would-be patient a small bag of multi-coloured candies and sent them home for two weeks with instructions—two blue in the morning, one yellow at night. Two weeks later, the patients brought back the bag, and a nurse counted through what was left to make sure they had taken the "pills" properly. The patients had to master the candy (and keep it away from children) before they got real drugs.

The MSF approach was controversial. AIDS clinicians from the West warned that without close laboratory monitoring there was no way to tell if the drugs were working or if patients were becoming resistant through poor adherence—raising the nightmarish scenario of thousands of Africans with some limited exposure to the drugs developing resistance to the main treatment options, and then passing on that resistant strains of the virus to sexual partners. The big pharmaceutical companies, meanwhile, were alarmed at this powerful advertisement for the generic drugs that so dramatically undercut their high-priced patented medicines; they warned that without the laboratory monitoring there was no way to be sure the copycat drugs really worked. MSF countered that they didn't need lab results to know people were taking the drugs correctly and the virus was being suppressed: patients who had been carried into clinics hours from death were, a month or two later, back in their fields tilling cassava, or back in the classroom teaching. They stayed healthy, too. And, the renegade medics said, as treatment expanded and public pressure grew, the diagnostic equipment—such as machines to calculate CD4 counts—was becoming cheaper all the time.

The MSF data were something of a bombshell dropped into the already feverish atmosphere of the Nairobi conference, where many impassioned African delegates were debating how their countries would possibly afford the brand-name drugs made in the West or the equipment needed to measure viral loads. Over the next couple of years, governments in most of the countries where MSF took their streamlined model of treatment in "low resource settings" (the development-world euphemism for poverty) were quick to see the impact and adopt the model for a national strategy.

Finally, in late 2003, the World Health Organization announced a plan, called "3 by 5," to put three million people in the developing world on AIDS treatment by 2005, effectively ending the debate about whether to try to treat Africans. But Eric Goemaere and his colleagues at MSF were not finished. They took a look at the map: in 2003, there were thirty-five armed conflicts under way in Africa, most of them chronic, long-term, intrastate battles over land and resources. Millions of people were displaced by war, and millions more were living in the middle of conflict zones. Where people were being treated for AIDS at all, it was in peaceful and stable places. But what about the three million civilians living in war zones? Nobody was talking about AIDS in situations of chronic conflict like that in eastern Congo. "You can't strike off whole areas of Africa because they are in conflict," Eric Goemaere told me with disgust.

There is no question that treatment is hard to administer in war zones, which typically lack health infrastructure and medical personnel.

# "With treatment you're converting the dying to the living."

The populations are unstable, fleeing from fighting or looting. People on the run or in makeshift camps have no access to condoms; rape may be common, and women in particular are often obliged to trade sex for food, shelter or the chance to cross a bridge or a border. And there are real questions about whether people in a war zone can follow a daily drug regimen, given the instability and violence in which they live. But on the other hand, Goemaere and his colleagues saw all kinds of spin-offs. An AIDS project in a war zone can bring hope, in a wonderfully visible and tangible form, to bleak places; it can reduce HIV-related illness and death and so take considerable pressure off whatever medical facilities are operating; it can help re-establish a health infrastructure; and if a program starts during a war, it is in a good position to expand quickly when the fighting ends and refugees start to stream home again.

But like Eric Goemaere's first clinic in Khayelitsha, MSF needed a place to test the theory and that led the organization to Bukavu. It is a teeming city of pitted red-dirt roads, filled with women in bright print wraps carrying plastic tubs of mangoes on their heads and young men hawking piles of ancient second-hand shoes. MSF had been running a sanitation project there since the 1990s, and the project had expanded into HIV prevention. In 2003, the hilly, crowded town was ringed by no fewer than six militia groups, camped just beyond the city limits—Congolese rebels fighting the government, and soldiers from neighbouring Burundi, Uganda and Rwanda, who were all using the war as a pretext to raid Congo and loot its mineral wealth. Bukavu's population was swollen by refugees; drunken teenage soldiers at checkpoints all over town demanded bribes to let people pass; and the brewery at the edge of town was the only business that operated with any regularity.

CHRISTINE AMISI

The fishing, trading, frequently displaced people of lakeside Bukavu are believed to have one the highest HIV infection rates in Congo—around 5 per cent of adults. But the city was two thousand kilometres from the capital, Kinshasa, and a million miles from the transitional government installed there. The Ministry of Health had nothing but nominal ties to Bukavu—it had not paid staff or provided equipment in more than a decade. And there was no AIDS treatment, although the disease was killing more people in and around Bukavu than anywhere else in the country. From MSF's perspective it was the ideal site for an experiment.

That October, the MSF team rented an old house in a hilltop neighbourhood called Bagira. The house had no running water, no electricity and no glass in the windows, and the nearest laboratory to process tests such as CD4 counts was in Bujumbura, the Burundian capital, 130 kilometres away down the lake. But none of that fazed MSF's half-dozen medics and counsellors. They declared the AIDS clinic open.

Back then, Tina Amisi was working in obstetrics and gynecology at Bukavu's public hospital—looted so many times in the war that it lacked doorknobs and mattresses and was chronically short of even the most basic medications. She leapt at the chance to work for MSF. The salary was a draw, of course, but more than that, the clinic had all the necessary drugs and equipment. This was a chance to do real medicine, the kind she had dreamed about in medical school, not the piecemeal, patchwork job she had been doing in Congo's public system. And Tina herself was a prize hire for MSF: a skilled and empathetic doctor; a Congolese national who spoke two regional languages as well as fluent French; a soft-voiced, unassuming young woman who would seem approachable to the clinic's patients, who were likely to be predominantly female.

There was one hitch: Tina's attitude toward people with HIV was not much different from that of other Congolese. "When I did my residency, I didn't want to go near the people with HIV," she confessed a couple of years after we first met. "I would see the diagnosis and think, 'Oh, they're just going to die.'" She said candidly that some of the problem was that

# "When the women tell me their stories,

AIDS patients, who always died in particularly painful and protracted ways, frustrated her as a doctor intent on curing the sick. But more than that, she shared her friends' and neighbours' distaste for and fear of the disease.

MSF, however, sent her to Antwerp for a three-week course on how to do ARV treatment, and when she returned to the clinic she soon found that she loved the work. "When in the hospital you have five patients with cryptococcal meningitis and three with toxoplasmosis, your resources are devoted to the dying," she said, describing two of the nastiest yet most common killers of people who have untreated AIDS. "But with treatment you're converting the dying to the living."

One thing about the job, however, started to make Tina a bit crazy: as MSF had anticipated, mostly women came for treatment. Every day Tina did their consultations, and heard how they had come to be infected. In some ways, none of what she heard was new. As a child growing up in the town of Katanga, in the centre of what was then Zaire, she had spent holidays in the village with her grandfather and his twelve wives, whom he beat routinely. She was a favoured child who got away with naughty questions. "I would ask my grandfather, 'Why have you married all these women?'" He didn't answer—he didn't have to. "They were his servants: They would go to work his fields every day, and then go to the market and sell, and take everything they earned back to my grandfather. When I was a kid, I thought it was normal. But then when my own father also took a second wife, I thought, What's going on here?" Her father went on taking new wives and then discarding them, leaving the women and their children to fend for themselves. By the time Tina was old enough to go away to college, she saw it as a way to make sure she never ended up as an embittered, discarded wife.

CHRISTINE AMISI

# who were raped
# I can hear their screams."

She also had vivid personal knowledge of the savagery of Congo's war. When she was in secondary school, she had seen students caught on the wrong side of the latest ethnic dispute tied to car bumpers and dragged away. And then there was the rape. Through the civil wars, sexual violence has been a standard weapon in the arsenal of every rebel group and of the national armed forces of Congo, Rwanda, Uganda and Burundi. Amnesty International says there has been more rape in Congo's wars than in any other conflict. It continues today, in the villages in the heart of the country still held by militias, and it has played a significant role in the spread of HIV. In just the first few weeks in her new job with MSF, Tina heard a dozen terrible stories. "When the women who were raped tell me their stories, I can hear their screams," she said with a shudder. "I can imagine how they resisted, these women raped by six men, or taken from their villages as sex slaves and raped by so many soldiers for two or three weeks."

She left the clinic each day feeling angry with men, and inevitably that anger spilled over into her relationship with Fefe. He had a trading business and was in the habit of coming and going as he pleased, and Tina trusted him. He had wooed her for years and he was a devoted husband. "But now I was listening to the women living with HIV, listening to their stories—'I am my husband's second wife, third wife'—and I'm not seeing any of these men in the consultation. These men going and doing all these things and it's the women who are paying for it," she recalled. "So I was very hard on my husband. I would see calls on his cellphone from numbers I didn't know and get suspicious. He thought it was crazy, that my behaviour had changed so much." They fought all the time, and Fefe wanted her to quit the job. "I said, 'I'm not leaving, I love this—

I love being with these people! They've been such victims of discrimination and it does me good to be with them.'" The argument went on for a year, until Tina found she was able to relax a bit with Fefe, and he adapted to his radicalized wife.

Slowly, the MSF project expanded its reach, each month adding a handful of patients to the rosters. Those who tested HIV-positive but were still healthy joined support groups and were given food parcels to help them eat nutritiously and stay well without drugs as long as possible. Those who were sick enough to need ARVs were given the medicines. Over and over again, Tina would send a wasted, wheezing woman out the clinic door with her first month's worth of drugs; four weeks later, the same woman would be back, but almost unrecognizable—plumper, more energetic, her cheeks rouged and her hair styled, eager to tell the doctor about the magical change in her life. Soon Tina and her colleagues noticed that a dating scene had developed in the waiting room among widows and widowers who knew there would be no awkward explanations required with someone they met at the AIDS clinic. Tina loved to eavesdrop on the flirting.

And then in May 2004, Bukavu came under attack again. It had always been a risk, one that Tina and Fefe recognized when they decided to stay in Congo, even though both had college educations and they could have done well elsewhere if they had left like so many others. But Bukavu was the home they loved, and they had gambled on the peace holding—a choice that seemed crazy as the rebels climbed over the wall into their yard.

Tina was weak with relief when her family was installed in the UN compound. But she was also desperate to leave again—to reach the MSF office and figure out how to get drugs to her patients. She couldn't guess how long this fighting would last—it might be the start of another round of conflict that would shut the city down for years. If her patients ran out of drugs, they would get sick again; if they interrupted their treatment, they could develop resistance to the drugs. HIV is a stunningly adaptable microbe, and it can develop immunity to the effect of ARVs after just a brief break in treatment.

And so Tina left the children with Fefe and walked back out, past the Kevlar-clad soldiers in blue helmets, a solitary figure not even as tall as the concrete barriers. It was a short walk to the MSF compound. She saw no one in the streets. At the office, she found that rebels had already looted it of everything edible, but they had left the drugs behind. With a pair of Congolese nurses who had also snuck back to the office, she set to work bundling together an emergency parcel of drugs to get each patient through a couple of months. She knew a trip to the clinic itself was madness—she would have to go back across the front line, where fighting raged, and all the stories of gang-rape echoed in her head. But two male MSF drivers who showed up at the office offered to try to take the drugs across the city. Fingers crossed, Tina sent them off.

The drivers made it—and a couple of local staff who lived close to the clinic had made it there as well. Over the next few days, MSF used the local radio station, which sometimes managed to get on air, to spread the message that the clinic was operating—in a manner of speaking. When fighting lulled in various areas, patients from those neighbourhoods would make hasty trips up the hill.

Tina, meanwhile, crept back through the deserted streets to the UN compound and her family. The next day they joined a UN-escorted convoy that took them over the border to Rwanda. She is blasé about it all, with the sanguine Congolese attitude to the recurring, now normalized, violence. Compared to the time Rwandan soldiers attacked her and her in-laws, firing bullets at their car "like rain," she told me casually, "that time was not so bad." The worst thing, she added, was knowing how terrifying it was for her small sons.

Ten days later, the Congolese army had fought off the rebels and restored calm to Bukavu, and Tina and the rest of the MSF staff came back. And they were heartened by what they found: the radio messages, the word-of-mouth network and the emergency drug parcels had worked amazingly well. Drug adherence had barely dropped while the clinic was closed. Only five patients ran out of drugs for more than four days, and none showed any adverse effects. And best of all, while thousands of people had fled Bukavu or been driven out during the fighting, not a single one of their patients was lost: everyone showed up again when the clinic reopened.

At the two-year mark, MSF took a look at the treatment results in the clinic. Seven per cent of their patients had died—a typical result for an African clinic, even in areas without conflict, since many people put off coming for treatment until their immune system is so hopelessly destroyed that not even the "miracle" ARVs can save them. Patients had, in the long term, a 97 per cent adherence rate—taking their pills correctly and on time—which is higher than the rate at most treatment sites in North America. Only 5 per cent of them had been "lost to follow-up," that is, stopped showing up and become untraceable—again, a number about on par with North America, and remarkable for a war zone. It is testament to the commitment of the people on the drugs, Tina said. "I think the ones we lost were ones who lived far away, or who were soldiers who didn't tell their commanders they were positive and then got transferred away." MSF's point about treatment in developing countries was made more clearly in Bukavu than anywhere else: if AIDS could be treated here, it could be treated anywhere. And at Tina's clinic, the disease was treated well.

The fighting in eastern Congo continues today, but the clinic on the hill has stayed open. Tina and her colleagues have helped the government hospital in town start treating AIDS too, supplying a CD4-count machine and coaching staff on how to diagnose and monitor patients. MSF has opened up several more ARV sites around the city. But Tina goes on working in the clinic, and people seek her out now, in the cafés and markets in Bukavu—her patients, once so sick, now flourishing, and others who know she works with AIDS and want quiet information on how they can get help. She is still dismayed by the stories her patients tell, by the rape and the multiple partners, and intensely frustrated that so little is being done to change any of it. "But I tell my patients, 'We can do something for you. There are drugs and we can give them to you.' And that gives me great joy."

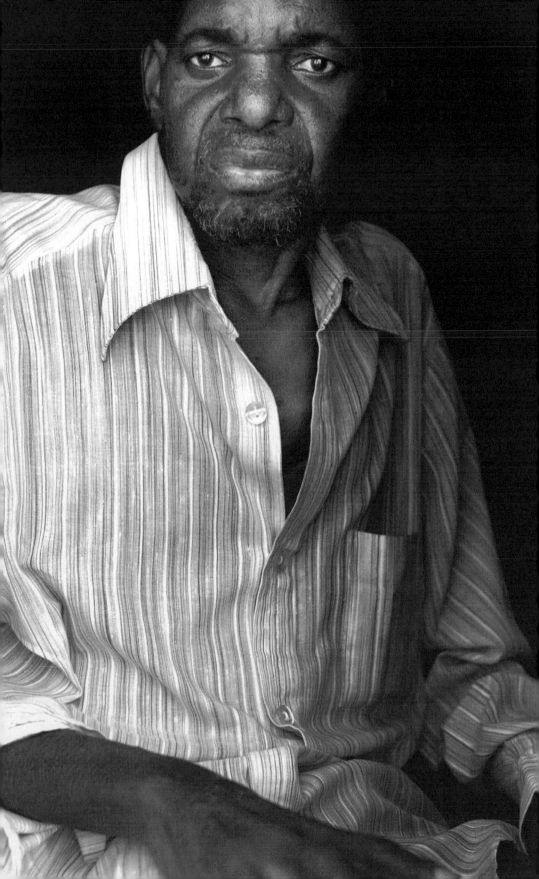

# NINE

# ManuelCossa

W hen Manuel Cossa came home from the mines, he brought a pair of green flip-flops, a battered pair of trousers, a white collared shirt worn and washed almost to transparency. And a wrenching, tearing cough that left him bent double, with tears in the corners of his wide eyes.

It was painfully little to show for a life spent in gruelling labour underground, and not the way Manuel imagined he would come home. Men who went to work in the mines used to return on visits with smart city clothes and gifts for their families—mattresses, enamel cooking pots and perhaps portable stereos. When they came home to Mozambique for good, after a decade or more in South Africa, it was with a fat packet of wages that they used to put sturdy tin roofs on their houses, to buy dark wooden tables and chairs with stiff upholstery, to put a cement floor in the latrine in the yard.

But these days, more and more of the miners come home without any gifts, without any savings, without any cash. They come home like Manuel did: thin and worn and racked with pain. Or they don't come home at all.

I met Manuel in Xai Xai, a sleepy town set between the Indian Ocean and the muddy Limpopo River in central Mozambique, some two hundred kilometres north of the capital, Maputo. A great many of the men from

Xai Xai (pronounced *Shy* Shy) work in the mines in South Africa, and the menfolk were gone from most of the houses. Manuel, however, was home. He couldn't get up to greet me from the green plastic chair where he sat stiff with pain, but he invited me to sit, and I joined his wife, Philomena, on a woven grass mat in their neatly swept yard. He spoke slowly in Shangaan, his words punctuated by the terrible fits of coughing that made Philomena and me flinch, and he told me how a boy from a farming town ends up spending his life underground digging for gold in a city far away.

When Manuel turned eighteen in 1967, he became eligible for conscription into the army of the Portuguese colonial rulers, which was fighting the rebel Front for the Liberation of Mozambique (FRELIMO). Manuel didn't want to fight, and so he went to the poky office maintained by a mining recruitment service right there in his small town. Within minutes he had a job—a job he couldn't begin to imagine in a country he had never seen.

When gold was discovered in 1866 beneath the ridge of earth that is now Johannesburg, white miners staked out the first jobs. But the gold was sparsely distributed through the earth—as far as five kilometres underground—and so a massive amount of dirt had to be hauled to the surface and sifted, and soon the mines were hungry for cheap black labour. Black people, driven off their land by white farmers and settlers, had begun to flood into the city in search of jobs. To keep control of the black population, and prevent permanent black settlements from developing, the government ordered the men to come alone and live in hostels right at the mines, leaving their families back in distant villages. The miners would work for a few years, and then—often when they were injured, worn out or in the early stages of the lung disease silicosis—be sent back to their rural homes, to be replaced by a new crop of young men. It was the beginning of South Africa's hated apartheid "pass system," which allowed only black labourers with passes into white areas, restricting the rest to regions designated for black occupancy.

The mines had a rapacious appetite for labour, which led to the development of a migrant flow that at its height drew more than 750,000 men from all of South Africa's bordering countries, plus Zambia, Angola, Malawi and as far away as Tanzania. Similar patterns developed across the region: men journeyed hundreds of kilometres from Malawi and Lesotho to work in the diamond mines at Kimberley; from Zimbabwe and Mozambique to the copper mines in Zambia; from Botswana to the coal mines of Zimbabwe. By the 1960s, South Africa's mines had work forces that were more than 80 per cent foreign—because the foreign men could be sent back across the borders when the mines were done with them, and because the mine bosses believed that some ethnic groups, such as the Basotho people of Lesotho, were easier to control than others. The men kept coming because the mines and the agricultural plantations were just about the only sources of waged labour available to black men in southern Africa through most of the last century.

Manuel was one of tens of thousands of Mozambicans who headed for the gold mines. As a boy, he had finished only three years of primary school before he had to help his father work their small patch of land. There was no work at home. "If I'd stayed here I could only have made grass baskets or floor mats. It helped me—I managed to feed my family."

He was gone for almost all of the next thirty-seven years, spending his nights seven or eight hundred metres underground, driving a cart through the humid, dimly lit tunnels along the veins of gold, picking up the rubble left by the blasting crew who worked days. He was a "scrap driver," one of just a handful of words he knows in English. He worked, most of those years, for West Rand Consolidated Mines and Stilfontein Gold Mining. The record of his employment, a bland list of new contracts every year or two, was so well worn it fell to pieces when he handed it to me. He smiled a bit when I asked him how he felt about the work in the mines, which are legendarily hot and dangerous (one in every twenty-five miners dies on the job, and fully half of miners have a permanent disability by the time they stop mining). "I liked it because they paid for it," he said simply. His top wage, after twenty-five years in the mine, was 60 rand, or $10 a day. But it wasn't easy, especially not in the early years. "In those days, a person could die like a dog and just vanish without anyone knowing where he was. It wasn't like today, when things are more organized and they have unions to protect people. But the white people didn't allow you to complain. It was like being a slave."

His contract was like all the other miners': he was allowed one home visit every eighteen months. "Sometimes my husband would come home for a month or six months and stay with me," Philomena said, with a fond glance at Manuel. But it was rarely that long, he explained: "You had to ask the company for leave to come home—sometimes you got ten days and sometimes a month." And of course he didn't get paid for those days away from work. But he was proud that he was not one of those men who left for decades. "I never stayed more than two years away without coming home."

Manuel was already a miner when Philomena was introduced to him by her family in the early 1970s, so she knew he would be going back to South Africa. "But I didn't know he'd be gone so long," she said wistfully. Even today she has little idea what his life was like there—she has "not one clue" about South Africa, she said. The lengthy absences were difficult for Manuel, and hard on his family. "I missed him," Philomena told me shyly, eyes fixed in her lap. "But I got used to it. I took care of the house and I did the farming and I knew my husband was working. Of course it's not a good thing to be apart so much time, but someone who goes away to work is going to bring something back. You can go to the fields around here and work and you'll get food, but no money to buy a bed or buy clothes—so what can you do?"

Manuel never earned enough to put up brick walls or a zinc roof, but the Cossa home has three separate buildings with reed and wattle walls. The family has proper wooden beds, rather than mats on the floor, and everyone has a few changes of clothes. One year he brought home a bicycle for his middle son, Mario, and a cellphone that his daughter, Elisa, likes to carry around—she charges it at the home of neighbours who have electricity.

When he left for the mines, Manuel travelled twelve hours west by shuddering, wheezing bus from Xai Xai on the lush Mozambican coast to the cool *highveld*. Through all his years in the mines, he lived in what's called a hostel, the mining industry's solution for housing the rotating crops of single men. The hostels are rows of rectangular rooms, each about six metres square, in which twenty men are each allotted a bunk and a cupboard. Hostels afford their residents no privacy; they are, Manuel said, one of the worst things about the job. After their shifts, there wasn't a great deal for the men to do. In the daytime, some of them played football in a rough field outside the hostel, and Manuel watched their matches. He did errands in the rough trading centre near the mine, and took a sewing class there, so that he could make a bit of extra money doing mending and alterations for other miners. There was a large open bar on the mine property that sold big cartons of potent sorghum beer. And there were women: none on the mine property itself, but plenty standing just outside the chain-link fence. Lots of them sitting in the shade of the low scrub trees in the fields across the road from the mine. And a great many, smiling and ready to drape an arm over a miner's shoulders, twine her leg with his, in the bars in the ramshackle informal settlement that served the mine. There, women sold sex for about $5—but when desperate, or when they looked ill, the price could be less than a dollar.

More than half a century ago, South African researchers linked the migrant labour system serving the gold mines to a large hike in the spread of syphilis and gonorrhea. In 1985, South Africa's Chamber of Mines—reflecting the apartheid government's paranoia about AIDS, which was beginning to be reported in other African countries—started testing foreign migrant workers for HIV. When a small group of Malawian miners tested positive, they were immediately expelled. For the next few years, the industry demanded tests of all foreign workers who wanted to come to South Africa, until opposition from unions and foreign governments forced a change in the policy. But by then the genie was out of the bottle: less than one per cent of pregnant women tested positive for HIV in South Africa in 1990, and almost 30 per cent were positive a decade later.

And it is no mystery why, says Mark Lurie, a professor of medicine and community health at Brown University in the United States who has

"I felt bad when
"But at the hospital
had it—some young
lifted my spirits: I'm not

made an extensive study of the mining industry in South Africa. "It doesn't take a rocket scientist to figure out that if you wanted to create an HIV epidemic, you would take as many young men as you could away from their families, isolate them in single-sex hostels and give them easy access to sex workers and alcohol. Then, to spread the disease around the country, you'd send them home every once in a while to their wives and girlfriends. The whole subcontinent is connected by people's movement, and infectious disease follows the movement of people."

Lurie has found that male migrant workers are two and a half times more likely to be infected with HIV than non-migrants. The hostels are grim, visits home are rare, the beer and the women are affordable on a miner's comparatively good salary—and, like long-haul trucking, the job is dangerous, giving many men a feeling that they don't need to worry about risk from HIV because they could die any day in a cave-in. Lurie told me that health educators find it difficult to persuade men who work surrounded by such visible danger to worry about a microscopic virus. Many South African mines report that nearly 30 per cent of their workforce is infected; studies of the women who work the bars or the open-air brothels in the fields outside the mine fence show they have HIV infection rates as high as 80 per cent.

Yet there is also a more insidious way in which migrant labour pushes up infection rates. The problem is not just what happens at the mines but also what happens back home. Lurie has tracked "discordant couples"—pairs where one person has HIV and the other doesn't. In two-thirds of couples, it is the migrant man who is infected—men who

MANUEL COSSA

I got the result," she said.
I met so many people who
some old—that it
the only one who has it."

buy sex in the years they are away, enjoying the anonymity of the city and behaving in a way they likely wouldn't if subjected to the scrutiny of family and neighbours. But in a solid third of the discordant pairs, it is the woman who is HIV-positive—because, of course, the women left at home also have other partners, seeking companionship, sex and often economic support. Many miners strike up long-term relationships with women who live or work in the mining towns, and may start using some of their wages to support those "town wives"; then they may cut back on visits home, or on the money they send. And so the women back in the village take what's called in isiZulu *ishende*—a man on the side, someone who contributes to the running of the household with school fees or food. All of this widens the circle of infection.

When I met Manuel, he had been home from South Africa for only a couple of weeks. He had been sick off and on for months, and at the mine he had grown so ill that worried friends insisted he take a bus back to Mozambique. (There is a particular, unspoken dread of dying far from home—if family cannot raise the money to bring a body home, a man will be buried in unknown ground far away from his ancestors and those who would tend his grave.) Manuel came home to Xai Xai in October 2005, arriving, Philomena said, "with empty hands." He was thin and gasping and nauseous; he could not walk without help. She went to her church and borrowed 11,000 meticais (40 cents) to pay for him to see the doctor at the local hospital. There, after a long wait on a narrow bench, Manuel was diagnosed with tuberculosis and advised to have an HIV test. Both he and Philomena tested positive.

Manuel seemed calm about the news, perhaps because his pain and fever were occupying most of his thoughts; I sensed he wasn't surprised. "A lot of my friends got ill. There are a lot who died."

Philomena, a gentle woman with an open face and a quiet laugh, seemed more shocked. "I felt bad when I got the result," she said, hands folded in her lap. "But at the hospital I met so many people who had it—some young, some old—that it lifted my spirits: I'm not the only one who has it."

Not the only one, indeed. An estimated 1.9 million Mozambicans, of a population of eighteen million, are living with HIV/AIDS. The adult infection rate in the central provinces, source of most of the miners, is 20 per cent, the highest in the country. Mozambique is spectacularly ill equipped to respond to a problem on this scale. The government is struggling, with little money and even less trained staff, to rebuild a health system that was neglected by the Portuguese and destroyed in the savage civil war that evicted the colonizers. In 2004, there were just 450 doctors working in the entire public health system. In May that year the government announced a national ARV treatment program but, only days after beginning, admitted the goal was hopelessly ambitious. "It is simply impossible to imagine that we can distribute ARVs countrywide," said Francisco Songane, the health minister. "We do not have the capacity to do that. We do not have the trained manpower or the infrastructure to handle such a massive program."

The best intentions cannot make a health system out of nothing—and for all that it is often held up these days as a rare African success story, Mozambique is still the sixth-poorest country in the world. After the peace deal in 1992 and the first democratic elections, the former Marxists of FRELIMO became the government and embraced a free-market program drawn up by the World Bank. The country has had remarkable economic growth—an average of 8 per cent per year—since that transition to democracy. But the numbers don't tell the whole story: the development is concentrated around Maputo in the south, in a couple of enormous industrial projects. A few hours outside the capital, life looks much like it did thirty years ago. Only 660,000 of Mozambique's eighteen million people have formal jobs.

And so the young men continue to make their way to the regional mining recruitment offices and then on to South Africa just like Manuel did. His oldest son, José, left at the age of twenty—he hoped to avoid work underground, but only the mines provide the vital work visa. Their second son, Mario, had no work at home but told me, "I would prefer to suffer here" rather than become a miner.

By the time Manuel came home from South Africa for the last time, he had been troubled by suppurating abscesses on his bony legs for more than a year. He got medicine from the mine doctor, but the lesions didn't heal. He tried the doctor in town, with no more luck. Finally, he went to an *inyanga,* a traditional healer from Mozambique who was working near the mine. The man made him a remedy, and that healed the sores, Manuel said.

At no time did the mine ever suggest an HIV test. This was a story I heard over and over again in Xai Xai and other villages of central Mozambique. I met Julius Inande, so weak he could not walk when he was relieved of his job and sent home from the Driefontein gold mine, unable to control his diarrhea or close his mouth because of the sores. I met Antonio Titus, who at thirty-four could not have weighed more than 25 kilograms; he tried to hide his wasted body in a football jersey that enveloped him like a robe. None of them was ever offered an HIV test, and they had a grim suspicion about why: If a man is sent home with a terminal illness, the mine owes him a package of disability benefits, but if he goes on a "temporary" sick leave, the mine contractually owes him nothing.

Manuel, Julius, Antonio and all the others were the sole wage earners in their families, and the loss of their salaries was devastating. Manuel had no pension and received no sick pay. The family had quickly spent the cash he had brought home from South Africa on the hospital visits, and Philomena found herself trying to feed her family on the unripe vegetables in the garden. In counselling sessions at the hospital, Manuel and Philomena were encouraged to eat well because good nutrition would bolster their immune systems—a bit ironic, Philomena pointed out, "since now we don't have the money even for soap." Their daughter, Elisa, was in Grade 10 and doing well, hoping to be a nurse—but now there was no money to pay the $10 a term to keep her in school, no money for fees for the youngest of their five children, Manuel, to stay in Grade 3, and none for their grandson, Manuelito, to start school at all.

Because mining remains the backbone of South Africa's economy, and because South Africa is the core of the continent's economy (Johannesburg and the mines around it produce 9 per cent of the GDP for all of Africa), the relationship between AIDS and mining is not just a social or medical issue but an economic one. In a 2006 assessment of the South African economy, for example, the Economist Intelligence Unit listed HIV/AIDS before any other factor (a volatile currency, powerful unions) as the one to watch in terms of its impact on growth. The big mining companies have been forced to acknowledge that the disease is pushing up the cost of operations—through absenteeism, funeral costs, lowered productivity due to illness, poor staff morale—adding, they say, $10 to the price of each ounce of gold they mine.

In Manuel's last years of work, the companies faced up to the fact that a third of their workforce was infected with a fatal illness. They began to take action, and some South African mining companies have emerged as the global leaders in corporate responsibility for AIDS. They began with comprehensive education programs and condom distribution, but cold economic reality suggested that they were going to have to move quickly on treatment. In 2003, before the South African government had begun public treatment, Anglo American, one of the largest mining firms, rolled out an ARV program that is unmatched in either efficiency or comprehensiveness by any other public or private effort worldwide. These interventions, which involve education, condom distribution and treatment, lowered the cost of AIDS from $10 to $4 an ounce of mined gold, Anglo said. Dr. Brian Brink, Anglo's vice-president for medical services, said the reduction of absenteeism compensates for three-quarters of the cost of the ARV treatment program—and since most mines already provide primary health care to their workers, the reduced burden on those facilities pays for the rest.

The other solution was family housing, which Professor Mark Lurie estimates could lower HIV infections by as much as 40 per cent. The mines had long resisted this innovation—because of the cost of building houses and of all the services such as schools and clinics that would be needed to serve the families that moved into them—but finally began to give in to the twin pressures of unions and AIDS. In 2005, BHP Billiton moved some of its miners into private or family housing, and turned old hostels into "community centres" to house orphans left by miners and hospices to provide palliative care for the dying. The National Union of Mineworkers demanded greater "living out" allowances so that miners could afford to accommodate their families near the mines or at least rent private accommodation.

But the commitment to these interventions varies wildly between companies; Manuel never saw evidence of any of them, save for some rudimentary safer-sex demonstrations in the bars, and Mark Lurie noted that the vast majority of miners still live in single-sex hostels.

Back home in Mozambique, Manuel learned about ARVs in his hospital counselling sessions. On the day he spent with me, however, he wasn't sure whether the hospital had the drugs or might arrange for him to get them. His torn scrap of paper from the local clinic said he had oral thrush and the skin cancer Kaposi's sarcoma; the inside of his eyelids were chalk white, a sign of severe anemia, which is also common in people with HIV. When he produced his plastic bag of pills, I saw that he had been given vitamins and the antibiotic cotrimoxazole—but no ARVs.

Manuel and Philomena were gracious with my questions, but our conversations about AIDS—about how they had come to be infected, and about fidelity in the course of their long marriage—were circuitous and oblique. "Life in South Africa is very tough, but it's not just a matter of relations with a woman," Manuel said cryptically. "I think you can get HIV through an apple or an orange or an injection or anything. Not necessarily through relations with a woman."

Philomena said that it was "possible" Manuel had become infected in South Africa, but then she added, her eyes fixed on mine, "He was a serious man when we met and he's always been a good man." Because Manuel's illness was so much more advanced than Philomena's, who said she felt quite well, he had likely been infected before passing HIV to his wife, although it is also possible that she was the first to be infected. In the soft light of late afternoon, looking into the middle distance, Manuel told me he was sure that Philomena always "waited" for him when he was away. Whatever suspicions they had about how HIV got to their family, the time for accusations was past.

Though he was in obvious pain, Manuel and Philomena laughed together when they told the story of their first meeting and how they quickly decided to marry. "I went to see her and thought, she's the right one for me," he said. Then he just had to hope she would agree: "When you're concentrating like that you can even forget about food." But Philomena was quick to accept his proposal: "I wanted to build a family with him."

They did build a family, and she grew their food and raised their children while he earned money to house them and bring precious presents back from the city. And, Philomena said, she was glad he had come home again. No matter what he had brought with him.

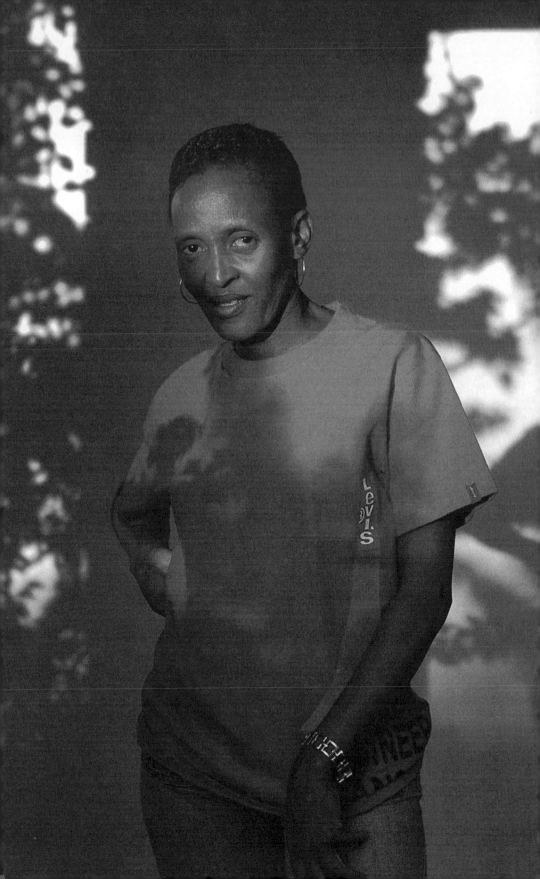

# TEN

# CynthiaLeshomo

ynthia Leshomo was born to be a beauty queen. Her default facial expression is a pout. She rolls her eyes at the foibles of lesser mortals. She is exhausted by the needs of her adoring public. No one, she is quite certain, really understands the demands that are placed upon Miss HIV Stigma-Free.

But then, hers is a particularly challenging tiara to wear. The Miss Stigma-Free pageant was launched in 2003 by AIDS organizations in Botswana's capital, Gaborone, with the goal of trying to ease the shame and perhaps inject a touch of glamour into living openly with HIV. In a country with an epidemic as severe as Botswana's, this was no small task.

The first contest drew a modest, somewhat skeptical audience, and the inaugural Miss HIV Stigma-Free was built like a linebacker. She was no sparkling conversationalist, but she was unfazed by talking about her life with HIV, and so she won plenty of attention both at home and abroad. By the time Cynthia saw posters advertising the third competition in 2005, it had grown into a big, glitzy affair.

She was convinced this was the route she had long sought to fame and fortune. Cindy, as she is known to her friends, filled out an entry form and began to hatch her strategy. She started by checking out her competition. Gaborone is Botswana's biggest city, but it functions like a village, and it wasn't difficult to learn who else was aiming to be Miss Stigma-Free. A couple of the other eleven contestants worried her slightly: some had gone public about living with HIV long before she had, and one had been a runner-up in the pageant the year before.

On the night of the contest, in muggy late February, five hundred people packed into a ballroom on the manicured grounds of the Royal Palm Hotel at the edge of the city. Music pulsed and klieg lights on the stage left the contestants with beads of sweat across their foreheads. First came casual wear; Cindy took the occasion to show off her long legs and high, round bum. Then questions from the judges about life with HIV: "Let's fight the stigma associated with AIDS, but not people with AIDS," Cindy said through a wide smile. Then traditional wear—and this was her moment.

Cindy walked slowly down the catwalk in a knee-length brown wool dress, carrying a clay water pot on her shoulder, swaying her hips. At the end of the runway, she sank gracefully to her knees, lowered the pot and reached inside. She lifted out a bottle of mineral water and a pill container. And there, in front of the crowd, Cynthia Leshomo took her ARVs.

She swallowed the tablets, gave the audience her most winning smile, restored the pot to her shoulder and glided back up the catwalk. There was still the evening-wear round to follow, but Cindy knew—as the stillness of the crowd was broken suddenly by wild cheers—that the crown was hers.

And indeed, an hour later, the flower coronet was placed on top of her long braids. Cindy clasped her hands to her cheeks in the beauty queen's universal expression of fetching disbelief. Stepping down from the stage, she embraced her older sister Tshenolo, and then turned to throw her long arms around Avo Avalos, the doctor who, a few years earlier, had told Cindy's family she had only hours to live. The doctor wept, the cameras flashed and the TV crews jostled for position. Cindy beamed, and turned to meet them.

Cindy is from Malokaganyane, a village in the arid south of Botswana near the border with South Africa. Born in 1970, she is the last but one of six children. Vivacious and sharp tongued, she was a ringleader in village games and she did well at school.

She has had, by the standards of the region, a life of opportunity. Her country is often heralded as an African success story: stable, peaceful and democratic since its independence, Botswana has some of the world's largest diamond deposits, and the government has channelled the mineral wealth into social spending. School was free when Cindy was growing up, and so was health care. Many people in Botswana work for the state; her mother was a school principal and her father a government driver.

The government paid for Cindy to travel to Pretoria to study for a college degree in commercial administration. She did well, although she never missed a party. She heard rumours about the spread of HIV, but she didn't worry too much. "I thought, 'I won't get it because I am young and beautiful and not of the class to be infected.'"

Botswana, in the mid-1990s, had a life expectancy higher than many nations in eastern Europe. But HIV was capitalizing on the most fundamental aspects of life in the country, and spreading with a speed that no one anticipated. The Batswana, as they are called, are a highly mobile people who traditionally divided their lives between a home in a village and a remote cattle post, tending to the herds that are the foundation of Tswana culture. By the late 1980s, Botswana was urbanizing quickly, and so people also moved between the city, where there was work, and the villages where they maintained their family ties, a way of life that incorporated multiple relationships. Cindy was no exception. An upper-middle-class family such as hers has cows—*everyone* in Botswana has cows—and as a girl she went sometimes to camp at the cattle post in the bush. But by the time she was in her late teens she was determined to leave Malokaganyane for one of the rapidly expanding cities.

After college she got a job as a legal secretary at a private law firm in Pretoria. She was happy to stay in the South African capital, where life was much more exciting than in sleepy Gaborone. She earned a good salary, enough to keep her in the latest shoes and leather handbags and dangly earrings. There were lots of boyfriends, lots of parties, lots of wild nights in newly-free South Africa. And then she started to get sick: black lesions appeared on her face, and she lost more and more weight off an already lanky frame. She saw a series of doctors, and each advised her to have an HIV test. She flatly refused. Pretty young women with college degrees didn't get HIV—the disease was for poor people, people back in the village with straw for a roof and chickens in the yard. Of course, deep down, she suspected HIV. "But there was so much stigma."

*Stigma* is one of the most used words in the AIDS pandemic, a two-syllable shorthand for the shame and fear that cling to this disease. Stigma is not, of course, unique to HIV—it is a common feature of incurable, transmissible and deadly illnesses; lepers are banished to colonies, and crimson warnings are smeared on the doors of people infected with a plague. But there is a particular distaste saved for those diseases where the sick are viewed as the authors of their own misfortune, and a particular shame that comes with a disease most often transmitted by sex. Because HIV infection in Africa passes primarily through sexual contact, people who admit to having HIV (even when they contracted it from their husbands or, as in Cindy's case, from relationships that are entirely socially acceptable) are perceived both by others and by themselves to be admitting to sin or violation of community mores. Stigma, with the blame it implies, gives people a way to distance themselves from risk: it happens to "them," not to me.

By 2000, when Cindy got sick and didn't get better, she was far from alone. Her country had the worst AIDS epidemic in the world: 37.5 per cent of pregnant women in Botswana were testing positive. For a country with a population of only 1.6 million people, it called survival into question. The president, Festus Mogae, spoke of "extinction."

In the early days of the epidemic in North America, when only gay men and heroin addicts had HIV, it was easy to shun people with the disease: these were marginalized groups, easily isolated, easily blamed. And even in Africa in the early years, only a small number of people had visible symptoms. But it is far more difficult, indeed largely impossible, to isolate a third of the population, or to argue that all of those people are guilty of something. And yet, in Botswana, the shame clung to AIDS in defiance of the 37.5 per cent prevalence rate. When the government surveyed the population in 2001, nearly two-thirds of the people said they would not buy vegetables from a vendor with HIV; nearly half said that a teacher with the virus should not be allowed to continue to teach.

Yet people weren't talking about it. Tswana culture is formal and conservative, reticent around both sex and death. If people referred to the new plague at all, it was as "that illness." When a friend or relative of Cindy's died, newspaper obituaries gave the cause of death as TB or influenza; people described the deceased only as "late." The gaudy condom billboards put up by international agencies around the cities were foreign, an embarrassment. "That was for others—it wasn't for me," Cindy explained, even though people her age were beginning to die in huge numbers. And even when she was tremendously ill, there was no way she was going to have an HIV test.

"All we were told is that you're going to die if you have HIV," she said. "If you died, you were buried the same day. People covered their faces in the mortuary when they went to collect a body." If she had it, Cindy figured, well, she'd die, but in the meantime, she wasn't putting herself or anyone else through the ordeal of living with that knowledge.

By late 2000, she was so sick that she had to go home to stay with her parents. Her mother took her to yet another doctor, and he too counselled HIV testing. This time, however, there was something different. "He showed me a bottle of Combivir"—a two-in-one antiretroviral pill—"and said, 'I am not saying you are HIV-positive but if ever you are, I will give you this bottle of Combivir and you'll be like Magic Johnson.'" This was a radical notion: that the treatment that could keep people with AIDS alive was available in Botswana. Available, that is, to people who could afford to pay $350 a month. Presented with the bottle of ARVs, Cindy agreed to have the test. When it came back positive, her mother immediately bought the first month's supply of drugs.

Botswana's leaders had been, for some time, paralyzed by the scale and spread of the epidemic in their country. But now President Mogae demanded drastic action. Crack teams of international consultants were brought in to design a plan, millions of dollars were put at their disposal, and in 2001, a year after Cindy started buying ARVs, Mogae announced

# Every time she swallowed
## about AIDS,
### now marked, stained,

the start of the first public AIDS treatment program in Africa. It was called Masa ("new dawn" in Setswana) and its goal was to provide every citizen of Botswana who needed AIDS treatment with free antiretrovirals. Although Botswana had the greatest percentage of infected people in Africa, it also had, unlike any of its neighbours, the money to buy the drugs and a solid health infrastructure to distribute them.

In addition to saving the lives of the sick, the Masa plan had another goal: ending stigma. Before Masa, most people thought as Cindy did: Why get tested if there is no treatment and no cure—if you will be sent home to die, shunned by your family and neighbours? Better to die of some unspecified combination of respiratory problems and diarrhea, and leave HIV out of it. Centres offering free HIV tests had been opened up all over the country, but in the absence of treatment, they were often empty. People wouldn't test if there was no treatment. The prevalence surveys suggested that 300,000 people were infected, yet by 2003 only 80,000 had tested.

This was a problem in plenty of other countries, too. It was seen as essential to get people to "know their status," on the grounds that if they were HIV-positive, they could take steps to stay healthy and protect their partners, and if they were negative, they could take measures to stay that way. The theory was that the availability of free treatment would motivate people—in the tens of thousands—to test for HIV. And when people with AIDS began to get well in large numbers, then the stigma would begin to fall away: as AIDS was transformed from a fatal to a chronic illness, there would be less to cause shame, less to fear. The eyes of the whole AIDS world were on Botswana, waiting to see just how well it would work.

It didn't. After a year of free treatment, the numbers of people seeking HIV tests had barely crept upwards. Some people were seeking out the

CYNTHIA LESHOMO

# a tablet, she thought about how she was spoiled.

treatment—but they were the desperately sick people who could not keep the secret any more. Treatment hadn't ended stigma. It had barely dented it.

If any of the high-priced consultants who drew up Botswana's AIDS plan had talked to Cindy, they might have seen this coming. Yes, she had her Combivir, but a bottle of pills didn't soothe the pain of being told she had a fatal illness at the age of thirty. Magic Johnson notwithstanding, she was *infected* with something, something she couldn't get rid of, something she caught having sex. She quit her job in Pretoria and lurked around her parents' house, feeling, she said, "like a black sheep, like I was cursed." Every time she swallowed a tablet, she thought about AIDS, about how she was now marked, stained, spoiled. The drugs soon made her well, but she still didn't tell her friends what she had. Here was the lesson for the architects of Masa: ARVs could make a person well, but they didn't end the shame of AIDS. Before long, Cindy was taking the medication money her mother gave her and going back to Pretoria, blowing the cash on booze and parties. "I'm still waiting to die but I don't die. So I'm just going to have fun—I drank until I dropped."

Within weeks of stopping the pills, she was sick again: her hair was falling out in clumps, her skin was peeling off. She got so sick her family had to keep her in diapers, and she decided she couldn't wait any longer for a death that was dragging its feet. "I thought, 'I'm going to suffer and going to die'—I just wanted to bring that day." She made a concoction of bleach, fabric softener, detergent and all the pills in the house, and drank it down.

She was in a coma for three days. She awoke in hospital to the news that she had pneumonia, stomach tumours, tuberculosis and Kaposi's sarcoma. Her CD4 count was 8. Doctors told her family that this horrifying array of illnesses would almost certainly finish the job she had started with her poisonous homemade cocktail. Yet Cindy beat the cancer, and the tuberculosis; she got over the pneumonia and her lesions healed. "There's no one who went through what she went through and is still standing," Avo Avalos, her doctor, told me. "I was just lucky to facilitate her will to live. She's my inspiration."

Cindy said that when confronted with actual, imminent death, it didn't seem so appealing any more. And she was lucky to be young and strong enough that when she decided, with her usual single-mindedness, that she wanted to live, her body could still fight back. She was filled with the sense that her life was spared for a purpose: "I still have to do something in life."

Soon she was out of the hospital and back on ARVs—taking them religiously this time. Her CD4 count slowly climbed. In the newspaper one day, she noticed an advertisement: an organization called the Coping Centre for People Living with HIV/AIDS was looking for a receptionist, and would give priority to a person with HIV. Cindy got the job. "That was the turning point of my life. I met these people living with HIV and AIDS who accepted their status and were living life to the fullest. I thought, 'My God, why not me?'"

At the centre, she was soon given rudimentary training in public speaking, and she began to do small talks in workplaces, telling people how she was living healthily on ARVs. She loved the attention, and how people drank up what she had to say. She was the only college graduate who was publicly HIV-positive, and that made people listen. Now talking about HIV won her admiration, and that eroded the shame in a way ARVs never did. "I really had an impact on people."

Audiences were drawn by the frank way she talked about contracting the virus. "I used to be naughty," she said. "I used to change partners, I used to drink—I was young and vibrant and that was Cynthia." Her honesty gave her a certain authority in talking about behaviour change: she had changed, she said, but it is extremely difficult to persuade other people, for the simple reasons that none of the other options are nearly as much fun. "Just tell a kid to abstain—I can't. I didn't abstain. And I didn't use a condom."

Every beauty queen needs her cause, and Cindy threw herself into public education, focusing her advocacy efforts on rural areas. "In rural communities they still don't know anything about transmission of HIV. People don't have information and they end up dying." Now, when she addressed a crowd at a village school or church, or in a *kgotla,* the traditional meeting place, people seized on the opportunity to ask this honest young woman all the things they really wanted to know. "People in rural areas ask me, 'How did you get infected?' And 'Do you have sex?'" Yes, she told them. "'I'm a human being, I do have sex, but in a safer way.' They want to know, at funerals, do you cook the meal? I tell them that transmission of HIV is not through food." There are many, many people who need to hear her message, she said.

Today some stop her in the streets, approach her at the mall, strike up conversations in the mini-bus taxi: everyone has seen her on TV. "They tell me I'm a role model, an inspiration." She often misses work because Miss Stigma-Free duties call; she serves as a treatment buddy to many people with HIV, accompanies those newly diagnosed to their first appointments at the clinic. She glides like a princess through the infectious disease centre in downtown Gaborone, mouthing "hello" left and right, her cellphone pressed to her ear.

Because she is so well known, she said, lots of people turn up at her house for counselling. That's how she met her boyfriend, Carlos, who was sent by friends to see her after he tested positive. Cindy giggled when I asked—of course it's against the rules to date your counselling client, even when he's tall and dreadlocked and handsome in a smouldering sort of way. "But I'm a human being." These days she lives with him in his mother's house in a suburb at the edge of the capital, close to the big Riverside mall where she goes to keep an eye on the latest fashion trends.

Cindy said there is ever greater demand on her as more people get on to treatment. When Masa failed to boost the number of people seeking HIV tests, the government took another radical step: in early 2004 it introduced the first-ever policy of routine HIV testing. Now health workers offer an HIV test to anyone who comes into contact with the health system—whether for tuberculosis or meningitis that may be related to AIDS, or an ear infection or a spider bite. People can decline the test, but researchers suspected that most would agree to take it. And they were correct: in the eighteen months after the new policy was introduced, 202,000 people were tested—a 134 per cent increase over the previous period. By late 2006, the country had seventy thousand people on treatment, about 85 per cent of those who need it, one of the highest ratios in the developing world. Finally, Cindy said, the normalization of testing and the sheer volume of people on treatment have served to erode some of the shame. "It's better now—for most people the stigma is not that strong. They're coming out and talking about it."

The Miss HIV Stigma-Free pageant was originally envisioned as an annual affair, but after Cindy won, organizers realized that far more women were living openly with HIV than were men, and they decided to find a Mr. Stigma-Free instead—so she retains the title today. She revels in the fame her status has brought her, and yet she also has a clear sense of what the disease has cost her. If she were HIV-negative, she said, she would have stayed in South Africa and furthered her studies, but because she can get free AIDS drugs only in Botswana, she is stuck there. She reckons she could have a lucrative career in communications, if she could reach a market outside her small country. "Then I would be in a position to maintain myself. I want to study to be a motivational speaker like Oprah, and speak on issues of HIV/AIDS—I could make it to the top. I would have my own house, my own car, my own talk show, and be helping the nation."

She has learned to speak the modest language of the pageant queen. "Today I am the happiest person if I save one soul," she told me earnestly. The recognition, she added, means nothing. "I never thought I'd be famous like I am today," she said in one breath, before adding in the next, "You know, at the end of the day I'm still myself. I'm still Cynthia."

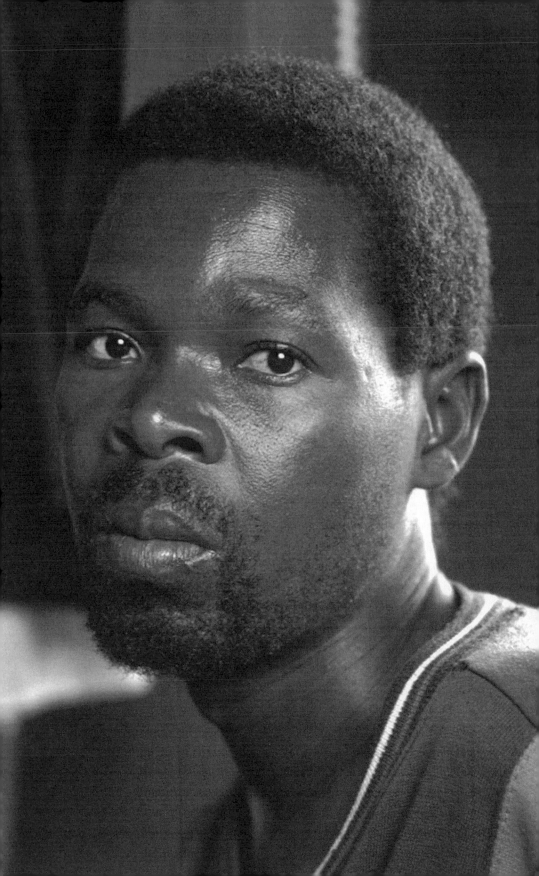

# ELEVEN

# Mfanimpela Thlabatse

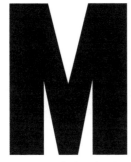fanimpela Thlabatse and I had met before.

On a sweltering March day in 2004, I had accompanied Siphiwe Hlophe on her rounds through Swazi villages. Toward the end of the day, she parked her white truck at the end of a dirt road and we started to walk, shooing the goats that ran beside us and nipped at my linen trousers. We leapt from rock to rock over a small stream and climbed over a cattle barrier made of branches. I struggled to keep up with Siphiwe, who, despite her heavy curves, was much more deft at this than I. We stopped in front of a small cement house with a tin roof, and climbed the stone steps.

Inside, a woman lay beneath a scratchy wool blanket on a low bed, gasping for breath in the last days of her life. Siphiwe knelt beside her, talking quietly, and I hung back in the doorway. When we had been in the house for a couple of minutes, my vision adjusted to the dim light, and I noticed two children sitting against the back wall. Their eyes never left their mother.

We stayed for twenty minutes or so—there was nothing Siphiwe could do, except refill the woman's tin cup of water and pat her hand. Back outside, I had met the woman's husband, Mfanimpela. He was working on their small plot of land, wearing a wide straw hat and dark green Wellington boots. His broad shoulders curved with muscle in a yellow tank top. He stood in the centre of a field of the fat heads of lettuce he would sell in town for a little cash to feed his family, and he raised a hand in greeting. Siphiwe chatted with him briefly, offered a few encouraging words, but when we reached the truck she was silent and grim.

Now, eighteen months later, I was back in Swaziland and coming to the end of another day spent with Siphiwe. We were headed toward town when she said she wanted to make one last stop. At the end of a road we parked and set out on a trail, and it quickly started to feel familiar—the stream, the cattle barrier. When we arrived at the rough stone steps, I thought, "I know this house."

And I was puzzled. There was no way the woman we had come to see a year and a half earlier could still be alive. With a wince, I thought of the children—perhaps we had come to check on one of them?

But this time it was Mfanimpela who lay on the bed. He was sweat-slicked and wheezing and lying under that same blanket that had covered his wife a year and a half before. And he was alone. Siphiwe had heard rumours that he was ill; this was how she had feared she might find him.

Mfanimpela courteously struggled upright when we came in, and tried to make conversation. He asked Siphiwe for news from town. He had a transistor radio tuned to soccer—Bafana Bafana, the South African national team that most Swazis have adopted as their own, was playing that day. Hunting for something to say, I inquired about the score. He was wearing the same yellow shirt I remembered, but now it hung from his shoulders. His town clothes—a shirt and an ancient necktie—hung over a pole in the corner, the remnant of another life.

Some things in Swaziland had changed since my last visit to this house: the country was making a halting effort to roll out ARV treatment. The drugs were being distributed from AIDS clinics at the hospitals in Mbabane and Manzini. But Mfanimpela had no money to go to the city. Since he had become too sick, a few weeks before, to work in the garden, he had had no money at all.

This time there was something Siphiwe could do: she whipped out her cellphone, called the Swapol office in the city and arranged for someone to come in a car the next morning to collect Mfanimpela and accompany him to the clinic. She didn't linger, but told him kindly that he must hold on while he made his way up the waiting list for ARVs.

I couldn't bring myself to ask Mfanimpela about his wife or the children, but when Siphiwe and I were making our way back down the path, I did ask her. "They all died, between April and August," she said baldly. "One after the other."

Mfanimpela had to give the children paupers' burials, she added, because after he buried his wife there was no money left for more funerals. I understood the shame this must have caused him.

Mfanimpela was thirty-four that day we met again—a few months older than I.

And he had outlived his entire family.

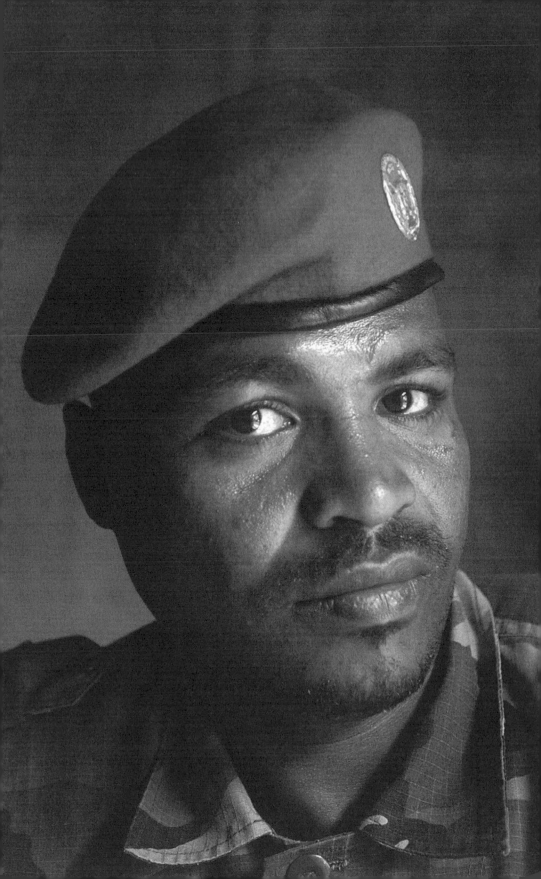

# TWELVE

# AndualemAyalew

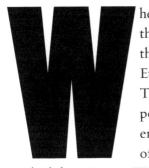hen Andualem Ayalew was a boy of seven or eight, the army came to his village: they were soldiers of the Derg, the Marxist dictatorship that then ruled Ethiopia, big burly men in fatigues and red berets. They laughed and spoke loudly, they moved with a power and a confidence Andualem had never encountered in the men who farmed in the village of Gachit. He lurked with the other children and watched them in awe. "We were riveted," he said. "They were the most fascinating thing we had ever seen." By the time the soldiers moved on, after a few days billeted there, he had decided he was going to become a soldier too—a commando with a red beret and a gun on his hip and black boots that gleamed.

In 1992, when Andualem was fifteen and had finished ninth grade, he persuaded the village elders to write a letter recommending him for military service. He set off for Mizan Taferi, a city fifty kilometres away, where the national army had a recruiting centre. There, the officers were a bit suspicious of his age—a man had to be eighteen to enlist—but his timing was good. After the seventeen harsh years of civil war, the alliance of rebels had toppled the Derg, formed a new government and was drafting an army intended to be representative of all the country's ethnic groups. Since Andualem came from the small Me-eyenit minority, he was good for their numbers. They took him without demanding any more proof of identification than the elders' letter.

Already a strapping young man, he excelled at the training. He passed the gruelling tests—days in the desert without food, whole weeks of forced marches—and he was selected for the commando unit, just as he had hoped. Soon he had the boots and the beret, and he felt people watching him walk just the way he had once watched the soldiers in Gachit. Military wages weren't great—200 birr a month, or $23, for a new recruit—but they were steady. He got on well with his commanders and had a wide network of friends among his fellow soldiers.

Over the next couple of years, he fought in small engagements with rebel groups challenging the new government, but this was a comparatively peaceful time in Ethiopia. Andualem was promoted to be a trainer of commandos, while he continued his education through a correspondence program and earned a high-school diploma. He sent money to his parents and five siblings in Gachit. When he went back to visit, everyone could see he had done well.

And then came the war with Eritrea. Once considered part of Ethiopia, the small northern territory of Eritrea had agitated for independence since 1962, and finally broke away in 1993 after the toppling of the junta. Following the split, the countries disagreed over currency and trade issues (Eritrea took Ethiopia's Red Sea coastline with it); the border remained undemarcated and, in several key places, disputed. In May 1998, skirmishes on that border escalated into full-scale fighting. Ethiopia, a highly militarized country with more than 300,000 regular personnel in its armed forces and a weapons budget of nearly a billion dollars, mounted a massive attack.

Andualem was ordered to ready himself for the front. Shortly before his unit was shipped north, the men were given a comprehensive medical screening that included an HIV test. There had been vague talk about this new disease among the troops for the past couple of years, but it was no surprise to him that his test came back negative: he was a healthy man.

Within weeks he found himself on a military base amid the rocks and dust of Tigray in the northern border region. His unit was posted near villages where the number of shops and bars soon swelled with the infusion of cash from soldiers—and new villages emerged as well, whole camps set up by prostitutes who accompanied the troops to the front.

I met Andualem through Ethiopian friends who knew I was interested in the way conflict and military forces have spread HIV. They told me they had heard of a fellow with an extraordinary story and would try to track him down for me. And so, one warm day in Addis Ababa in May 2006, a huge man in fatigues strode up to me at a busy intersection and nearly crushed the bones in my hands in greeting; several hours later, over a café table covered in emptied Coke bottles, he was well into his tale and telling me about the prostitutes who thronged to the border war.

"They were following soldiers from all over the country," Andualem recalled. After a few months at the northern base, he was given four days' leave, and spent it in Adinebri, one of those villages. "At that time we didn't know much—we had these misconceptions, for example that a fat person didn't have HIV. There was no HIV education from the military. I knew HIV existed but I had this misconception that it affected a person visibly as soon as they were infected. Plus I had tested negative and I was so fit and healthy and was doing so much physical activity that I couldn't believe it could attack me." So he spent his leave in the company of a sex worker, whom he remembers well. "She was beautiful. A fat one." A short time after he returned to the base, he developed gonorrhea, but that was easily treated by the medics. He never thought for a moment that he might have caught anything else.

In June 2000 he was sent to the front. In the trenches, he was only a few hundred metres from the Eritreans. The sun beat down hard, the dust rose in a constant, swirling cloud, and the crashing noise never let up. On his fifteenth day in combat, he was hit with shrapnel from a mortar. It tore into his groin and the soft skin of his lower belly. Medics on the scene packed the wound, and he was evacuated to a field hospital, where he had a series of surgeries over the next three months. Then he spent eight more weeks recovering at Bella Military Hospital in the capital. "They were picking pieces of shrapnel out of me for months," he said with a grin.

# "If I'd really thought it
# I probably
# That's human nature,

By the time the doctors were done with him, the war was over— Ethiopia mounted an offensive and occupied a quarter of Eritrea, displacing 650,000 civilians, and the Eritreans were forced to withdraw from the border and accept a ceasefire. So Andualem rejoined his unit at a rural base, where the men were about to start another round of training. He was promoted to 2nd lieutenant. But right about then, he said, things started to seem strange. "Fifteen days after I returned to my unit, we went back into intensive training, walking two hundred kilometres on foot with no food, in the middle of nowhere. You would kill frogs, or snakes—you'd eat anything you find." Andualem used to revel in these feats of endurance, but now he found them terrifyingly difficult. He lost weight on the marches, and he didn't gain it back afterwards. He suffered repeated bouts of diarrhea. He sweated uncontrollably. He barely had the strength to walk.

After the training, his unit was shipped down to Addis Ababa, where the government was using the army to quell pro-democracy demonstrations by university students. Andualem had years of experience in these kinds of engagements, but the ugly clashes with the crowds in the streets of the capital left him shaken and exhausted.

And so in early 2001, he went back to the clinic at the military hospital in the capital and asked for another HIV test. He admitted with a grin that he was sure the results would be negative again—"if I'd really thought it might come back positive, I probably wouldn't have gone. That's human nature, isn't it?" While he wanted to know what was wrong, he was also thinking he needed a route out of the gruelling demands of the commando unit for a while, until he built his strength back up. He was planning to apply for training abroad; China, for example, took Ethiopian

ANDUALEM AYALEW

# might come back positive, wouldn't have gone. isn't it?"

soldiers for advanced courses, and so did Israel. But any soldier sent on such a trip had to test HIV-negative first.

He waited in line to leave a vial of blood, and went back a few days later for his results, already imagining what it would be like to travel outside of Ethiopia. A sombre counsellor told him the test was positive. He suggested Andualem give up alcohol and try to eat well.

The lieutenant's knowledge of the disease had not progressed much. Most soldiers knew just one thing about HIV, he said: "The disease will reduce you to bones with no flesh—and you'll die." As he stepped into the teeming streets outside the hospital, he could see only one option. "I wanted to commit suicide." He'd be dead soon, anyway; there was no reason to prolong the suffering.

But he quelled the thoughts of suicide and instead went looking for an old friend, Birhanu Mengiste, an educated man who Andualem thought might know more about HIV. And indeed Birhanu calmed him, telling Andualem that people did not have to be afraid to come near him, and that he might not die right away. He returned to the barracks, and over the next few weeks he told his dreadful news to a couple of friends. They were shocked: he was six-foot-six and still brawny. It seemed so unlikely. All the same, they pledged their full support.

Andualem's HIV test results were confidential—the military medical service would not alert his unit. But he was worried about his physical capacity and decided to confide in his commanding officer. "I was suicidal, I had to tell him. I was crying, I felt so awful. I needed some assistance, and I told him—so I could be given lighter duties and a better diet." The two had a good relationship, and so he felt safe asking for support. Yet instead of the assistance and encouragement he had anticipated, the officer recoiled in horror. "He said, 'We should arrest you. Or detain you.'" And he didn't keep the secret, quickly sending the news up the chain of command.

There was no immediate impact but relations with his commander went from bad to worse. "He was *not* supportive," Andualem said. "He told higher officials I'm not working properly. He was determined to fire me." In September 2001, he found himself dismissed—although not through the usual formal military procedure where a delinquent soldier is called to account before a board of investigation. His commanding officer simply walked up one day and ordered him to remove his uniform, to unlace his boots. "Gather your things and go," the officer said, pointing toward the gate, then turned and strode away. Andualem, the consummate soldier, followed orders: he left his uniform folded on a bench, red beret on top, shiny black boots side by side below. Men in his unit hastily took up a collection and stuffed a few hundred birr in his pocket; a couple of them walked him to the gate. Then Andualem found himself standing alone and barefoot on the other side of the barbed-wire fence, outside the structure of the military for the first time in his adult life.

Over the next few days he made his way south to the city of Awasa, where Ethiopia's senior generals were meeting, hoping to appeal his dismissal to them in person. But his health crashed under the stress. He wandered the streets feverish and half-crazed. He couldn't bear to go far from the military base; he crept up each night to sleep on the veranda of the building where the senior officers worked. When morning came he would try repeatedly to get their attention. They stepped with distaste around the indigent man claiming ill treatment, writing him off as a madman. He could not think where else to go: he had no money, and he couldn't go back to his family in Gachit. "How could I return to my mother and father in this situation? I had been helping them financially, and how could I face them like this?" He certainly couldn't tell them he had HIV. "In that rural area, they don't know anything about HIV/AIDS. They throw stones at people who are suspected of being infected. They think HIV can be transmitted just by looking at a person. Dying of AIDS is a curse."

Finally he heard about a local AIDS organization in Awasa and made his way there. The staff took him to a shelter, where he was fed and nursed back to physical health. He learned that people with HIV don't necessarily look sick—that, in fact, the plump prostitute could well have been infected—and that having an untreated sexually transmitted infection such as gonorrhea increases, tenfold, the likelihood of contracting HIV. He learned that if he had used condoms in the brothels near the front he would likely never have contracted the virus (although no one raised the possibility that he might have been infected by blood or needles after he was wounded.) He learned that he might live, not just for months, but for years yet.

As he began to feel better, Andualem thought often of the friends he had left behind in his barracks. They didn't know any of this: they didn't carry condoms, they contracted sexually transmitted infections all the time and they sought out the fleshy prostitutes, believing they were safe. He began to feel an urgent need to share what he had learned. He made his way back to Addis Ababa and called a couple of men from his old squad. They brought him bits and pieces of the commando uniform, until he was fully kitted up. And then Andualem presented himself at the offices of a division—not his own—and said he had something to say about AIDS. He asked the officers to assemble their troops. "I said, 'They will listen to me when they won't listen to other people, because I am one of them.'" His logic was not lost on the officers, and within days, Andualem found himself holding a microphone and standing in front of several hundred soldiers in fatigues, sitting in rows on a parade ground in the sun. He told them a simple story.

"I knew I was HIV negative, and because I was ignorant, I slept with a girl—a beautiful girl, a fat one, so I thought she didn't have AIDS. And I was exposed. Physically, I'm okay now. But you have to use condoms properly." Condoms are crucial, he said, and he demonstrated how to use them on a wooden model penis.

It was the beginning of his new career. He was invited to bring his wooden penis to one detachment and then the next. "You know ABC?"

Andualem asked me, referring to the "Abstinence/Be faithful to one partner/use a Condom" principle that was pioneered in Uganda in the 1980s. "ABC" has been championed by PEPFAR, the major funder of HIV/AIDS initiatives in Africa, and today it is the bedrock of most HIV-prevention campaigns across the continent. But Andualem found the emphasis on abstinence unrealistic. "In the military, A and B are not used so much," he said with a frank grin. "So I talk about C. I just try to tell the men to use condoms, that if they don't they will be infected with HIV. I try to tell them to use condoms when they drink, because that's when they will be exposed. In a fair way I try to express that they will be just like me unless they are very careful. I tell them to take a voluntary test. I remind them they've seen people return from hospital who were once very fat and grown very thin—at the present time most of the beds in all the military hospitals are occupied by HIV-positive patients. I tell them these facts."

And, he said, the soldiers listen. "They believe me because I was one of them. I talk like they do. When other educators come, they don't believe them. With me, they say, 'This guy is one of us.'" He told me this with enormous pride, adding that he feels his new role is just as important for Ethiopia's security as the one he played as a commando. "Saving another life is heroic. It is courageous."

Over the next four years, Andualem gave more than five hundred of these talks. He was paid 30 or 40 birr (about $4) each time, barely enough to survive. And he wasn't always well received: in February 2004, when he arrived at a base, he was detained by the military police. They refused to believe his letter of invitation from the commanding officer, which said he had HIV and requested that he come to do AIDS education. "They said nobody who looked like me could be infected." They concluded he was a spy, beat him and interrogated him, and held him in an underground trench for nine days until the officers who had invited him discovered where he was and convinced the police that he really was an AIDS educator.

Nevertheless, Andualem put aside all thought of finding other work, driven with a messianic fervour to bring his message to the country's military camps. "I think of myself as a candle," he said. "I am giving light to others, but we know it will burn out."

Andualem's experience is in many ways a reflection of the larger journey that Africa's armed forces have made with HIV: the initial response was fear and rejection, but out of sheer necessity, militaries have had to take bold steps on AIDS, with the result that in many countries, including Ethiopia, they have emerged as leaders in the response to the disease.

The problem for Africa's defence forces began much like Andualem's did. For a whole host of reasons, soldiers are among those at highest risk of infection with HIV—as Brig.-Gen. Pieter Oelofse, the director of medicine in the South African National Defence Force, explained to me in Pretoria a few months before I met Andualem. "They deploy at age nineteen or twenty, they are young, healthy people with all the normal levels of hormones a person should have, and the effect of those hormones is not shied away from, if I can put it like that. They think 'it's not going to happen to me'—whether it's getting shot or snake bite or HIV/AIDS." They are often far away from their families or regular sexual partners and "those desires don't suddenly go away because you're not at home. You put all these things in a pot—young, healthy, invulnerable, trained to kill the enemy—and the longer you're away from home the more difficult it is to stay in your room," he said. "What comes out of that pot is high-risk behaviour. Add a few drops of alcohol to high risk and it doubles." In fact, studies by the Institute for Security Studies, in Pretoria, have found that military infection rates in Africa are up to twice those in the wider population.

Africa's militaries are deployed for border conflicts, insurgencies at home and peacekeeping missions across the continent and outside it, and those movements, combined with high-risk sexual behaviour, make soldiers a key vector for HIV. And because they are often—as Andualem and his commando unit were—among the few people with steady wages, soldiers' camps draw large groups of commercial sex workers as well as poor women seeking, if not to enter the profession full time, at least a short-term liaison with a man who will provide regular meals. In addition, military forces have repeatedly been implicated in rape, either attacking civilian women or demanding sex in exchange for protection or safe passage. Soldiers are exposed to HIV in all these ways, and when they go on leave they carry the virus back to their wives and villages.

Even as HIV preys on military behaviour, it undermines military strength. In 2005, Uganda acknowledged that despite the fact that its military was fighting a protracted civil war with rebels in the north, it was losing far more soldiers to AIDS than it was to conflict. In South Africa, seven out of every ten deaths in the armed forces are AIDS related, and by 2006, with a quarter of uniformed soldiers infected, the disease had undermined the country's ability to play its continental peacekeeping role. "We've come to a point in our combat readiness where if we have to get involved in many more new missions, we will have trouble to fill the gaps," Brigadier-General Oelofse said bluntly. He and generals from other countries began to meet to discuss the ramifications for state sovereignty.

The threat to military readiness also has grave implications beyond the borders of individual states. In 2000, the UN Security Council recognized HIV as a threat to global stability, the first time the council had ever deliberated on a health issue. Former U.S. secretary of state Colin Powell, shortly before he left the post, called AIDS one of the chief threats to global security. A 2005 study by the U.S. Council on Foreign Relations called the pandemic a greater threat than terrorism, citing its effect of weakening economies, government structures, military and police forces, and social cohesion. And 2006 research by American academics looking at 112 countries concluded that those with the highest HIV prevalence rates are also those with the greatest incidence of conflict and human-rights abuses, because the weakest states respond poorly to the health crisis and because HIV erodes economic, social and political stability.

"Militaries were forced to confront this directly, and they are well ahead of many sectors in their own societies—often they had a greater response than national governments," Martin Rupiya, an expert on African armed forces at the Institute for Security Studies, told me. "Military readiness is key to national security, so they made AIDS a priority. And then, because of how militaries are organized and resourced, they were better able to take charge—of prevention, care, treatment, even research." Indeed, I had seen this first-hand across Africa. Sierra Leone's military, for example, developed the first workplace HIV policy in the country; Eritrea made a condom pouch part of the standard uniform. As Rupiya pointed out, that classic military ethos of discipline and following commands is an excellent way to fight AIDS: it ensures blanket distribution of condoms, regular AIDS testing and that HIV-positive soldiers take their medication consistently.

For Ethiopia, the first hint of a problem came at the start of the war with Eritrea, when all soldiers being deployed to the front were screened, as Andualem was, for HIV. The Ethiopian government won't release the prevalence rates found by those tests, but a retired general told me it was much higher than the overall population's, and, even more shocking to the leadership, infection was not confined to rank-and-file soldiers: some of the most senior officers tested positive, too.

It took several years for this information to produce a response— the years in which Andualem was battling to raise awareness. But slowly the Ethiopian military began prevention education targeted at soldiers through comic strips and radio dramas, sent mobile test centres around camps and bases, and gave condoms to all soldiers going on leave.

Today, militaries will not accept new recruits who are HIV-positive— but what to do about personnel already infected? As the number of people living with HIV climbs, armed forces have realized they cannot simply dismiss any soldier who tests positive—Andualem told me that no Ethiopian soldier has had an experience like his in recent years. Instead, many militaries have moved quickly on treatment and care. Long before Ethiopia began any ARV treatment in its public system, the military was paying to put sick soldiers on the drugs; the retired general frankly called it "cost-effective." And research from South Africa has found that soldiers can thrive on ARVs even when deployed in conflict settings. Now the country wants to challenge a UN regulation that bars soldiers with HIV from serving as peacekeepers: there is no reason not to deploy those who are healthy on treatment, provided they have a good supply of drugs with them, Brigadier-General Oelofse said.

# Two large framed pictures
# Andualem in uniform on the
# the military, and another
# wedding day, he in a
# she in a cream dress,

In 2003, Andualem went to Gondor, in Amhara province in the north, to give one of his talks to a large collection of troops. He stayed with his old friend Birhanu Mengiste, to whom he had first turned after learning he had HIV. While the two men sat chatting one evening, Birhanu's nineteen-year-old daughter listened with awe from the doorway. Tigist (her name, common in Ethiopia, means "patience") had never heard someone speak as frankly about AIDS as the soldier did. After he left for Addis Ababa, she asked her father to accompany her to a clinic for an HIV test. It was positive. So was a second test a few weeks later. Tigist said the results were a shock, even though she had been troubled by persistent minor infections during the past year. Her father, too, was stunned, although he had been hearing about more and more young people with the virus in their city. But, much as he had comforted Andualem two years earlier, he now reassured Tigist that she was not about to die. And indeed, in the years since he first spoke of AIDS with the lieutenant, the government had begun its first steps in its national AIDS treatment program, offering ARVs through public clinics.

Through the next few months, Tigist kept thinking about Andualem, how comfortable he seemed in his own skin and with this disease that she had hesitated to tell anyone she had. Her father soon had matchmaking on his mind: he could imagine no better husband for his infected daughter than the one man he knew who was courageous enough to live openly with HIV, and he asked Andualem to come back to Gondor to talk to Tigist. "After I heard the news, I was soothing her, telling her she can live a very long life," the soldier said. Andualem himself had been thinking it might be time to marry, and not only was Tigist pretty and charming—he, too, saw the advantage in their shared HIV status: so much less explaining and fear to cope with. They were married that year, and she moved with him to Addis Ababa.

He could not offer the sort of life she would have had as the wife of a commando earning 850 birr ($95) a month, as he had been before he was discharged from the army—instead he knew he was lucky if he brought home 250 birr. They rented a one-room house in an industrial neighbourhood outside the capital—big enough for a single bed with a magenta sateen cover, four wood chairs, and a mat on the floor with a few green cushions where they entertain guests. A bare electric light bulb dangled from the ceiling, which was covered in burlap sacking. There was a pit toilet out back, and Tigist cooked on coals in the courtyard. Two large framed pictures decorated their walls: Andualem in uniform on the day of his induction into the military, and another of the couple on their wedding day, he in a dove-grey suit, she in a cream dress, both of them beaming.

When I met Tigist, she was twenty-three and still visibly awed by her husband, who is twice her size; she was also able to giggle at his more self-important moments. He was in the habit of bringing people back to the house—soldiers newly diagnosed with HIV, community leaders who wanted to hear his story—and she sat quietly at the side of the room, roasting green coffee beans in the traditional ritual. They had recently had a visit from Andualem's family. Initially horrified when they heard of his

HIV infection in a media report, they had learned more about AIDS from the government's public-education campaign, and were delighted, he said, to come to Addis and see him healthy and married.

Tigist had not been so well. In early 2006, she suffered a tenacious attack of herpes zoster, lesions and swelling. Her CD4 count began a free fall—and doctors at the military hospital, where she and Andualem still qualify for treatment despite his nebulous discharge status, told her she must start antiretrovirals quickly. The drugs are free, but taxis into the clinic cost them 20 birr ($2.50) each visit, money they cannot afford. "We're relying on donations from friends," Andualem said, frustrated and embarrassed that he cannot provide better for his young wife. "If I end up in bed she won't have anything." By mid-2006, Andualem's CD4 count was holding steady at 500. He figured his need for ARVs was still a long way off, and the couple was talking about perhaps having children, once the ARV treatment had suppressed Tigist's viral load to undetectable levels, eliminating most of the risk to a baby.

In December 2005 Andualem was summoned to parliament, where the prime minister gave him a medal of national recognition for his efforts against AIDS. But the armed forces have not taken him back. He believes he has grounds to sue for unfair dismissal, or at least to regain the pension he would be receiving if he had been discharged through the normal route, but he does not have the money to hire a lawyer.

Despite the dismissal, which rankles constantly, Andualem still wears his uniform every day—he said it only makes sense. "Back then I was defending the sovereignty of the country, now I am still defending my nation." He sees no irony in the fact that he now puts all his energy and time into providing a service—largely a free service—to an institution that has treated him badly, his years of gruelling service notwithstanding. "If you pay back something or someone who has done wrong to you with something done well—if you pay back a bad with a good—that is a good thing, that is praised by God," he said, then added, with the wisdom of a veteran soldier, "In your lifetime if you spend all your time fighting, you will not survive."

His new career as an educator is nothing like the life of adventure he imagined when he walked into the military recruiting centre in 1992. He knows that if he had kept quiet about his HIV infection, he might have kept his job, and its salary. Yet Andualem said he rarely regrets his decision. "I feel good when I think that I have saved so many lives, and when I take my friends to get tested. I leave the regret behind and focus on that. After all the difficult things I have lived through, saving lives is now the most important thing."

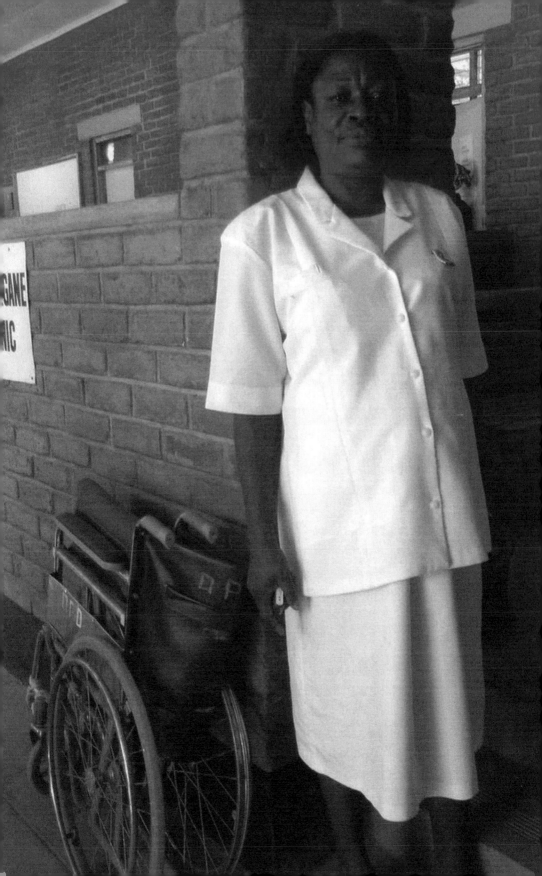

# THIRTEEN

# AliceKadzanja

t began a couple of years after she graduated from nursing school in 1980. A rumour went round the clinic where she worked that a fellow nursing sister had been diagnosed with AIDS. "People were running away from her," Alice Kadzanja recalled, "saying, 'She's HIV! She's HIV!'" Then another nurse fell ill, not long after, and then so many more. The grim running tally she keeps in her head has reached about two thousand. Two thousand nurses that she worked with or studied with or knew of—all of them killed by AIDS.

"Through the 1990s nurses were disappearing," Alice said, gazing down a crowded hospital hallway through small copper-framed spectacles perched on the end of her nose. "And it got worse and worse. It's not just nurses. Even professors. Or you would ask, 'Where is the cleaner?' They all died. And we are still losing nurses—the government is blaming emigration to rich countries. But in fact, they die."

This goes some way toward explaining the state of the clinic where Alice works today. Zomba Central Hospital, in southern Malawi, is one of the main medical centres in the country. Zomba is the poorest district in the fourth-poorest country in the world, and one of the worst hit by AIDS. Nearly twenty per cent of adults have the virus, and three-quarters of admissions to the hospital are HIV related. Zomba Central has three hundred beds, and it runs at 400 per cent occupancy: that means two or three skeletal patients in each old iron bed, and many more on the floor. It means sick babies tucked under

# "It got worse and worse. Even professors. "Where is the cleaner?"

benches and women in labour left alone in a fly-filled ward. Alice remembers all the niceties of bedside nursing she learned in college, fluffing pillows, wiping sweaty foreheads and offering encouraging words—but there's no time for any of that now: she is one of just six registered nurses in the hospital.

Alice herself came perilously close to being one of Malawi's lost nurses, although the sight of her today—towering, imperious, like a rugby player in a crisp white uniform—makes that hard to believe. "I'm strong like anything," she told me not long after we met at Zomba Central in mid-2005. "You'll never see me reporting sick."

But in June 2002, she was thin and weak, plagued with pneumonia and coughing up blood. Malawi's public hospitals had no ARVs then, but one could buy the drugs privately, for a hefty fee. Alice, then forty-four, was a research nurse for an international project, and she earned a good salary, $225 a month. So she juggled the family budget and bought the pills. In a matter of weeks, the lung infections were gone and she was back at work, healthy and strong. But all around her, doctors and nurses and technicians kept dying, and it was no mystery what killed them.

Small and impoverished Malawi left it tragically late, like so many other countries in southern Africa, to organize a concerted response to HIV. There were years of denial and paralysis and fumbling. But finally, by the time Alice fell ill, the country had faced up to the size of the problem and was fully engaged. Stephen Lewis, the UN special envoy on AIDS in Africa, has called Malawi "a nation obsessed," so focused are its government and its citizens on the response to AIDS. Government ministers worked out a detailed, multi-pronged strategy developed in conjunction with Britain and other key donors to tackle prevention of infection, block mother-to-child transmission, care for the sick and orphaned and provide antiretroviral therapy to keep people alive.

ALICE KADZANJA

# It's not just nurses.
# Or you would ask,
# They all died."

They pledged to use the best education strategies, import the cheapest generic drugs and mobilize the widest possible net of community care-givers. They would bring in experts on supply chains of drugs and control of tuberculosis. And they had money to fund it all: aware of the scale of the crisis in Malawi, and impressed with the national plan, the Global Fund promised $36 million, and other donors made similarly generous pledges. Britain chose the country to pilot interventions that might help across the continent, such as a $200-million infusion to boost health-care salaries in an effort to get and keep nurses and other staff in the health service.

And yet despite this obsessive drive, and the steady flow of cash, Malawi has not won the fight. Not even close. By 2005, ten people were dying of AIDS every hour.

I went to Malawi once or twice a year from 2002 onwards, and I saw the Herculean efforts being made, and the rare degree of international assis-tance, and I wanted to know why they were having so little impact on the rate of death. A few days after I met Alice, I went to see Biswick Mwale, a debonair and jovial workaholic doctor who heads Malawi's National AIDS Commission. I put the question to him, and he threw up his hands in frus-tration. "As much as we want to do scale-up, there are no bodies," he said. "People can't translate money into action when there are no people."

The impact of AIDS on Malawi's public system has been crushing. "We have only 10 per cent of the physicians we need," Health Minister Hetherwick Ntaba has said, "and only about a third of the nurses." In 2005, this nation of twelve million people had just two thousand nurses and a hundred doctors working in all its public hospitals. It had a total of eleven obstetrician-gynecologists. The vacancy rate for surgeons was 85 per cent, for pathologists, 100 per cent (that is, the public health service didn't have a single one). The Ministry of Health said that a solid two-thirds of its jobs were unfilled—and that assumes a level of normal staffing so lean as to be unthinkable in a Western hospital.

So next I went to see Anthony Harries, the government's technical advisor in HIV care and support, in his office in the eerily quiet Health Ministry building on the edge of the capital. He told me the health service had a 2 per cent mortality rate. That didn't sound too bad—until he talked me through the math. "With 2 per cent mortality, compound it over ten years and you are losing 25 to 30 per cent of your health-care workers to death. And before they die, they are sick and can't work."

This critical lack of human resources, or "capacity" as it is baldly known in the AIDS world, is not unique to Malawi—it is felt across the continent. When the World Health Organization announced in June 2005 that it would fall badly short of its "3 by 5" target, the primary cause cited was lack of skilled staff. Every single country reported long waiting lists of people desperate to start ARV treatment, but said the health system simply did not have the doctors, nurses, counsellors or pharmacists to treat them.

The cycle is pernicious. Malawi loses 2.5 per cent of its primary-school teachers to AIDS every year. Few are replaced. Children stop going to school when they are folded into a giant class of 150 pupils or simply have no teacher at all. Then fewer children move on to secondary school, fewer graduate, and there are fewer candidates for the medical or nursing schools to become the clinicians who might have put those primary teachers with AIDS on ARVs. "We can't find the students for the medical schools because they're not finishing secondary school," Anthony Harries said. And that cycle is not limited to health-care workers. Teachers, police officers, technocrats and agricultural extension workers are dying as fast as all those nurses Alice knew. Malawi's civil service—one of the few sources of employment in a country this poor—has been decimated. In 2002 AIDS was the leading cause of death, and more than three-quarters of the jobs for secondary-school teachers were vacant; half of the positions in the national police service were empty.

A couple of days after I met Alice at Zomba Central, she and I sat down in a patch of sun in the open-air waiting room, finally quiet at four o'clock, and she told me her story. Her husband, Johnny, is a college administrator. Shortly after they were married, she began to suspect him of "going around." In 1994, when she was still breastfeeding their youngest child, she developed a painful case of shingles. Alice knew that healthy people don't just get shingles, and that it was ubiquitous in people with HIV. She stopped breastfeeding that day and went to a private lab to try to get an HIV test. At the lab, staff told her, "But there's no medicine, why does it matter? If we tell you yes, we'll just make you depressed." They sent her away.

So Alice went home and told Johnny that if they were going to have sex again, they would have to use a condom. He flatly rejected that idea, sneering that he would just go to "bar girls" instead—"Why would I bother with an old cockroach like you?" Alice flinched as she recounted his words. She knew, and she will tell anyone who asks, that he had infected her. "I was a virgin when we married, so he couldn't blame me." Johnny didn't get tested for HIV until 2002, after he had twice had tuberculosis. He started ARVs himself, and "soon he was very strong and very fat," she said. "He thought he was healed, and so he started moving all about again. I said to him, 'You know you're HIV-positive and you're going to spray it.'" But he went right on spending his salary on bar girls. Alice saw it happening all around her: educated people with jobs like hers kept getting sick—her husband's colleagues at the college, the teachers at her children's schools, her co-workers at the hospital. Her own two brothers and her sister, all of them educated, died of AIDS before the end of the 1990s. The people who ought to know better, she told me, take the biggest risks of all.

AIDS in Africa is often understood as a disease of poverty—of hungry young women who sell sex for food, slum dwellers who can't afford condoms, and subsistence farmers who can't pay for medical treatment. And this is accurate. But that picture is not the full one: AIDS is also a disease of wealth, and therein lie some of the roots of Malawi's problem. Population surveys across East Africa have found that the rates of HIV infection are more than three times higher for people living in the best-off households than for those in the poorest. A door-to-door survey in Malawi found women in the wealthiest bracket had nearly double the infection rates of those with the lowest incomes. Why? People who have a bit of disposable cash can afford to pay for the services of commercial sex workers, or maintain a girlfriend in the city as well as a wife back in the village, or have sex with an occasional partner and in return pay her school fees or buy her a cellphone.

Years of research has made clear that Africans do not, in the course of their lives, have a greater number of sexual partners than North Americans or Europeans. But where people in the West follow patterns of serial monogamy, moving from one partner to the next in relationships of varying length with limited overlap, many sub-Saharan Africans have the same number of partners in what are called concurrent sexual networks, where some or all of the partners overlap. Because of the way HIV works, those networks greatly increase the odds of infection. An estimated 40 per cent of HIV transmission occurs when the people transmitting the virus are in the initial six weeks of infection—when their blood teems with the virus, before their bodies muster an immune response and pushes the level of HIV back down for several years. Say the civil servant husband gets HIV from his girlfriend in the city. A few weeks later, as the presence of the virus peaks in his system, he goes home and has sex with his wife. She gets infected. Then when her husband goes back to the city, and while she has the peak level of virus in *her* system, she has sex with her local boyfriend—who is then at much higher risk of infection. And so are the boyfriend's other partners.

In Malawi, like much of the rest of sub-Saharan Africa, the bulk of the population is subsistence farmers, who live in villages in a religious, tight-knit society with more limited opportunities, other than polygamy, for concurrent sexual networks. But the relatively small percentage of people who are educated and living in one of the handful of urban centres have some money, and often that means more partners. So while AIDS has attacked the entire country, its impact was felt first and hardest by educated people— the ones on whom the government had built its response to the disease.

ALICE KADZANJA

Up against all of this, Malawi has done its best. The country is land-locked, dependent on rain-fed agriculture in a region plagued by drought and still recovering from thirty years of quietly repressive dictatorship—but it has nevertheless had some astonishing successes in its response to AIDS. By the end of 2006, some sixty thousand people were on ARVs—up from fewer than a thousand three years earlier. But by that point, a quarter of a million people were so sick that they needed the drugs immediately; eighty-five thousand more people would need them the next year, and every year thereafter. The response to AIDS had to be dramatically scaled up, and that takes people.

The most urgent matter was to get HIV-infected health-care workers to test for HIV and to start those already ill on ARVs so they could return to health and work. And yet, as Alice explained, that is not as easy as it sounds. "The nurses are reluctant to test," she said with a sigh. "Here in Malawi, women of my age who hear they are HIV-positive, they get so depressed." And the shame of the disease is still so great that many continue to deny any possibility that they could be infected, even as they develop signs they recognize, just as Alice did her shingles infection. That stigma frustrates her enormously, and she has made it a personal mission to cajole and bully her colleagues into getting tested.

In November 2004, she went to work for Dignitas International, a Canadian humanitarian organization that was setting up shop at Zomba Central Hospital in an effort to try to shore up the collapsing health system. Alice got the job of nurse in charge of the Tisungane Clinic (the name means "coming together to help one another" in Chichewa), which was focused on getting people on to treatment. After a couple of months in the job, she nervously approached the kind, young Canadian doctor running the project and confided that she herself had HIV. She was dreading a negative reaction, but instead he told her she could be their best advertisement, and she took the role to heart.

One crisp spring morning in 2005, I watched her get out of a shared mini-bus taxi, arriving for work, and lean back through the window, lecturing the driver even as he started to pull away. "There is no reason for you to die, since we've got medicine," she scolded him. "Look at me, I'm also HIV-positive, I'm on ARVs, I'm strong, I can take care of my children!"

Smoothing her white skirt as she stepped into the hospital, she shook her head. "These people, they tell me, 'You don't look like one of them' . . ." Inside the clinic, the low wooden benches were filled with thin, coughing, grim-faced patients. Alice herded one group into a room and, in her deep, gruff voice, began their education. She told them how a person gets HIV: from sex and blood products and mothers passing it to their babies. She told them how the virus works, keeping their body from fighting off the bad germs they catch. And she told them about antiretrovirals: how they must take a pill at six o'clock every morning and six o'clock every evening, every single day, to make them well again. "Why," one young man asked her, "should I take the pill? It won't cure me, will it?" Alice tsked. No, she said, it won't get rid of the virus altogether. "But it snatches the key to your cells out of the virus's hand, so it can't get inside. Your virus stays, but the drugs make it very weak so it can't multiply." Surely you know, she pointed out slyly, what it's like to be too weak to have sex? The group laughed, a little shy. Next she told them that they must use condoms when they had sex, and that prompted a ripple of rebellion from the men, who muttered about "eating a sweet with the wrapper on." Alice snorted in frustration: she'd heard *that* many times before. Once again, she explained about spreading the virus, and the risk of getting cross-infected, with another strain of HIV.

Then she went back to her office and started calling the names—reading the charts, taking the temperatures, counting out the pills. By mid-afternoon, her desk was littered with the foil caps of the big drug bottles she had emptied into patients' pill vials. She scolded, joked, teased, hectored: take the

"eating a sweet with the
Alice snorted in
that many times before.

tablets at six in the morning, six in the evening, don't come back to see me unless you can't move your arms and legs any more. "I enjoy working here because I'm able to advise—I know the drugs and the side effects, especially the first two weeks of prickly pain," she confided over a cup of milky tea when the last of the patients was gone. "I reassure them—one day you will pick up. This first-hand experience makes me a better nurse."

Every day there are more people in the waiting room at Tisungane, as word spreads about the clinic. The effect of the drugs is not lost on other hospital staff. They see people who, a few weeks before, lay in the wards at the edge of death, and now come bicycling into town to pick up pills. Every week or two, another nurse takes Alice aside and asks if she can sign up to get the drugs discreetly. At Tisungane, all health staff are given priority and moved to the top of the waiting list, and that is unofficial policy in most public sector clinics across the country as well.

Getting nurses on to drugs is one key intervention. In addition, Malawi has made its treatment program as simple and standardized as possible. Using the model pioneered by Médecins Sans Frontières, public clinics rely on symptomatic diagnoses, not laboratory tests; even privately funded efforts like Tisungane can rarely get a CD4 count, because they can't find a laboratory technician to do it. Malawi uses only one drug (the Triomune triple-therapy tablet that Alice doles out all day), which may not be the ideal combination for every patient but means that health-care workers can be quickly trained in just one protocol. And patients, once stabilized, are told to come back only every three months for follow-up rather than every two weeks or month as they might in North America or Europe. There is a price to pay for this, the Health Ministry's Anthony Harries acknowledged. "But otherwise how do we cope?"

There is additional help to be had from the British grant, which was used to increase the salaries of most health-care workers by about 50 per cent. A nurse's annual wage rose to $2,850 a year, a doctor's to $3,500. The goal was to try to lure twelve hundred trained nurses who had fled the public system back to work—in 2000, Malawi lost the equivalent of a whole year of graduates from its nursing colleges to the United Kingdom, and many of those who stayed behind deserted the public system. As I looked around the wards at Zomba Central, it wasn't hard to understand why: the massive workload, the appalling conditions (few hospitals can keep latex gloves in stock, for example), the fact that before ARVs there was nothing they could do for most patients—all that for $100 a month?

Alice earns $430 at the Dignitas clinic, a good monthly salary in Malawi, but even so, she said, "I'm failing to manage." She has a daughter and a son in college, whose tuition she covers by raising chickens; a daughter hunting for odd jobs to pay for college and who dreams of studying in England; it costs $650 a year to keep the youngest two in secondary school; plus she is supporting her sister's two orphans. From the day of her diagnosis, her husband, Johnny, had gone on living with her but contributed nothing to family maintenance; nonetheless, Alice felt she could not divorce him, because divorce is a scandalous thing in Malawi. Then in 2006, he threw her and the children out, installing the bar girl-cum-wife in the family home instead. Alice scrambled, with loans from friends, to rent a small room to house the children.

Even the boosted public sector wages leave staff struggling, and the exodus has not slowed. Although Britain adopted a policy forbidding its public National Health Service from recruiting staff in developing countries with personnel shortages, private facilities in the U.K. go right on hiring them. Malawian nurses move to London or Birmingham and work for a few months in nursing homes before making the jump to more regular full-time work in the public health service. They can earn fifteen times the salary they had in Malawi; the money they send back is often the only source of income for a vast network of relatives. And the calm, tidy British hospitals, where Malawians join a shift of fifteen or twenty nurses, are another world after Zomba Central.

Alice understands the temptation. She won't leave Malawi now, because she wants to keep a close eye on her children, but when they are finished school she thinks she might try Britain. While Malawi's government pleads with nurses to stay, Alice thinks that unfair. Her colleagues who leave for England have orphaned nieces and nephews to feed and put through school, she said, and they have no choice.

Higher salaries, and getting nurses and doctors on drugs, help Malawi in the short term, but the longer-term problem is the need to train more people for these jobs. The Global Fund gave the country an additional $27 million in 2004 for "health system strengthening," but it takes four years to train a registered nurse or a pharmacist, and eight to train a doctor. In the meantime, the National AIDS Commission's Biswick Mwale told me, only one thing will get Malawi through this crisis: importing personnel. It makes for a strange twist in thinking about foreign aid. For decades, the mantra has been "teach a man to fish": don't send teachers and nurses, but rather build a teacher's college or design a public health strategy. But what Malawi needs now, Mwale said, is bodies. Worry about teaching us to fish later, he said bluntly.

That's how Alice sees Dignitas, with its two expatriate doctors: a vital boost to get them past the crisis. "Without Dignitas there is no way this clinic would go." The doctors, in turn, told me that they wouldn't have half as many people in the waiting room if Alice didn't drag them in—from the wards and the markets and the taxis, putting herself forward as fearsome proof of what an HIV test and ARVs can do.

The next time I stopped in to eavesdrop on one of Alice's counselling sessions at Tisungane, a school principal, a soldier, a church clerk and two nursing assistants were in the circle. All of them were badly needed at their jobs. Alice picked up their charts, and a large bottle of Triomune, and peered over her glasses to decide who to see first. One by one, she plans to save them all.

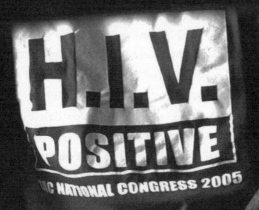

# FOURTEEN

# ZackieAchmat

There was euphoria in the air. In Cape Town back in 1990, Zackie Achmat said, the world looked very good indeed. After decades of bloody struggle, South Africa's last apartheid government was bowing to the inevitable. President P. W. Botha agreed to negotiate a transition to democracy. The legendary African National Congress leader Nelson Mandela walked free after twenty-seven years in prison. The ban on the ANC was lifted, and it began to seem possible that after all those dark years, the party might soon rule the country.

By rights, Zackie should have shared in that jubilation. He had endured jail and beatings as a member of the ANC. He'd fought apartheid for fifteen years, from the time he was a child growing up in a mixed-race Muslim neighbourhood outside Cape Town. His parents were factory workers— not radical, but they had left-wing leanings, and his mother was a shop steward in one of the strongest unions. The Achmats are Cape Malay, a unique ethnicity of people descended from Malaysian slaves imported in the 1600s and 1700s to work the white-owned sugar planta-tions. They were classed as "coloured" under apartheid, and so lived better than the black "natives," but were still denied most of the rights of whites. That precarious in-between position had, as the white government intended, the effect of keeping many coloureds from radical activism.

"The doctor gave me
he recalled.
He retreated into his
rented every movie he had

Zackie was a teenager when the country erupted in the wave of opposition that would eventually bring down white rule, and he was disgusted
by his community's diffidence—coloured children, for example, backed
out of the school boycotts in 1976. So Zackie, at age fourteen, made a bold
entrance into activism: he burned down his school, ensuring no one could
go to class. Nobody was hurt in the fire, but it resulted in the first of his
seven arrests by the apartheid police.

It was also the start of his personal battle. "Things really changed in
1976," he told me, "a combination of sexuality and rebelling against parents
and principles and, for good measure, police. It just became a blur of
rebellion, teenage rebellion, which for me became sustained." He quit school
and left home at sixteen. Things were tense there anyway: his devout
Muslim parents were horrified that their son thought he might be gay.

Zackie spent much of the next ten years underground, organizing
cells of the outlawed ANC and training new members of the resistance.
Sometimes the security services caught him, and he carried his activism
into prison; in 1980, he joined a hunger strike that won key concessions
for political prisoners, including beds and books. Those were exhilarating
years, full of comradeship and vital purpose—but they were also marked by
times of fear and great hardship. Unable to work while he was on the run,
Zackie sometimes sold sex to older men for cash.

But by 1990, it began to look like change was coming. He remembers
it as a time of giddy joy. Then, that February, he had a routine medical

## six months to live," He was twenty-seven. house, drew the curtains, ever wanted to see, and waited to die.

appointment, and asked his doctor to test him for HIV. The virus was still largely unknown in South Africa: the apartheid state had made a concerted effort to cordon the country off as AIDS spread in other African nations, and less than one per cent of the South African population was infected. But Zackie's community of gay men, many of whom travelled frequently to Europe or North America, was beginning to be seriously affected. Several of his friends had died. His test came back positive.

"The doctor gave me six months to live," he recalled. He was twenty-seven. He retreated into his house, drew the curtains, rented every movie he had ever wanted to see, and waited to die.

But at the end of six months, he felt as well as he ever had. Zackie opened the windows, turned off the VCR and decided he might as well go back to activism.

There were a great many things to do in the new South Africa. He founded an organization called the National Coalition for Gay and Lesbian Equality, and fought for formal protection for gay rights in the new constitution. He also joined early efforts by people with HIV—in those days, mostly gay men fighting to end discrimination against those infected—and went to work for a fledgling organization called the AIDS Law Project.

For the next seven years, Zackie stayed well. He was, he would learn, a "slow progressor": HIV reacts differently in everyone that it infects, and in Zackie's body, the virus took a long time to establish enough of a toehold to do much damage. Those were glorious years, as Mandela was sworn in as president and the country adopted a constitution that protected not only gay rights but also the social and economic rights that Zackie championed. Black boys dated white girls (and white boys) and home-grown *kwaito* music rocked at every party. Zackie was now getting paid for his activism, he had a new boyfriend, he bought a lovely house in a once white-only neighbourhood by the sea. He pushed thoughts of HIV to the back of his mind.

Then, in 1998, he started to get sick. He developed systemic candidiasis, the fungal infection better known as thrush. White scum coated his throat and tongue; the pain kept him from swallowing. He could not eat, and he was sure he would die. His doctor told him about the antibiotic fluconazole (marketed by the multinational drug company Pfizer as Diflucan), which easily dispatches most cases of thrush. But it cost $14 for each daily dose, a substantial amount of money in South Africa, where the average monthly income was only $300. Zackie bought what he could, and friends helped him out, too. Within a week or two, he was well.

A short time later, however, his friend Simon Nkoli, a leader in the fight against apartheid who also had HIV, died after contracting thrush. He could not afford Diflucan. Zackie started asking questions—and he learned that a generic version of the drug, made in Thailand or India, cost just 75 cents a day, but was not sold in South Africa because the country's laws protected Pfizer's patent. He was outraged by the rank injustice of it, and at Simon's funeral, Zackie announced that he would start a campaign to make drugs available to poor South Africans.

Even in 1998, when three million people in South Africa were living with HIV/AIDS, fewer than 100 of them were open about being infected. A woman named Gugu Dlamini had recently been beaten to death by a mob of her neighbours near Durban after she revealed on a radio program that she was HIV-positive. Nevertheless, Zackie declared publicly that he had the virus. He and a few activists created a group they called the Treatment Action Campaign, or TAC, to target the large pharmaceutical companies. Soon their ranks began to swell. "We exposed profiteering from medicines in a way that hadn't been done before, at a time when so few people were on the medicines," he recalled. "And we struck such a chord that even whites said, 'Good for you guys.'"

TAC's initial goal was to force the international drug companies to lower the prices of patented medicines to treat opportunistic infections such as thrush and tuberculosis (the leading cause of death for HIV-positive people in Africa). But as TAC members met in Zackie's living room, they decided to add antiretrovirals to their fight. From friends in North America, they knew that the cocktail of drugs was keeping people with AIDS alive and well. But those drugs cost $1,200 a month. The price was too high for the public health system, which was lurching through the monumental task of rebuilding after apartheid. And certainly too high for almost everyone to pay themselves.

Zackie decided to lay his body on the line. "I will not take expensive treatment until all ordinary South Africans can get it on the public health system," he said in front of reporters at a government hearing on health services in December 1999. "That probably means I will die a horrible death, even though medical science has made it unnecessary." He knew the risk inherent in his pledge, but felt he had to take it. "It's wrong to be able to buy life."

He never imagined the reverberations his stand would have. Zackie—a gay, atheist, full-time rabble-rouser and one-time sex worker—was an unlikely public hero. But he caught the imagination of South Africans, especially poor black South Africans who were the vast majority of those infected with HIV/AIDS. They were taken with the drama of his drug strike and his scrappy courage. TAC's membership continued to grow, and more and more people came to rallies wearing the white-and-purple T-shirts emblazoned "HIV POSITIVE" that Zackie had made iconic.

The campaign had early victories. TAC started with babies. What company could withstand charges of profiteering on babies? Forty thousand children were being born infected with HIV in South Africa each year because their mothers could not afford the $50 for a few doses of the antiretroviral AZT, which would lower the risk of transmission by at least half. GlaxoSmithKline said the price it charged for the drug reflected the years of research and development costs that went into making it; TAC said the company was banking a profit far beyond what was reasonable. Zackie led crowds on marches to the company's headquarters, bellowing into the megaphone about corporate greed.

TAC had government support in this campaign. "If you want to fight for affordable treatment," said Nkosazana Dlamini-Zuma, then the health minister, then I will be with you all the way." She signed her name to a TAC-led demand for lower-priced AZT. Then, even more promising, she rewrote the Medicines Act to allow the government to purchase or permit the production of cheaper generic versions of patented essential drugs—to break patents, because of the urgency of the crisis. TAC was jubilant: this would cut drug prices enough to allow for a national treatment program.

But the pharmaceutical industry was determined to stop South Africa—and any other developing country that had similar ambitions— from breaking patents. GlaxoSmithKline, Bristol-Myers Squibb and thirty-eight other big drug companies sued the government, and in the U.S. the industry aggressively lobbied the Clinton administration, which obligingly threatened trade sanctions if South Africa went ahead with changing the law. South Africa's government, desperate to generate economic growth in its efforts to rebuild the country, in turn bowed to U.S. pressure and dropped the new legislation.

Zackie and his colleagues were disgusted. They turned up the heat, with more and more demonstrations. And in the United States they enlisted the help of sympathetic activists, veterans of organizations such as the legendary ACT UP (the AIDS Coalition To Unleash Power, which pioneered the "die-in" in the 1980s), to follow presidential candidate Al Gore on the campaign trail and wave banners that accused the government and American greed of killing South Africans. It made for embarrassing headlines; the United States withdrew the threat of sanctions. Pharmaceutical companies, sensing a public-relations disaster in what the media presented as a lawsuit against Nelson Mandela and dying babies, expressed a willingness to negotiate on providing lower-cost medicines. TAC anticipated victory on all fronts.

And then it all went hideously wrong. Telling me this tale four years later, Zackie grimaced with pain at the memory. "Then the government went mad."

On October 20, 1999, South Africa's newly sworn-in president, Thabo Mbeki, gave a speech in which he said that AZT was toxic. Now that, to an extent, is true: AZT is a powerful drug, hard on the liver, and it often causes unpleasant side effects. But since the alternative is dying, those are risks most people with HIV are willing to take. Mbeki, however, seemed to be suggesting that the drug was poison and people shouldn't take it.

And that was just the beginning.

Mbeki was then widely regarded as Africa's greatest statesman. The son of a prominent African National Congress leader, he grew up in exile, studied in Britain and did military training in the U.S.S.R. Aloof and icily intelligent, he is a cut-throat politician, and at the end of Mandela's five-year term as president, he emerged as the anointed successor. He took office in 1999 and spoke with great passion about the need for an "African Renaissance," for Africans to solve African problems. He decried the poor governance on the continent, corruption and the misuse of aid, and he led his fellow African leaders in creating a new framework for development assistance, emphasizing good government, trade and investment. He was soon the darling of the G8 leaders. He continued Mandela's use of South Africa's revitalized military as continental peacekeepers, intervening everywhere from Burundi to Côte d'Ivoire. He pushed the domestic agenda of extending water, electricity, houses and schools into once-isolated black South Africa, while wooing foreign business interests and pitching the country as an ideal climate for investment. He did not have Mandela's mass appeal, but he was a popular president.

Under Mandela, the ANC had done little on AIDS; in its first years in power, the epidemic was just one more problem the party inherited after apartheid. But Mbeki, as Mandela's deputy, had shown an intense interest in the disease. In 1997, he championed a product called Virodene, made by a South African firm that claimed it could kill

HIV—and at just $6 a month, it was vastly cheaper than the $1,200 monthly cost of ARVs. Virodene's makers said that South Africa's Medicines Control Council wouldn't license it because the council was discouraged by Western pharmaceutical companies from considering a local alternative. Mbeki, sympathetic to their argument, pushed the council to approve human trials. It quickly emerged that Virodene not only couldn't kill HIV, it contained a highly toxic industrial solvent, dimethyl-formamide, which can cause fatal liver damage. Production was quickly cancelled, and Mbeki was slammed in the press, accused of being obsessed with "African solutions" at the expense of common sense.

The Virodene incident may have contributed to his wariness of drug-based responses to AIDS, but it did nothing to diminish his interest in anti-establishment scientific views. A colleague gave him a copy of an unpublished manuscript called "Debating AZT," by a South African lawyer named Anthony Brink, who said AZT, not AIDS, was causing people to "waste away." Mbeki was intrigued, and contacted a murky group of scientists in California who had been insisting since the early 1980s that AIDS was not caused by a virus, and not transmitted by sex, but was rather the result of other factors, including malnutrition and recreational drugs used by gay men. They alleged there was an AIDS "industry"—a scheme hatched by the pharmaceutical industry to create a billion-dollar market for drugs to treat a harmless virus. The Internet, of which Mbeki was an early proponent, is tailor-made for such conspiracy-spinning, and the denialists set up websites to spread their views that antiretrovirals are "poison" and kill the people who take them.

Soon the president was inviting scientists whose views were widely and fiercely disputed in the West to sit on his advisory panel on AIDS alongside mainstream researchers. Experts working at the forefront of virology found that they were expected to debate the existence of HIV with researchers who held outlandish views on the subject. There was more public criticism, and in April 2000 Mbeki penned an impassioned letter to President Bill Clinton and United Nations Secretary-General Kofi Annan saying there was an "orchestrated campaign of condemnation" of his association with the dissidents, whom he compared to once-persecuted anti-apartheid activists or medieval "heretics" burned at the stake. But, he said, "a simple superimposition of Western experience on African reality would be absurd and illogical."

In July, the International AIDS Conference came to South Africa. Mbeki was to deliver the keynote address—the first time an African leader would speak about the pandemic in such a forum. Some participants ostentatiously walked out before he took the stage, in protest at his inclusion of denialists on his advisory panel. Many of those who stayed were dismayed by what he had to say: he acknowledged that AIDS was spreading on the continent, but he also questioned the accuracy of HIV tests, and mentioned ARVs only to say that they required further research. He said poverty, not AIDS, was the great killer, and suggested that the furor around AIDS was a means of drawing attention away from more difficult questions of inequity. His tone left much of his audience uneasy. Then, in September, Mbeki told *Time* magazine that "a whole variety of things can cause the immune system to collapse." He said ARVs could "poison" people who took them. His statements contradicted the positions of everyone from the World Health Organization to South Africa's own Medicines Control Council. At home and abroad, the response was bewilderment: What could Africa's most reputable leader possibly be thinking?

It was a mystery then, and it remains one today. Mbeki refuses to do media interviews on this subject. As the years have passed, he has largely refused to address the issue at all. That leaves Zackie—and indeed South Africa and the rest of the world—to speculate. Part of Mbeki's suspicion may lie in his experience of the fight against apartheid, when the white government sponsored medical research into biological weapons that would target the black population. From that perspective—when science fiction was real life—it isn't too much of a stretch to think that drug companies would deliberately misrepresent AIDS.

Mbeki has also been intensely critical of Western characterizations of blackness and black sexuality. In a lecture he gave at the University of Fort Hare in 2001, he said that those who hyped AIDS in Africa were "convinced that we are but natural-born, promiscuous carriers of germs, unique in the world [and] they proclaim that our continent is doomed to an inevitable mortal end because of our unconquerable devotion to the sin of lust." Zackie said he understands Mbeki's rage, but not where it has led him. "That Western picture of Africa is wrong, of course," he said. "But you cannot let other people's perceptions and prejudices draw your policy."

There is a certain sympathy for Mbeki's position among South Africa's new black elite, also veterans of the fight against apartheid. Mbeki has a key ally in Manto Tshabalala-Msimang, who was once the chief of health services for the ANC exile operation in Tanzania. Mbeki made her his health minister, and she was soon stridently arguing his line on AIDS. When TAC was lobbying for public access to AZT so HIV-positive women did not infect their babies, she said she could not in good conscience "poison" a pregnant woman with the drug. Instead of antiretrovirals, she said, people with HIV should look to traditional African wisdom and preserve their health with a diet of garlic, lemon, olive oil, beet root and African potatoes.

Now TAC was fighting on two fronts: against the big pharmaceutical companies, the enemy they expected, and another they had never imagined. "It's like your parents withholding medicine from you when you're a kid," Zackie said. "We never expected to fight the government. I mean, the love we had for them . . ."

TAC put that love aside and stepped up its campaign. In late 2000, Zackie and a friend flew to Thailand, bought five thousand generic fluconazole pills for 28 cents each and publicly carried them into South Africa. The government detained them on smuggling charges. Drug companies were caving in to the TAC pressure—Pfizer said it would provide Diflucan free in government clinics, and other companies began to take similar steps, offering discounts of up to 90 per cent off their initial prices. By the summer of 2001, Boehringer Ingelheim was offering pregnant women free nevirapine, a drug that proved even more successful than AZT in blocking transmission of HIV to babies. But the government was proving a harder target. It refused, for example, to accept the nevirapine—making the reasonable argument that it couldn't plan a public health program based on the charity of a drug company. But it made no counter offer, and TAC leaders sensed stubbornness at the root of the decision.

They considered their options and decided it was time to try South Africa's new court system. Gathering a coalition of community groups, they petitioned the constitutional court, alleging that to deprive pregnant women of a medication that would save their children's lives was unconstitutional. South Africa's highest legal body stunned the Mbeki administration by agreeing, ruling that the government had to provide the drug to pregnant women.

Still, Mbeki's team stalled. Now they said that most of the country's hospitals lacked the infrastructure to deliver nevirapine. It was certainly true that the apartheid rulers had neglected health centres in all but the major cities. However, providing nevirapine for pregnant women is not a complex medical procedure. A woman needs to take one pill when she goes into labour, and the baby is given the drug in syrup form shortly after birth. Nevertheless, the government said it wasn't possible. Mbeki's ministers argued that the courts should not be writing health policy—but at the same time, they gave signs that anger at the upstart TAC activists, one of the few voices critical of the widely admired ANC government, lay behind their intransigence. In early 2002, for example, the provincial health authority in KwaZulu-Natal was awarded $72 million by the Global Fund to pay for an ARV treatment program—but the health minister refused to allow the regional government to accept the money.

The fight started to divide ANC supporters, who had been united for so many years in their opposition to apartheid. The unions, a traditional bastion of ANC support, took TAC's side. A handful of high-profile politicians defected too. (In one of the darker ironies of this story, it was an open secret that more than a few HIV-positive members of parliament were on "toxic" ARVs paid for by their government health plans.) Through all this, Zackie's renown grew, and TAC emerged as the strongest social force in post-apartheid South Africa. He stayed on the drug strike; his was a constant voice of articulate criticism at home, while he was recognized abroad both for the courage of his convictions and as a back-handed way of expressing disapproval of the Mbeki government. He was the guest of honour at the Elton John AIDS Foundation annual ball; he was recognized by the Global Health Council in Washington; *Time* Europe selected him its annual "Hero." And, finally, he won the support of the most influential person in South Africa.

In July 2002, Nelson Mandela went to visit Zackie at his home in Cape Town, and they toured the Khayelitsha clinic where Médecins Sans Frontières had four hundred people on ARVs. Mandela had come to a belated realization of the horrific scale of the AIDS crisis in his country, and signalled his distance from his own party by publicly embracing Zackie; in one of the seminal moments in the fight against AIDS in his country, he wore an "HIV POSITIVE" T-shirt in front of the television cameras.

The government was unmoved by Mandela's intercession. So TAC took the gloves off and in March 2003 launched a campaign of civil disobedience, occupying police stations across the country and demanding that Health Minister Tshabalala-Msimang and Trade Minister Alec Erwin be arrested for culpable homicide. Activists put up "Wanted" posters plastered with the ministers' faces. Crowds of six hundred—the number of people then dying of AIDS in South Africa every single day—occupied offices and ministries. They were huge protests, with broad public support. The government was enraged and fought back, claiming that TAC was in the pay of the pharmaceutical companies and trying to infiltrate trade unions—in other words, trying to undermine the party's core support base.

Zackie was leading the demonstrations and every press conference, defiant and loud—but he was profoundly ill. His viral load was critically high, and every week he contracted a new infection—bacterial, fungal, viral. "I can't remember how many times I vomited. Diarrhea was just a natural part of life for me." He had oral thrush, skin thrush, constant respiratory infections that left him gasping. The worst part was that the nausea and dizziness meant he could no longer concentrate well enough to read a single page. All his life his greatest joy had been reading, but now he could no longer get through an email. He conserved his limited shreds of concentration for TAC memos and speeches; the rest of the time he could barely get out of bed.

Yet he gave no hint of this in public. "An activist has to be strong. I couldn't say, 'Sorry I don't want to do this interview now.'" He looks back on film and TV footage from those years with amazement: there he is, mustering his articulate rage for the rallies and the press conferences, and the cheering crowds have no idea that he's been brought to the demonstration straight from bed, his fever blazing.

The health minister mocked him at public meetings with little jabs about his health, and the worst part was that Zackie knew he didn't have to be so sick. Many of his close friends were on ARVs, living healthy lives, and brimming with energy. He could have bought the drugs himself. Friends and family were begging him to drop the drug strike. But until the government agreed to make ARVS available nationally, he would stick to his promise.

I had seen Zackie in action at the protests, and after months of requests finally managed to sit down with him in July of 2003. He was charming and voluble, putting up a good front. Yet he was also clearly very ill, his once-golden skin now grey. "Did I ever think it would be this long?" His expressive face twisted in disbelief. "Never. Never."

All through our lunch in a downtown Johannesburg café, people approached to give him gentle words of encouragement or thanks, and afterwards, I went around the corner to the bustling TAC office to try to get a better sense of this devotion he inspired. There I met Rose Thame, who was fifty-one and had been infected with HIV on one of the three times she was raped near her home in the desperately poor and violent Johannesburg township of Orange Farm. Once sickly and reclusive, she had found new courage from her association with TAC. "Zackie is my role model," she told me. She saw no irony in that description, in the idea that a self-professed "fag activist" might be a role model for a stout grandmother with a pocketbook and a small mohair hat. Rose was terribly worried about him. "He cannot die," she fretted. "If he dies, those who won't release the drugs will be responsible."

Edwin Cameron was also watching with alarm. Cameron is a judge on South Africa's highest court and had been living openly with HIV since 1999. A long-time friend of Zackie's, he disapproved of his strike. "There's no point in his dying," Cameron told me. "His death would serve an instrumental purpose in highlighting the lack of access to drugs—but that would be totally outweighed by the loss of leadership." Even Mandela urged Zackie to end his strike.

There was so much Zackie wanted to be doing: he had enrolled in law school at the University of Cape Town, with the goal of becoming a judge himself—he had a new fascination with the constitution and the courts, thanks to the TAC petitions—but he was too sick to go to class. He wanted to write a novel, but he couldn't focus long enough to read haiku. But how could he back down, when people such as Rose Thame still couldn't get the drugs? "I meet these women who say, 'I hang on because I know you're not taking your medicines,'" he said that day at lunch. "If I decided to take them, I would have to explain myself to those people. Not to the media, or to Thabo Mbeki." He laughed and added, "Though I don't want to kill myself for Thabo Mbeki. I can't think of a dumber thing to do."

A month later, however, he was given an order he could not refuse. TAC held its national congress in Durban in early August 2003. The agenda was heavy with serious matters—the civil disobedience effort, the progress of a national treatment-education campaign. But at the start of the meeting, treasurer Mark Heywood stood up on the dais beside Zackie and the other members of the executive, and made a motion. "TAC is about ensuring people live," he said to a sea of people in "HIV POSITIVE" T-shirts. "Zackie must take his medicines." Speakers rose from the floor to affirm the motion. "You must take the drugs, Zackie, because we need you to be around to fight," one woman said. It went to a vote, and the decision was unanimous: Zackie Achmat's own organization ordered him to end his strike.

A few days later, Zackie marched with thousands of other TAC members to the site of South Africa's first-ever national AIDS conference. Many key members of government were inside. Zackie faced the crowd. "I have decided to take my medicines," he said. The response was a deafening roar. "I am not going to die because they want us to die." The crowd broke into songs and dancing.

It wasn't just that Zackie would live: there was a public benefit in having such a high-profile person take the "poisonous" drugs and get well. "It is high time that South Africans see that these drugs are lifesavers," said Dr. Kgosi Letlape, chair of South Africa's Medical Association. Yet in the media, Zackie's decision to take the pills was characterized as the end of "an unsuccessful effort to force the government to give its people the medicine." That was a bitter spin to have to live with.

But just four days later, South Africa's cabinet, in a stunning reversal, announced that it would begin steps to make ARVs available in public clinics. The cabinet promised an operational plan by the end of September, and, in details that would not have made headlines anywhere but South Africa, it stated the mainstream view that HIV causes AIDS and can be treated with ARVs. Conditions in South Africa had changed dramatically in the five years of Zackie's strike: drugs that cost $1,500 a month were now between $120 and $240, and the government said the new pricing allowed it to make an "enhanced response" to AIDS.

The announcement was hailed at home and abroad. Mandela pronounced himself "overjoyed." Mbeki and his government, of course, made no mention of TAC's role in their decision, and even though TAC members knew more about ARVs and how to help people take them safely than anyone else in the country, the government did not invite the organization to help plan the drug rollout.

At Zackie's house, meanwhile, drama was playing out on a more intimate scale. After a couple of weeks of medical checks—to suppress the opportunistic infections and establish his baseline blood counts—he was ready. One day in early September he held in his palm his first Triomune, the generic combination pill. He felt a cold tickle of trepidation—after all those years of listening to the health minister rant about poison, he had momentary qualms. "I thought, 'What if I turn green or something?'" he later recalled with a laugh. Or what if he was one of that small number of people for whom antiretrovirals simply don't work?

He swallowed. The strike was done. Five days later, he was on his hands and knees scrubbing his kitchen floor. "I hadn't cleaned my own home in four years!" he said, still giddy with the memory. "And more importantly within a week I had read an eight-hundred-page book—a history of the Spanish Civil War. And my energy flow was back. I was capable of holding a thought, speaking, engaging, being nice. And within two weeks I was almost a whole human being."

Within weeks of starting ARVs, Zackie was going flat out. Despite the government cold shoulder, TAC mobilized teams to go into communities across the country—rural villages and crowded city townships—to teach people about the drugs and how they work, how to take them properly and how drug resistance happens. At the same time, the WHO's "3 by 5" effort was now under way and activists the world over wanted the advice of this best-known treatment organization.

Meanwhile, though, the health minister continued to insist on prescribing beet root and lemons as the best treatment, implicitly undermining the drugs. She publicly embraced a coterie of "healers" who claimed to be able to treat AIDS with vitamins, herbs and magnets. Soon TAC was back in court, successfully suing one of the self-professed healers, Mathias Rath, for defamation; Rath, who claimed to be curing people with vitamins, had accused TAC of poisoning people and being a front maintained by pharmaceutical companies.

As the months slipped by it became clear that despite the cabinet-backed plan, the health ministry was not in any rush to get the drugs out. One year along, only eight thousand people were receiving the medication in public facilities. Five months after that, in January 2005, that figure was up to thirty-three thousand—but even so, comparatively wealthy South Africa had no more people on treatment than its much poorer neighbours such as Zambia. The country still suffered from critical staff and laboratory shortages, but the pace was so slow that there was obviously more at issue than just a lack of nurses. "At the very highest levels it seems there is still a suspicion of HIV treatment," Jim Yong Kim, who headed the WHO's AIDS division and designed the "3 by 5" plan, told me then. "To succeed you've got to have political buy-in from the very top—you can't have the president and the health minister ambivalent about scaling-up care. The epidemic is fundamentally dropping the life expectancy of Thabo Mbeki's people. He has to get personally involved and hold people accountable. He has to say, 'Okay, how many did we get this week, why are we going so slowly?' If he did that, South Africa could get to 500,000 in a matter of months—they have so much more capacity than any other country in Africa."

Kim's words were unusually blunt for a diplomat, and when I quoted him in the newspaper the government was furious. But he spoke about South Africa with frustration born of great affection. "This is a government full of warriors for social justice, and I couldn't admire them more in terms of what they've done to push forward social justice for South Africa, especially black South Africans," he said. "That's why I'm stunned that they seemingly do not understand the social justice implications of full access to HIV treatment. What is more basic than the right not to die if there is available treatment?"

TAC's battle culminated in a showdown when the International AIDS Conference was held in Toronto eighteen months later, in August 2006. By then, 180,000 people were on public treatment in South Africa, by far the highest figure in Africa but still less than one in six of the people who needed the drugs, and far fewer than there could have been if the government were pushing the program. In a conference plenary session, with the health minister smirking in the audience, TAC leader Mark Heywood used his address to call for her resignation; silent TAC members took the stage behind him with posters decrying the government's failure to make ARVs more widely available. Closing the conference, Stephen Lewis, the UN special envoy on AIDS in Africa, also broke diplomatic ranks and said the South African government had been "obtuse, dilatory and negligent" in delaying treatment. A few days later, eighty-one prominent international scientists signed a public letter to President Mbeki asking him to fire the minister, saying her "pseudo-scientific views" were an embarrassment to his government. More and more senior ANC figures said publicly that the situation had to change.

And finally it did. In October, when Mbeki was distracted by other crises in his government and the health minister was off sick, the deputy health minister, Nozizwe Madlala-Routledge, stepped to the fore and said the government had "been in denial at the very highest levels" about the success of AIDS programs. In a move that left South Africans agog, she singled out the government's most powerful critic for credit. "We need as a country to thank Zackie Achmat," she said. "He risked his own life so that treatment with antiretrovirals could be made free of charge in our public health facilities."

Zackie and the TAC handled the about-face gracefully, pledging to work with the government on a new plan to accelerate treatment access. Just a week earlier, Zackie and forty TAC colleagues had been arrested demanding that the health minister step down; now, the deputy

# than the right not to die?"

president, Phumzile Mlambo-Ngcuka, went to AIDS activists to pledge that the government would get ARVs to 650,000 people by 2011—and she did it standing arm in arm with Zackie. "I haven't been this optimistic since the early 1990s," he told me a few days later.

None of this, however, changes how many lives had been lost during the long years of the fight, and how many more would be lost before 2011; Zackie trembles with anger when he talks about it. He told me, a few months before the government reversal, that he is sure Mbeki and his inner circle will one day have to answer charges of crimes against humanity for their handling of the issue. He wishes, in fact, that the TAC had fought harder, and earlier, perhaps with civil disobedience that might have resulted in mass jailings. "The tragedy for me is that we put our party loyalty ahead of people's lives."

Today Zackie is a hero not just in South Africa but across the continent, his name invoked a bit breathlessly by people living with HIV in countries where the battle for treatment is still young. He claims the adulation irritates him, but he cannot resist a microphone, or a crowd. He jokes that without AIDS he'd likely have been unemployed, but told me that the fight has brought him—and others—as much as it has cost. "AIDS has in many ways opened my eyes to whole new things. I think it's a unique opportunity to deal with gender relations, openly. It's a unique opportunity to deal with global corporate governance, the role of pharmaceutical companies."

Mostly, though, he wishes he had never had to do any of it. "A million people have died in our country already," he said. "You don't want to be a hero on a base of skulls."

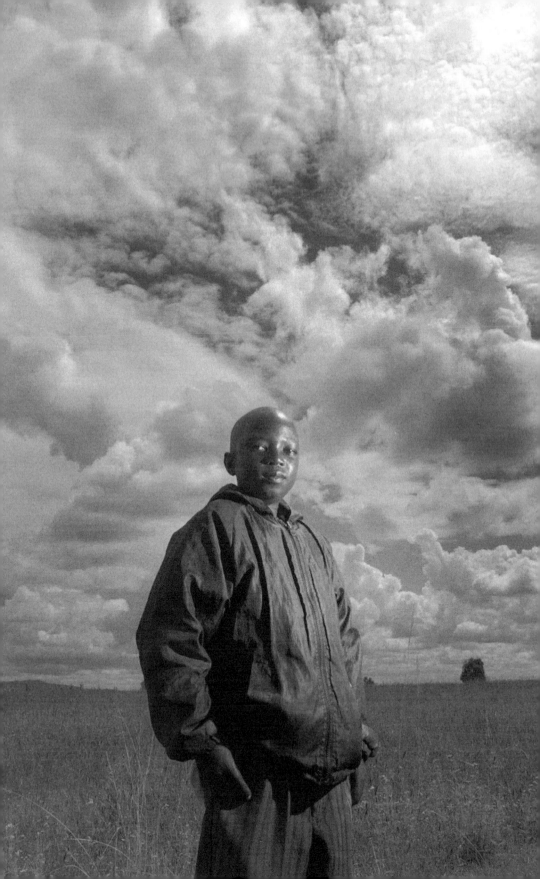

# FIFTEEN

# LefaKhoele

t is, Lefa Khoele said, manifestly unfair: He is much, *much* smarter than the other children. But he doesn't get to study history or geography. "I'm *more* clever than they are, the ones in Grade 7. That's where I should be." Instead he is in Grade 3, where the other pupils are all *babies.*

Each year since he was seven, Lefa has been too sick to write the end-of-year examinations. So he could not be promoted up a grade, and when the new school year started he had to return to Grade 3. There are some good things about Grade 3: in home economics, they learn about gardening, and he has grown some rather splendid pumpkins. But still. Grade 3.

At twelve, Lefa is the same size as the seven-year-olds in his class, so he doesn't look out of place. But when he opens his mouth, he's brash and cocky, and it seems improbable that such a caustic personality could be packed into his small body.

He lives with his grandparents in the village of Khola, in the green lowlands of central Lesotho, a tiny mountain nation that sits surrounded by South Africa on the tip of the continent. On the days when Lefa can catch his breath, he joins the other boys after school to herd the cows past fields of brilliant yellow mustard and maize, through the ravines that stream with runoff from the snow in the mountains.

Lefa's grandparents, Paulus and Julia, have the nicest house in the village—it is made of cement, rather than the usual piecemeal stones, and it has a solid tin roof and five big rooms. It was built with the wages Paulus earned over forty years of digging coal in a South African mine. There is a wire fence outside, to keep the cows out of the vegetable patch, and inside there is a sitting room painted peacock blue, with framed pictures of the Last Supper on the walls and some sturdy wooden chairs. They have a stove, a fridge, a television and a portable stereo: enormous luxury, by the standards of Khola. The village, like most in the country, has no electric service, so the appliances have been adapted to run on gas, but it has been years since the family had the money to buy any. So the fridge is used for storage, and the stereo is coated in dust.

In Lefa's room, beside a bed heaped with traditional woollen blankets, sits a wide, low table, and it is covered in bottles: tablets, syrups, salves, ointments. On the shelf nearby, wrapped in plastic for safekeeping, is the little booklet that holds his medical records. The covers on Lefa's book (three books, really, stapled together) are worn soft and floppy. In the pages, the messy scrawl of a half-dozen doctors tells his story. The record begins in March of 1993 with "Home delivery," and the next few pages hold the ghostly presence of Lefa's mother. Justina Khoele brought her baby down from the hills to a clinic for a first visit when he was three days old. He received a round of immunizations; a nurse weighed him at 3.4 kilograms and noted, "Suckling well." Justina was a young woman trying to do everything right.

The pages fill up fast after that initial entry: Lefa was sick every few months until the age of two. Then there is a gap, and his grandmother recalled that he was mostly fine for the next five years. The pages of the health record get crowded again from 1999: Lefa was repeatedly diagnosed with tuberculosis, diarrhea and skin infections such as ringworm. He began to miss a lot of school.

Around the same time, his father got sick, too. Gerard was a miner like his own father—like a third of the men in Lesotho in the 1990s. He had a few years of education, so he was spared the worst work of digging, and often got to work aboveground as a clerk. But at the age of thirty-nine, he came home unwell, suffering from painful hands and feet, his mother,

Julia, said—what may have been HIV-related nerve damage, although Gerard was never tested. He did get diagnosed with tuberculosis, but the treatment didn't work. He died in 1999.

Lefa doesn't remember much about his father—just that when he came home from the gold mine on visits, he brought clothes and food and, for his son, plastic guns and cars. His mother is a clearer memory. When he was a small boy, he said, she was full of energy, working in the garden, sweeping the polished cement floor, washing their clothes in basins she filled from the village hand pump. And singing as she worked. But not long after Gerard died, Justina got sick too. She had headaches and seizures and what, from Julia's description, sounds like tuberculosis, although she was never treated for it. Soon Julia had to take over the gardening and the cooking she had happily relinquished to her daughter-in-law a decade earlier.

Even when she lay in bed most of the day, Lefa told me, his mother still sang. There was, he said, one hymn she loved the most, and she was teaching it to him: he sang a bit of the melody in Sesotho, his voice high and clear, then he told me the gist of it: "We meet hard things in life and Jesus looks after us." His mother was singing it in bed one day when she began to cry. Alarmed, Lefa summoned his grandfather. His mother smiled at them through her tears, and said to Lefa, "Your grandfather will have to teach you the song." She died that evening, after gently reminding her small son that he must mind his grandparents.

Paulus and Julia now had Lefa and his older brother, Naledi, to take care of, so they took in a lodger, and Paulus invested their savings in a tractor that he could hire out for plowing around Khola. Naledi went off to secondary school and seemed all right.

But Lefa didn't grow, and it was more and more of a struggle for him to herd the cows or help in the yard. He spent weeks in bed. He began to dream about his parents: "In my dreams I see pictures of them. I see them, ask them what they want, and then I wake up." On nights when he was very ill, he would creep into his grandparents' bed and wake Julia up, asking her to sing that hymn. Julia in turn would wake Paulus, and together they would sing to the wheezing boy. When he could manage it, Lefa sang too.

There were a great many deaths in Khola around this time. Not people Paulus's age, in his early seventies, or Julia's, in her mid-sixties, but young people—mothers, and men who came back from the mines. And babies. Lesotho's HIV infection rate hit 28.9 per cent. That meant sick people in every small stone house in Maseru, the one major town, and in the snowy highlands, and in the sloping foothills. But Lesotho is so poor, and so isolated, that the plague devoured the Basotho people almost unremarked by the outside world. Few people within the country spoke about it either. AIDS came cloaked in fear and shame.

It wasn't lost on Julia that Lefa's symptoms, while unusual in a child his age, were not unlike the illness that was taking so many lives. "We only knew about HIV from what people said. It described Lefa." But she didn't take him on the long trek into the city to be tested. If the chatty grandson whom she loved so fiercely did have *that* disease, well, there was nothing anyone could do. And that didn't bear thinking about.

Huge strides have been made in getting adults in Africa on to treatment in recent years, but children—who need different drugs and different tests but who could not educate themselves—were almost entirely overlooked. By 2006, 2.6 million children in the world had HIV/AIDS, and 1,400 of them died each day.

More than 90 per cent of all children with the virus contract it from their mothers at birth. Those infections are easily avoided: used together, a single dose of nevirapine given to the mother in labour and baby at birth, a Caesarean delivery and formula feeding lower the risk of passing the virus to a baby to less than 2 per cent. Because it's so simple, fewer than three hundred children were born with HIV in all rich countries combined in 2005. But less than 10 per cent of African women get those interventions (in fact, most aren't even tested for HIV) and so 700,000 children are born infected in Africa each year.

Of those 2.6 million children worldwide with HIV/AIDS, 90 per cent are Africans. Half die before they are two, and most of the rest before age five. "Children have an immature immunological system, which means HIV hits them harder," Chewe Luo, a Zambian pediatrician who heads the

UNICEF AIDS team, explained to me. Adults may live a long time with the virus, but the disease pattern in children is much more aggressive. However, clinicians can't diagnose AIDS in children based on symptoms, as they do in adults in much of Africa, because children with AIDS turn up in clinics, just as Lefa did, with respiratory infections and diarrhea and rashes— all of which are also common in kids *without* HIV. To control the disease, children have to be tested when they are very young. But while adults and older children can be screened for HIV antibodies using a blood or saliva test that costs less than $2, those tests don't work on children under eighteen months; they may still harbour their mother's antibodies, which means they can test positive without actually being infected. Babies need a test called DNA polymerase chain reaction, which looks for the virus itself. But it requires expertise, sophisticated laboratory equipment and, at $120 per test, big budgets—none of which are available in a country such as Lesotho.

Cheaper interventions are not necessarily accessible either. Giving the antibiotic cotrimoxizole to babies born to HIV-positive women, and to those who are definitely infected, in what's called prophylactic treatment (where the child takes the drug every day to ward off infections) can cut mortality by almost half. The drug costs at most 3 cents a day—but in 2006, less than one per cent of infected children in Africa were getting it, because of a combination of patent restrictions, poor planning and those children's limited access to health care.

Then there are the ARVs. Children need antiretrovirals early, often as infants. But small children can't swallow pills, and few ARVs are made in syrup form. The syrups that do exist are five times more expensive than the tablet equivalent and usually require refrigeration. They have an appalling taste, bitter and metallic, which is a significant problem if one is trying to persuade an eight-month-old to swallow a capful several times every day. There are few dosing guidelines for infants and children so health workers have to chop up pills made for adults. "Breaking adult tablets is looking for trouble," Dr. Luo said. "Drug resistance is an issue: if you under-dose a child you are compromising that child's future." Whereas an adult with HIV can be given a supply of drugs and sent away for months, a child's treatment has to be continually recalculated as he or she grows. Then a tired mom or granny has to keep straight a jumble of broken tablets.

The few existing pediatric AIDS drugs are vastly more expensive than those for adults—the most common combinations cost as much as five times more, and the less common drugs, for children with drug resistance, cost as much as twelve times more than the same treatment for adults. And this isn't going to change: pharmaceutical companies have little incentive to develop or produce the pediatric medications because there are so few HIV-positive children in the developed world, where there is a market of parents or health systems willing to pay high prices for drugs. The first fixed-dose combination of an ARV made specifically for kids didn't come on the market until mid-2006. By that point, just one in twenty children who needed treatment was getting it. And of 8,000 desperately ill kids in Lesotho, just 261 had drugs.

By the time he was eleven, Lefa was a very sick child. Quite often he couldn't hear and couldn't speak. He didn't eat. He was racked with cough; his urine was ochre-coloured. In February 2006 Julia took him, as she had so many times before, to the clinic in Kolo, the nearest to their home (the trip required a two-hour walk and a half-hour by taxi, which cost a precious $4). She was hoping that maybe this time he would be given a different kind of tablet that might make him a bit better. There was no new tablet—but a sharp-eyed nurse named Rosina Phate had an idea. "Bring him back next week," she told Julia. "A new doctor is coming."

Lesotho should have been an easy place, by African standards, to mount an effective response to AIDS. It is tiny; culturally, ethnically and linguistically homogeneous; peaceful and democratic; and it has a government that is passionately committed to fighting this disease. And yet the rollout of both prevention methods and ARV treatment has been achingly slow. The world woke up to the imminent disappearance of Lesotho in 2004, and a great many international actors rushed to set up programs there, offering both technical assistance and a flood of cash, but that could not make up for the lack of nurses, doctors, health educators and pharmacists—or erode the shame and myths that were still keeping people from getting tested or using condoms or seeking treatment. Two years into a national treatment project, in mid-2006, just 5,200 people were on ARVs. There were only forty practising physicians in the entire country, almost all of them expatriates who didn't speak Sesotho.

That caught the attention of Médecins Sans Frontières. By now, the aid agency already had seventy thousand people on AIDS treatment in twenty-nine countries in the developing world, and was hesitant to start any more projects—drugs for life for that many people is a massive commitment, both moral and financial. But Lesotho was crying out for the MSF approach. Despite the crippling lack of health-care staff, treatment was centred in a handful of hospitals and supervised by doctors. So, rather than sending very ill people on a journey to hospital that could take hours—requiring money they simply did not have—MSF started nurse-oriented community-based care in rural areas. The organization imported a pair of doctors and a couple of nurses to travel in teams each day out to fourteen rural clinics to see patients and coach the local nurses on treating AIDS right there.

And so one February day, a South African doctor named Prinitha Pillay arrived at the little stone clinic in Kolo—the new doctor that Lefa and his grandmother had been told to come back and see. Pillay ran her eyes over the crowd of people waiting outside the clinic, huddled in blankets despite the summer heat, and stopped at Lefa. He wore pin-striped trousers like a 1920s gangster, and when she walked over to him he immediately reached up to help himself to her sunglasses.

"Looking at him, I knew he must be HIV-positive, but I couldn't understand how he could even be alive," she told me a few months later. For a child with AIDS to make it to the age of twelve with no access to treatment of any kind is nothing short of astounding. Pillay took blood to measure Lefa's CD4 count and sent it to the hospital in the city. The next week the lab returned the result: an almost unfathomable 2. He had a respiratory infection, a hugely enlarged liver, a massive spleen and, by the sound of it, chronic lung disease. As Pillay talked to his grandmother about his health history, Lefa, already worn out at nine in the morning, fell asleep in his chair.

# "Looking at him, I knew but I understand how

"He was incredibly sick and in stage 4, the final stage of the disease," Pillay recalled when I visited the clinic a few months later. "He was on the downward slide." But he was nonetheless feisty and mischievous and entirely charming.

Although Pillay met Lefa on the first operational day of MSF's Lesotho project, when there were gaping needs everywhere she looked, and although she knows how complicated it is to treat children—and even though he was so sick he had an absurdly low chance of survival—she decided that he would be their first patient. He had made it to twelve, against outrageous odds, and it was high time he got a little help.

Pillay broke the news to Julia that Lefa had AIDS, and the grandmother assumed this meant he would die. But Pillay told her that, just as she had hoped for so long, there *was* a new tablet, and something could be done. Julia had never heard of anyone getting treated for AIDS; when people in Khola got sick, they lay in darkened rooms at home until they died. But this whip-thin, fast-talking doctor was counting tablets into a case for her, telling her which ones Lefa would have to take each morning and which at night.

Yet she sent the boy and his grandmother away, Pillay wondered to herself if even the drugs would do it. She feared his immune system was just too worn out.

A month later, back in Kolo for a clinic day, she looked out the window and saw Lefa charging up the hill. His face was fuller, he stayed awake, he laughed more—the lusty chuckle that is such a surprise coming from his little boy's body. When he stepped on the scale and found he had tipped over the 25-kilogram mark, he ran through the clinic like a prizefighter, pumping his arms in the air and accepting hugs from all the staff. He took

# he must be HIV-positive, couldn't he could even be alive."

over the counting of his pills into the plastic case himself. "Nevirapine" and "efavirenz" were among his first words of English. Julia sat in a corner of the crowded clinic, watching her grandson with pride. "He was not like this before," she told me quietly.

Children with HIV typically experience developmental delays—because they are stuck in bed, like Lefa, when other kids are learning, and because the virus targets the central nervous system, which impairs their growth and acquisition of skills such as speech. Some of this can be remedied: kids who have been on treatment for a year or two may catch up on motor skills and gain considerable weight. Prinitha Pillay told me that Lefa is unlikely to grow a great deal more, because his bones had already fused before he got the drugs, and that his lungs have sustained permanent damage from a series of infections. But she thought he might make rapid leaps in maturity.

Lefa himself had no interest in talking about AIDS. Instead, he was making plans for the future, although the subject presented something of a conundrum. When I asked him what he wanted to do when he finished school, he paused for an uncharacteristic moment of reflection. "I want to work for the police," he began. "I want to catch thieves." He considered this, then added, "Maybe I will be a doctor. And I think another thing I could do is be prime minister. I'd use my salary and give all the people food. I'd help them to plant maize and pumpkin and watermelon and then sell it."

His short-term agenda is much clearer. "I will live and I will go to school."

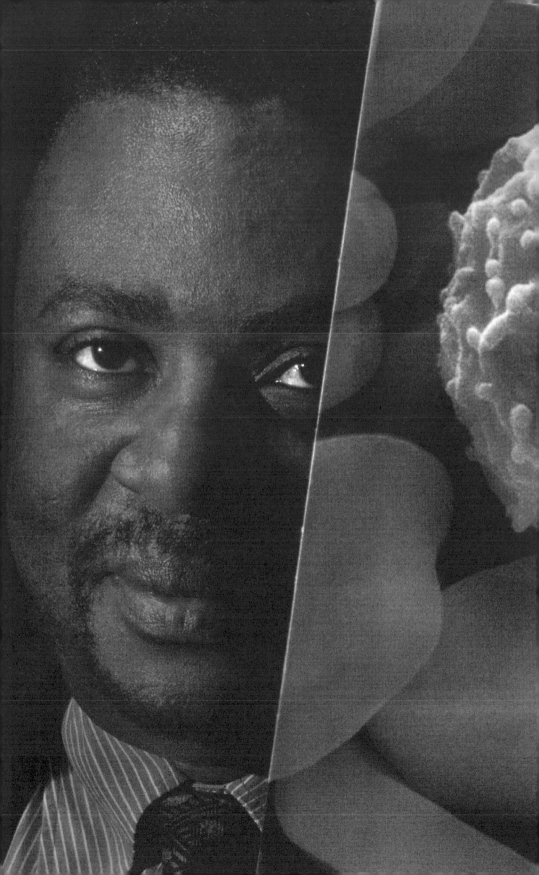

# 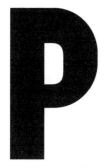PontianoKaleebu

ontiano Kaleebu speaks of HIV with reluctant admiration. He has spent his entire working life with the virus, and yet, he says, he doubts he has the full measure of his foe. It is a long, slow dance in which he and HIV are engaged; on the good days, Pontiano sees the incremental steps forward. On the bad ones, the virus seems always out of reach, with one more manoeuvre in its arsenal, one more way to keep from giving up its secrets. But Pontiano has a vision, of a world without AIDS—some days he thinks he might see it in his lifetime. Certainly, he can imagine it for his children. And most days, that is enough to keep him going.

In medical school at Uganda's Makerere University in the 1980s, where he studied a few years after Lydia Mungherera, Pontiano had plans to be a pediatrician. He had a twinkly sense of humour and a warmth that drew children to him, and he thought he would enjoy clinical medicine. But a year of internship in a Kampala hospital had him rethinking a lifelong plan to be a doctor. "It was monotonous," he confessed. "There were long hours of working, but you could see that the following day you were doing the same thing." After the internship, he found a post as researcher at the Uganda Virus Research Institute and quickly realized that he liked research much better. "Every day that comes there is something new, there is something exciting," he said, enthusiasm undimmed by twenty years in the field. "With every experiment, you are looking forward to something."

The Virus Research Institute was founded in 1936 at Entebbe, on the shores of Lake Victoria forty-five kilometres outside the Ugandan capital. For the first fifty years, its researchers worked on yellow fever and other tropical bugs. But around the time that Pontiano finished his medical studies, something else was brewing on the shores of the lake. For the practical portion of his final exam, he was required to diagnose a wasted patient with a severe respiratory infection and unhealed abscesses on his skin. Pontiano correctly concluded that this was Slim, the new disease spreading among fishermen and traders in villages along the lakeshore. And it wasn't confined to fishermen. First one student in his class died, then another. "By the time I finished my internship, there were many: it went up that fast. Then it started to be my relatives and friends."

At twenty-eight, Pontiano went to work in the institute's collection of low white bungalows and joined a team considering this new germ. He introduced HIV into tissue cultures of healthy cells and watched through a microscope in horrified fascination as, within a day, the virus caused the cells to warp, swell and die. He and his fellow researchers turned to discussing a vaccine—it had been clear since the day HIV was identified that a vaccine was an imperative. Everyone working in AIDS knew that it would be possible to prevent some HIV infections by persuading people to change their behaviour—not to share needles, not to have unprotected sex. But with sex and drugs, just like smoking or seat belts, behaviour never changes completely. People being people, they go on taking risks. And in much of Africa, they can't get access to prevention materials such as condoms or the clean water to formula-feed babies. That leaves vaccination. Through history, it has proved to be the only way to halt most epidemics, and the only way humanity has ever deliberately eradicated a disease—first smallpox and, imminently, polio and perhaps measles.

A vaccine is, in essence, a trick: it is made up of all or part of a microbe, killed or altered so it can't cause infection, and introduced to the body, which thinks it is being attacked and provides an immune response—making proteins called antibodies to wipe out the invader. Then, if the person later runs into the real germ, the antibodies are on standby, primed to recognize and kill the virus. Pontiano and his colleagues were hunting for two types of vaccines against HIV. The first, called a therapeutic vaccine, would be for people already infected—it would stop the progress of the disease. The second, more conventional vaccine would prevent people from becoming infected by triggering their immune system to neutralize the virus when it entered their system. Both would help, and they knew that the latter kind, in particular, would have a massive effect on the spread of AIDS, the kind of impact that nothing in the global health arsenal today can hope to have.

I have followed the hunt for the AIDS vaccine through the years, struggling to unravel the complex science of it. Much of what I know I have learned from Pontiano, whose institute I first went to visit in the early days of African vaccine research and where, over the years, I have returned to hear the latest news. Pontiano is an unassuming and gentle man who delights in a joke and has a palpable interest in people—not what you might expect in a scientist who can get lost in a lab for hours. He has led Africa's efforts in the quest for a vaccine, in both the pure science and the equally complicated moral questions that accompany research in a place this poor and this desperately in need of solutions.

The search for a vaccine kicked off shortly after the discovery of the virus, in an era of supreme faith in technology. Margaret Heckler, the U.S. health and human services secretary under Ronald Reagan, said with great confidence in 1982, "We hope to have a vaccine ready for testing in about two years." She concluded, "Yet another terrible disease is about to yield to patience, persistence and outright genius."

More than two decades later, Pontiano says—and that's on a good day—that an HIV vaccine is still at least another ten years away. Producing a safe and effective vaccine typically takes fifteen years and costs at least $140 million, but even by the standards of vaccine development, HIV is a monstrous challenge. If molecular biologists had set out to design a virus that would stymie a vaccine, they could not have come up with a more pernicious specimen.

This bug thwarts the conventional approaches in vaccinology. A polio vaccine, for example, is made of a fragment of polio DNA, and when the body encounters it, the immune system makes antibodies that destroy it. If in the future the body confronts a real polio virus, the antibodies kill off the virus. But that simply doesn't work with HIV: first of all, the virus destroys the immune system—the very mechanism designed to fight it. Second, HIV can hide for more than a decade snuggled deep into the lymphatic system, attracting no notice at all. Third, it is a retrovirus, a genetic shape-shifter: it doesn't just kill cells, it inserts its own genetic material into the DNA of every cell, so that when they divide, HIV goes too. That means millions of viruses are constantly produced, and they mutate frenetically, so the immune system faces an endless stream of new forms of the virus that it cannot hope to subdue.

When HIV enters the bloodstream, the immune system does produce antibodies, but unlike the case with almost every other germ, those antibodies can't eradicate HIV. The second stage of the body's defence system, the T lymphocytes, better known as killer T cells, break down too—"We don't really know why they don't work," Pontiano said. Part of the problem is that HIV, once in a new host body, stealthily coats itself in sugars, so antibodies don't recognize it. A second factor is that the virus mutates so quickly that the killer T cells don't recognize it either. "But there is more to it, things we still don't know."

Vaccines come in several types. Polio vaccine is made from a live, weakened sample of the virus. Others, such as the flu shot, are made with a dead sample. The third type, including the vaccine for hepatitis, is "recombinant"—made of genetically engineered pieces of viral protein or DNA, delivered on their own or in a vector (a harmless virus or bacteria that carries the viral proteins into the body). Vaccines made with weakened HIV were ruled out after they were tested in monkeys and slowly infected the animals instead of protecting them: the rapidly mutating virus is too hard to control. Similarly, Pontiano explained, killed HIV is no good: if he were to kill it so completely that he was sure it was safe ("you know, by boiling it," he joked), it wouldn't do anything. So scientists focus these days on recombinant technology. Because the bits of artificial virus used in this sort of vaccine are missing key structural genes, the HIV cannot reproduce and there is no danger that it will infect the volunteers who test it.

In his first months at the institute in Entebbe, Pontiano recognized that—grim but true, he said—AIDS made it an exciting time to be a promising young scientist in Uganda: it was clear that HIV vaccine research was not going to be a short-term project. He decided that if he was going to work effectively on this effort he would need more skills. With funding from Britain's Overseas Development Administration and the WHO, he headed for London in 1989 and plunged into a Ph.D. in immunology and virology. His thesis concerned the differences between the various strains of HIV; he studied infected people to see whether they had what are called "broad neutralizing antibodies"—while the antibodies an infected person produces can't eradicate HIV, they can at least recognize it, and he wanted to know whether those antibodies responded to only the strain of the virus with which the person was infected or to all the different strains. (The latter, he proved.) This was just the sort of virological puzzle that fascinated him.

Plenty more were waiting for him when he went home to Uganda five years later. By then, nearly one in five adults had HIV/AIDS. "Many, many people I knew had died while I was away." But the vaccine trials he had been anticipating when he left were not under way. They hadn't even started.

It isn't just the sneaky machinations of the virus that make an HIV vaccine complex. There is also the problem of the variations in the virus itself. There are two different types of HIV, which have only 43 per cent of their genetic material in common—and within those types, there are many different subtypes, or "clades," which also differ in their makeup and cause the disease to progress in different ways. The more virulent HIV-1 has three strains; two are rare, but the third, called Group M, makes up the vast majority of infections globally. And it comes in nine distinct subtypes.

Almost all the HIV infections in North America and Europe, for example, are Group M, subtype B. Africa has every strain, but the great majority of infections in southern Africa are subtype C, while A and D dominate in East Africa.

Scientists don't know whether a vaccine made to target one subtype of the virus will work equally well against all the others. And until very recently, almost all the research—which originated in the universities and health institutes of the developed world—looked at subtype B, even though millions more people in the world have or are at risk of contracting C. Only in the past few years has research investigated whether a vaccine made to target one subtype will work against another—in other words, whether a vaccine made with bits of DNA from subtype C will stop infections in Uganda, where most people have A or D.

With the bulk of the pandemic, and the most urgent need for a vaccine, in Africa, it makes sense for vaccine research to take place there. That research, however, is a big-budget undertaking, requiring not only investment in the labs and equipment to design the products but also millions of dollars to run animal and human trials. No African facility initially had that kind of money, and few had the expertise or the infrastructure to do the sophisticated microbiology that this search requires. The institute in Entebbe was ready by the mid-1990s, Pontiano said, but it was difficult to persuade First World funding agencies of that. But eventually, simple scientific expedience made it necessary for the focus of vaccine research to swing to Africa. "If you want to move fast you have to go where the disease is," he said. Testing a vaccine requires thousands of people in a population with a reasonable chance of infection. Norway or Canada can't provide that.

In 1996, Pontiano was appointed a principal investigator for the first-ever vaccine trial in Africa, of a French-made vaccine candidate that put some of the genes responsible for the production of HIV proteins into a vector, a vehicle to carry it, in this case the canary pox that is also used as a vector in the vaccine for rabies. He was keen to dive into the work, anxious to get initial safety tests out of the way and move on to trials that might show whether the vaccine actually killed the virus.

But few people in Uganda shared his excitement. "AIDS Vaccine Could Start a New Epidemic" screamed the headline of a popular news-magazine. Prominent academics, abysmally ill informed about vaccinology, gave interviews in which they said the vaccine could easily morph into "full-blown AIDS" with no chance to stop it once it was injected; that it could cause physical mutations in the volunteers; that the people who received it could go out and have sex with "countless unsuspecting Ugandans" and spread this new plague. The country's colourful, populist media seized on the story, capitalizing on fears that a trial vaccine might inadvertently infect those who volunteered to test it. There were, Pontiano added, other, legitimate anxieties: What compensation would there be for anyone harmed by possible side efffects? Since the vaccine didn't use their subtype, were his volunteers simply "being exploited as guinea pigs"? Who would own the rights to the vaccine if it worked—that is, would Ugandans have access to it?

The public debate grew so heated that the normal regulatory approval channels, with a scientific and an ethical committee, were deemed insufficient: everyone in Uganda's government wanted the opportunity to scrutinize the research. In the end, no fewer than seven committees were struck, and international agencies were called upon to weigh in as well. Pontiano and his colleagues were summoned before the cabinet, and then various panels of parliamentarians, to explain their intentions—unheard of for a medical trial in Uganda. Pontiano chafed at the delays, but the minister of health counselled patience, telling him and his team that if they managed to get government on board, they would have vital and necessary protection from the public mudslinging. While negotiating with the ever-growing list of parties required to approve the trial, Pontiano attempted to press on with building the trial site and preparing the communities from which volunteers would come. It was, he said, like "building a ship and trying to sail it at the same time."

In the end, the researchers won the government over and got the community on board too, but they had lost precious years. The first of forty Ugandan volunteers was injected with the trial vaccine in 1999. But the vaccine didn't work. While it proved safe, causing no harmful side efffects, it provoked so little immune response in the volunteers in Uganda and in more advanced tests at other sites that it did not move on to a larger trial.

The perfect vaccine would block HIV infection in every single case. But that scenario, Pontiano said, is a fantasy. Because the need is so urgent and new trial vaccines take so long to develop, Pontiano will settle for results of 40 per cent efficacy in a vaccine: it must prompt an immune response in at least 40 per cent of infected people in an initial trial to justify moving forward to a large-scale study.

And what of other outcomes, besides the gold standard of 100 per cent protection? What if the vaccinated people get infected but don't get sick—that is, the virus is present in their systems but in minuscule, "safe" amounts? Or what if they get sick but not until thirty years have passed, instead of the ten that are common now? Or what if they are infected but don't pass the virus on to sexual partners? Did the vaccine "work"?

And this gets to the third complicating factor in HIV vaccine research. When Edward Jenner invented the first vaccine, for smallpox, in 1796, he simply took a healthy young boy, injected his prototype vaccine into his arm, waited a couple of weeks, exposed the child to smallpox and watched to see if he got sick. Happily, the ethics governing vaccine trials have progressed somewhat since then. The trial of a vaccine candidate, like any other drug, works like this: When laboratory trials on animals have shown a product to be safe, and ideally also to trigger some sort of immune response, the vaccine moves to being tested on people. A phase I trial is typically quite small, perhaps a few dozen people, ideally located in different parts of the world to test across ethnicities. This trial looks purely for safety: do volunteers experience any adverse effects? In phase II, which usually takes a couple of years, researchers look not only for safety but also for some sign of immune system reaction in the volunteers. Most trial HIV vaccines die right here: they do not provoke enough of a response in the volunteers' bodies to merit the considerable expense of going on to a larger trial.

Should a vaccine make it to phase III (as four in the world had by late 2006), a researcher wants to prove that, tested against a placebo, it provides protection against contracting the disease. This kind of trial takes years—volunteers must be followed for a long period to see whether the vaccine goes on protecting them, and by how much—and it presents significant ethical challenges as well. Researchers want to see if the vaccinated group has fewer infections than the placebo group after, say, two years. Ideally, to study this, they would send their volunteers out on the town with a budget for cocktails and the instructions to have a good time. But they can't, of course, do that with a fatal and infectious illness. Instead, volunteers—both those getting the vaccine and those receiving the placebo—are given extensive counselling in infection pre-vention, and access to condoms, or clean needles, or whatever protective measures may best safeguard them against the virus. But we know, Pontiano said, that while counselling and condoms bring the incidence rate—new infections—of the participants down below the level of the general population, it doesn't go down to zero: some people will still engage in activity that exposes them to the virus.

All of this makes an HIV vaccine trial an ethical minefield. Take the issue of informed consent. Many of Pontiano's would-be trial volunteers have only limited literacy and education, but he must explain concepts such as genetic engineering so that they understand what they are agreeing to do and why the vaccine cannot infect them with HIV. As well, the idea of "consent" works differently in many African communities than in the West. A community's traditional leader may need to approve trial partici-pation, as well as the individual volunteer. Pontiano has a chronic problem recruiting women, who may express initial enthusiasm but then have their participation vetoed by their husbands. Then there is the thorny question of what care to provide people who get infected in the course of a trial. Volunteers in the developed world get ARVs; the standard structure of a drug trial says that if a participant contracts the illness under study, he or she gets all possible care, courtesy of the trial. But when Pontiano started vaccine tests in Uganda in 1999, there was no public AIDS treatment in his country. That question has been resolved to some degree because of the scale-up of Uganda's treatment program, but limited access to ARVs is still an issue, as is the question of what kind of psychological and social support to offer a person who contracts an illness as heavily stigmatized as HIV/AIDS. Pontiano, however, has never felt this was enough to keep from doing a trial: in a public health emergency like AIDS in Uganda, he said, volunteers can make clear-eyed assessments about whether they are satisfied with the care he can offer them.

An additional ethical consideration, one that has preoccupied Pontiano since his first days in the field, is what access participants will have to a vaccine should one be discovered through their trial or any other. In the early days, most vaccine research was bankrolled by pharmaceutical companies or relied on proprietary information. It was a set-up for the same situation as happened with ARVs, which remained out of reach for people in the developing world for so long. What if a Western company found a successful vaccine—if the company charged First World prices for it, in the interests both of recouping research costs and generating profits, how would Ugandans afford it? How would it be distributed in Africa, even if that was the site of the greatest spread of the virus?

Cold economics has largely resolved that problem. Until recently, vaccine research has been badly underfunded—receiving less than 3 per cent of global AIDS spending in 2006—precisely because the bulk of the epidemic is in Africa. As with pediatric ARVs, there is no incentive for pharmaceutical companies to develop a product for which most of the market is poor people who can't pay for it. And vaccines, by their nature, are less profitable than drugs—a person would, ideally, need a dose of vaccine only once, compared with ARVs every day for life. When initial optimism about a vaccine began to fade in the late 1980s, attention shifted away from prevention and on to treatment, where there were exciting new developments, and AIDS activists focused on universal access to ARVs. Vaccine research languished in the small laboratories of academic institutions for almost a decade.

Toward the end of the 1990s, however, a few things happened. The

Clinton administration in the United States rekindled interest in a vaccine. In 1997, President Clinton himself committed the U.S. to finding a vaccine within a decade, in a speech reminiscent of John F. Kennedy's pledge to get a man on the moon. The U.S. National Institutes of Health started to invest in small biotech companies that were looking at vaccine technology. The Bill and Melinda Gates Foundation, which since 2004 has emerged as the most significant and influential funding body in the world of AIDS, made a vaccine for HIV a top priority, and had committed more than $450 million to the research effort two years later. And an innovative public-private partnership called the International AIDS Vaccine Initiative, or IAVI, began to raise money from national governments, charities and the private sector to bankroll the research that the pharmaceutical industry wasn't doing. IAVI invests in companies and academic labs, and helps with arranging clinical trials, regulatory approvals and distribution systems. The vaccine candidates it tests either are owned by the organization or are offered by their inventors with a contractual clause that says that any finished product must be priced within the reach of the poor, or else IAVI can take over production. That resolves the access question, and in 2002, IAVI set up its second trial site in Africa, at the Uganda Virus Research Institute in Entebbe, with Pontiano as its key collaborator.

It had taken years for this renewed interest and additional funding to move the vaccine out of the Petri dishes and into clinical trials. But finally, by 2003, Pontiano and his fellow researchers could evaluate different candidates based on the results in animal trials, and decide in which they wished to invest time and energy—a change from the early attitude of "test anything you can," he said. That year, African researchers began testing the first vaccine actually engineered in the developing world (at the University of Cape Town in partnership with the South African AIDS Vaccine Initiative), one made with bits of DNA from different strains of the virus.

Pontiano headed his second trial in 2003, this one for IAVI, of a vaccine candidate made from subtype A, prevalent in Uganda. This time, the regulatory approval process took him only half as long, with just two committees and one international expert working group. And he set out to woo the media from the beginning, conducting a charm offensive that included extensive education on vaccines and how trials work. It was all made easier, he said, by the fact that the first trial had gone well and several of the volunteers were happy to talk to the media and community groups about their positive experience. The institute's community advisory board designed a radio and poster recruitment campaign using the slogan "Imagine a world without AIDS." Most of the volunteers who turned up willing to get the injections were people who had lost friends to the disease, Pontiano said.

The vaccine for this second trial was created at Oxford University with a concept known as prime and boost: it used an initial priming shot of a vaccine made with naked HIV DNA, followed by a second shot of HIV genes embedded in a weakened pox virus as a vector. The theory was that the first shot would teach the body to recognize HIV, when harmless viral proteins were produced; the second shot would mobilize the killer T cells. Designers hoped the two injections together would elicit a larger immune response than the recombinant proteins or the vectors did on their own. The product had gone into testing two years earlier in Kenya, in the first trials of an AIDS vaccine specifically designed for Africans.

But this vaccine too was a failure. While it was safe, it didn't trigger enough of an immune response to merit further trials. And so, in 2006, Pontiano began another test: another prime-and-boost vaccine, with viral DNA inserted into a harmless vector called adeno-associated virus. This trial will run until mid-2007, with thirty volunteers in Uganda, and Pontiano hopes for a strong immune response. He is not at all convinced, however, that he will find it. "We have not had good vaccines," he said. "We cannot rely on small parts of the virus." A whole new field of vaccine design is needed, he said, one that generates a harmless synthetic copy of

PONTIANO KALEEBU

get protected?
longer than others?
We need these answers."

the virus that mimics it almost perfectly. "I think technology will lead us there." But it won't be fast.

And there is still a question of money. By 2006, the global AIDS vaccine effort was funded at $700 million a year—better but not yet the $1.2 billion that IAVI estimates is needed to do all the possible development, evaluation and regulatory work that could be going on.

While he supervises the trials, Pontiano also keeps his hands in the work he thinks holds the key to an eventual vaccine. For years, he has puzzled over the phenomenon of discordant couples, where one person has HIV and the other does not, despite repeated exposure. "There are more discordant couples than concordant positive ones—why is that?" he mused. It suggests that different bodies respond to HIV a number of different ways—he wants to know what those are. Similarly, he is fascinated by long-term non-progressors, people with HIV who don't get sick. It is essential, he said, to figure out what is unique about their immune system. "Why do some people get protected? Why do some live longer than others? We need these answers."

These kinds of questions bring Pontiano, now the deputy director of the virus institute, to his office in the small white bungalow by 8 a.m. on most days, before the heat has settled, and he is very often still there at 10 p.m. The home he shares with his wife, Elizabeth, and their children is a short walk away, so he tries to duck out for dinner or play with the kids when he needs a break. He works most weekends, too. His family, he said, understands, most of the time.

Today the bulk of vaccine research spending goes on subtype C—"the imbalance has been corrected," Pontiano said, in part, he added with an uncharacteristic bit of cynicism, because subtypes of the virus once confined to Africa increasingly show up in the West. But it also speaks to the developed world's greater comfort with doing this kind of work in a place like Uganda. "People said you can't do studies in developing countries, but IAVI has shown you can do it very well." The institute's staff has swollen to nearly nine hundred, with all the international partnerships and trial funding. Some things, however, have not become any easier. "People you really know come to you for HIV testing," Pontiano said with a wince, "and they are positive." He hates those conversations.

He also dreads the confrontations, which come from time to time, with his volunteers and his community advisory board. "How often will we come here and you tell us about failed vaccines?" one board member snapped not long ago as Pontiano updated them about yet another unsuccessful trial. He struggles to maintain the community's sense of momentum. "People should not look at this and say, 'If there is no vaccine it is a failure,'" he said. "As scientists, we know we are advancing, we see progress." With that in mind, he is working to recruit a large cohort of volunteers for a phase III trial, people who show they have a long-term commitment to coming back for follow-up; he wants them always on standby, in preparation for the day when he gets the call to test a vaccine that has, at last, shown a real response in human immune systems.

A world without AIDS, he said, "may not happen in our lifetime, but it is possible. It's not easy. But I think you cannot say, 'This will never happen.' I am a strong believer in science, that we are making a lot of advances in science, that with the knowledge we are gaining we can make big and surprising breakthroughs." It will take a massive international effort—more time, more people, more money—but it is possible, he said. And most days, that's enough to keep him going.

Some evenings, though, when he walks home and sees his children playing, "then I feel terrible. This disease has been with us for more than twenty years. I had hoped that by the time all my children became sexually active and mature it would be solved—but it won't be. We may not have a vaccine in ten years, in twenty years," he said.

And then, almost to himself, he added, "No, we have to, we have to. It's a challenge."

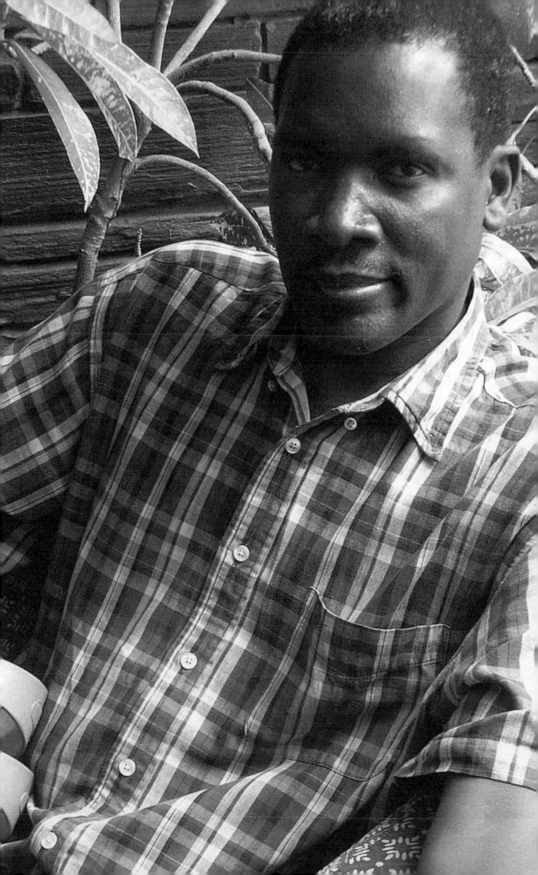

# SEVENTEEN

# WinstoneZulu

**T**he first time I met Winstone Zulu, he asked *me* the questions. How, he wanted to know, can your government, your country—you—just let us die?

"I have friends, married couples, who both have HIV and they can afford ARVs for only one of them," he said. His gaze was fierce. "So they're trying to figure out which one will take the drugs. Will their kids keep a mother or a father? What kind of choice is that?"

It had already been a grim day. I had met grandmothers swamped with orphans, pleading for help to buy food, and patients in an overcrowded clinic that lacked the most basic drugs. I had interviewed the minister of education, who told me about rural schools with 250 pupils and no teacher, and had a conversation with the minister of child welfare, who admitted, hushed but horrified, to an explosion in incidents of abuse of children by overstretched foster parents. Come evening, I had wound up in a plain meeting room in Lusaka, the capital of Zambia, with a dozen members of a local group of people living with HIV/AIDS. They were warm and thoughtful, and sick. They told me how they were waiting and waiting for the state to make ARVs available, but the government said it had no money—and in the meantime, another member failed to show up for each weekly meeting.

And there was Winstone, and his questions. He sat at the end of the table wearing a faded red-and-white "HIV POSITIVE" T-shirt.

The crutches he used to walk leaned against his chair. He had strong, handsome features and the honeyed voice of a late-night DJ. He was polite and gracious, but his disgust with the injustice of their situation lay like a sheen on his skin. "What are our lives worth?" he asked.

I had no answer, and I took refuge in my job, avoiding his eyes while I scribbled his words in my notebook.

Winstone was then buying his own ARVs, just managing on his salary as director of the group; his wife, Vivian, didn't yet need the drugs. "So my children keep both their parents. For now."

When Winstone spoke, his words made the crisis in Zambia searingly real—in a way that even the hungry grannies and the emaciated babies couldn't do.

I saw him often over the next few years. I sought him out whenever I returned to Zambia, and I bumped into him at AIDS conferences in different parts of the world—he is much in demand as a speaker. In bits and pieces, I learned about his astonishing life, and sometimes I felt the gentle sting of his wicked sense of humour. ("I see you've *also* got a sexually transmitted condition," he said to me, deadpan, when we met up in Zambia in 2006 and I was enormously pregnant.) And through him, I have come to understand the injustice of AIDS in a newly visceral way. The virus has exacted an almost inconceivable price from his life. And it never had to be that way. Winstone knows it. And it fills him with a clear, hot anger, something he keeps cloaked in good-natured wit. Most of the time. If it were me, I wonder, could I do the same?

Winstone learned of his HIV infection by accident. He was born in 1964 in Lusaka. He survived an attack of polio when he was three

# can your government, let us die?

("Bugs love me," he says), hence the crutches, which have etched cal-luses into his powerful arms. He had political ambitions and in 1990 won a scholarship for a six-month political science course in Leningrad. His visa application (much like Siphiwe Hlophe's) involved a routine medical, including an HIV test. He would never have tested otherwise, Winstone said. "I wasn't entirely naive about what it meant." A former girlfriend had died the year before—of AIDS, although no one said so at the time. So when he went for his test, "I was hoping against hope."

The hope was denied. Winstone headed home from the clinic, pass-ing garbage bins in the street emblazoned with the skull and crossbones and the words "AIDS Kills." For the next few days he sat in the small room he was renting with his brother Shadreck and wrote—dark, despairing poems about having his life so brutally truncated. After a week holed up at home, he thought he would try to find a place to pub-lish them before he died; he knew he was a good writer, and a collection of poems seemed as good a legacy as any other. A friend told him about a new centre for people with AIDS, called Kara Counselling, run by a Catholic priest. Winstone went there, hoping the staff might be able to help with his manuscript. They couldn't—but they did offer support for people newly diagnosed with HIV. The first counsellor with whom Winstone sat down told him he might live as long as another six years. "I thought, 'Well. I can use six years.'"

Four days after his test, he had his first conversation about HIV, with Shadreck. "His reaction was typical. He said, 'I think I might have it myself—it's no big deal.'" Alarmed, Winstone began to pester his broth-ers to go and test, but they resisted. Three months later, his brother Erasmus was dead at thirty-three. His wife died the next day. Then

# "What are our lives worth?" he asked.

another brother, Christopher, died a week later, at thirty-one. All three died of tuberculosis; they were all made vulnerable by an underlying HIV infection, for which they agreed to test only in the last days of their lives.

Kara, at the time, was an offshoot of a Zambian aid agency called Family Health Trust, and took its name from the building where the first office was located. But its founder, an Irish Jesuit named Michael Kelly, wanted to turn it into a free-standing AIDS service organization, and Winstone offered to help. It was an incredibly courageous decision: in 1991, not a single person in Zambia, or anywhere else in southern Africa, was openly living with HIV. "But I had this anger that this disease was killing so many people and no one was speaking or even showing the face of this disease. I decided, Look, this thing is going to kill me but I might as well use it to help people."

He started big: he went to *Good Morning, Zambia,* the most watched program on the national broadcaster. He sat down in the studio chair, the cameras went live, and he said he had the virus. Interviewers peppered him with questions: How did you get it? How do you feel? How did your parents and siblings react? Are you scared you're going to die? Televisions were, and are, scarce in Zambia, but news travels plenty fast by mouth, and by the time Winstone left the studio, it seemed as if everyone in the country knew he had HIV.

A few days later, Father Kelly took him to speak to a group of young seminarians. Then to a factory, where he addressed the workers. Soon he was the country's AIDS outreach effort, a campaign of one. He found it strangely comforting, despite the staring crowds and their probing questions. "I was feeling as if a burden was removed, the sense of worthlessness. One of the things that happens to you when you are HIV-positive is you lose all esteem." Winstone didn't feel so bad when he spoke before the crowds. And by standing up in front of them, he shattered the myth that a person infected would be visibly wasted and ill.

Before long, he had company. A young man named Simon, a year older than he at twenty-seven, agreed to join Winstone on his rounds of workplace education. Soon a third fellow, David, came too. Many people were reluctant to have them speak—"AIDS was bad for business," Winstone said—but they made their way through the industrial zones. Winstone began to accept invitations outside Lusaka, and spoke to groups of soldiers, teenagers and hospital patients around the country. Three more young men joined what was beginning to feel like a club, and they decided to move in together, renting a house in a poor, high-density neigh-bourhood on the edge of Lusaka—the kind of place where AIDS was having its worst effect, where they thought they could be most useful as activists. Before they moved, social workers they knew at the University of Zambia did a survey of the neighbours' attitudes. It wasn't encouraging: more than half said they would not eat with the men, and a third said they should stay away altogether. Nevertheless, Winstone and his pals moved in. And before too long, the neighbours softened—perhaps, Winstone speculated, because the men didn't *look* sick, or maybe it was the nuns they knew through Kara. If the nuns had tea and scones with them, could the men be that bad? Soon people from the street came by to borrow sugar, and some even stayed for a meal.

Winstone and his new friends did outreach workshops all day, and in the evenings watched videos or went to the bars in town for drinks. There was no hiding that they had HIV—they had all been on TV— and now he faced the judgment and public moralizing that would become a constant in his life. People tsked when they saw him order a beer; when Simon found a girlfriend, neighbours came right out and said that these men with HIV should not be having sex. "But we refused to die before we were actually dead," Winstone wrote about this time. "We believed in life before death and we did not want to live like monks in the mountains of Tibet."

Then it started. George, whose HIV infection was more advanced than the others', got sick and died at thirty-nine. "The rest of the team looked at each with the question: who is next?" Winstone wrote. By this point, most of the men were troubled with diarrhea; they kept a container of oral rehydration salts in the kitchen. (Rakish Simon kept a bottle of vodka alongside it.) Lawrence was the next to die. "He got so thin that you could actually count every bone in his body." The men fell into macabre humour about who would be next. "But inside, some, and maybe all of us, were scared shitless." In the end, Arthur was next.

Winstone threw himself into work at Kara. The agency began to offer testing and counselling, and opened a hospice, called Hope House, to provide dignified care to people dying of AIDS. And in the spirit of defying death, Winstone got married. Vivian, six years younger, was one of many people who had sought Winstone out after his first TV appearance. She had tested positive in 1989, although she had not told anyone. Winstone's tough, droll demeanour softens when he talks about her, her strength and her courage. "At the time I was thinking, 'It's wrong to get married, it's wrong to have children'"—other people certainly thought so, and he had those doubts himself. But he thought, too, that if he could persuade himself that he really had a right to the life he wanted, then maybe in time others would come to see it that way as well.

Vivian desperately wanted children. "Here the stigma of not having children is horrible," Winstone explained. "If you die without having kids you are going into the ancestors' world without leaving anyone. Your life is useless." But they agreed it would not be fair to pass the virus to a baby. Instead, they adopted a boy they named Michael, after Father Kelly. The child was born to Vivian's sister, who was single and struggling to raise him. People expressed their unsolicited approval: this, they told Winstone and Vivian, was the *right* way for people with HIV to have children.

As one of the first Africans to live publicly with HIV, Winstone was welcomed into the emerging international AIDS establishment, and given a rare opportunity to have a voice in how the global response to the pandemic unfolded. In 1994, he helped draft the Paris Declaration, which laid out the then-radical notion that people with HIV must be consulted about their care and treatment, and that they must be guaranteed legal protection from discrimination. He was part of the 1996 meeting in Como, Italy, at which UNAIDS was founded. And he helped to organize what was perhaps the most seminal AIDS gathering of the past twenty years: the 1996 conference in Vancouver where David Ho announced that he had successfully suppressed HIV using his cocktail of antiretrovirals. Winstone was in the audience when Ho presented. He didn't quite understand the implications at first—he needed to decipher the technical jargon—but when he did, he felt the first rush of hope since his diagnosis.

Except, of course, that no one in Zambia had the cocktail. The next year, Winstone came down with TB. He was treated, and recovered, but he knew he needed the new drugs. "I thought, 'If I'm thirty-three and I have TB there must be something terribly wrong with my immunity.'" He enlisted the help of friends in AIDS organizations abroad, who sent him pills donated by patients in the developed world who no longer needed them, and Winstone began ARV therapy. The drugs had side effects—nausea and numbness—but he ceased to be plagued by the rashes and infections he had had for years. Soon he felt fine.

And then a crazy thing happened. At the 1998 AIDS conference, held in Geneva, Winstone encountered a group of the so-called AIDS dissidents, who staged a hunger strike at the global gathering. They insisted that HIV did not exist and that the idea of AIDS was being peddled by Western drug companies and scientists in their pay. Winstone stopped to listen, intrigued that people of such passionate conviction were being ignored or dismissed as lunatics by everyone else at the meeting. "I was looking for an escape. For me the idea was, 'If these guys are proven to be right then I'm off the hook.' I was seduced by the promise of the idea."

He didn't feel he knew enough to judge whether the dissidents were right or wrong. But among their ranks were Nobel Prize–winning scientists such as Kary Mullis, who had won the award for chemistry in

1993. It seemed to Winstone that the dissidents were asking valid questions that no one from the world of mainstream AIDS thinking was willing to take on. "They were people questioning things. They didn't have solutions—but these were real questions. For example, why is one child of an infected woman born with HIV and not another?" And then he heard that the dissidents had an additional supporter: Winstone had been a committed member of an African National Congress solidarity organization during the years Thabo Mbeki lived in exile in Zambia, and now he learned that Mbeki, South Africa's new president, was also expressing doubts about the validity of mainstream thinking on HIV. "Here was Thabo Mbeki, my hero—when Thabo Mbeki questioned it, I was sold."

Winstone resigned from his various posts with AIDS organizations, and in February 2000 he stopped taking ARVs. "I really believed them—that AZT was doing me harm." Vivian asked him gently if he was sure this was a good idea; he was firm. "I said, 'Yes. I met these Nobel Prize winners who said this is wrong.'"

The dissidents were thrilled: attracting one of Africa's best-known activists to their fringe cause was a coup. By the time the next International AIDS Conference rolled around, in Durban in 2000, Winstone was firmly in their camp. Mbeki used the meeting to make clear the breadth of his skepticism about AIDS; outside the conference venue, thousands of people with HIV hurled abuse at the dissidents, accusing them of murder—it was the kind of protest Winstone usually led.

His stance caught Mbeki's attention, and the president invited him to join the panel of experts he had struck to investigate the truth about HIV and its treatment (Winstone was the only non-scientist). He remembers the panel meetings as fraught, each side convinced that the other was responsible for the deaths of hundreds of thousands of people. He listened to microbiologist Peter Duesberg, a respected researcher from the University of California at Berkeley, who argued that HIV was simply a harmless "passenger virus." AIDS in the developed world was an illness brought on by long-term recreational drug use, Duesberg said, while the African pandemic was simply old diseases lumped under a new name. There were doctors from Australia who argued persuasively that HIV had never been isolated, and Mullis, who said he had yet to see proof that HIV caused AIDS. Could they all just be crackpots?

"For ten years I've lived with HIV," Winstone told reporters after the first meeting of the panel, "and for ten years I've preached the main line. To hear that I could be wrong is good news. If you were in my shoes, you could understand. . . . These ideas from the other side will find fertile ground in Africa because the conventional thinking hasn't been much use."

By March 2001, Winstone was sick again. He was covered in fungal infections and lesions that would not heal. His toenails dropped off. Soon he had to use a wheelchair. He heard the news that one of the dissidents he had met on the panel had died of AIDS. Mbeki, meanwhile, was saying AIDS was a disease of poverty, yet Winstone could see that all around him in Zambia, well-educated and comparatively well-off people were hardest hit by the disease. So he began to reconsider. "What saved me was that I didn't feel too ashamed to go back and ask for real advice."

By then, he could no more deny his own illness than he could what was happening around him: all but one of his five brothers had died. His sister Rebecca died. Her husband died. His cousins, nephews, nieces died. All his friends from the early years at Kara were gone. This wasn't an old disease under a new name: something extraordinary and terrible was happening in Zambia. "I went back on my medicines." When Winstone had stopped taking the ARVs, his CD4 count was 536. When he went back on the same combination two years later, the count was 34. But once again, the drugs worked: within a month, he was out of the wheelchair. And back to activism.

One issue, in particular, now obsessed him: the "twin epidemics" of tuberculosis and HIV. TB had taken the lives of his HIV-positive brothers, sister and three sisters-in-law, and the vicious impact on his family wasn't particularly unusual—more people with HIV die of TB than any other infection. Nearly two billion people around the world carry the TB bacillus; it lies harmless and dormant in most of them, but having HIV more than doubles the likelihood that a person will develop the disease. Two-thirds of people with TB in sub-Saharan Africa are HIV-positive, and in Zambia, three-quarters of new tuberculosis cases are in people with HIV.

When Winstone himself had begun to show signs of tuberculosis four years earlier—chest pains, night sweats and weight loss—he recognized them from his brothers' experience. He went to the hospital for an X-ray and a sputum test, but a week later, staff told him he didn't have TB. Winstone was unconvinced. He started to share the drugs of his last surviving brother, Danny, who was then on TB treatment, and in just three days he was feeling better. He went back to the hospital, telling staff he was sure he had TB. They tested him again. This time, they took four months to deliver the results—and in fact, he did have TB. "I could be dead now if I'd waited for them to diagnose it." It may have been incompetence, he said, but it is equally possible that well-intentioned staff were simply misled by the notoriously inaccurate diagnostic tests, which were invented more than seventy years ago. The sputum test he had catches, at best, half the cases of active TB, a fact Winstone finds outrageous. "We need new diagnostics—you can't defeat TB without detecting it," he said. "It's the most infectious of the opportunistic infections. If you have TB, chances are you'll infect fifteen or twenty people before it's detected." Yet there is little investment in TB treatment because it is viewed in the rich world as an old-fashioned, fading disease. In fact TB incidence is exploding, but since, as with HIV, 95 per cent of people with tuberculosis live in developing countries, it's not nearly as sexy a subject for researchers as, say, bird flu.

His brother Danny died of a second bout of TB in 2003, because the antibiotics were out of stock in Zambia's clinics. "He was twenty-nine—I was nine years older," Winstone said. "Danny should really have lived and I should have died." By the time Danny died, Winstone was speaking about HIV and TB around the world; more driven than ever, he lobbied senators in Washington and members of parliament in London and lent his chiselled features to billboard campaigns and educational videos under the slogan "Winstone Zulu Is Alive." Alive, of course, because he got the drugs. "If my brothers had survived TB, they might have lived long enough to access HIV drugs like me."

Effective treatment for TB could change the way people think about HIV/AIDS, Winstone said. The response to AIDS is undermined by the abstract nature of the syndrome—the idea that something is slowly and invisibly weakening the body's ability to fight off infection. When he speaks to audiences in Europe or North America, people talk about feeling paralysis in the face of the statistics—the twenty-eight million people in Africa with an incurable illness. "Many people just want to look away because the problem looks so insurmountable. They think, how can we deal with this? But if you say, 'Hey, wait: the biggest killer of people living with HIV in Africa and many other developing regions is tuberculosis—and if you give them drugs that cost $10, you can save someone's life, and you can avoid having more orphans'—then people see it differently."

In 2003 Winstone and Vivian moved to Kabwe in the Copperbelt in the north, to open a Kara counselling centre, AIDS hospice and program for orphaned street kids. Kabwe is a mining town, but its once-vibrant economy had been choked by a World Bank–engineered privatization of the mines and railways that caused thousands of people to lose their jobs. Now young women stood on the trucking route in and out of town, selling sex for as little as $1 per encounter.

At the new Kara centre, Winstone organized a support group: it grew from ten members the first week to eighty-three the third. He was delighted to see people coming forward, but also amazed at the pace of growth. A staff member suggested they ask the group to test for HIV. Only twenty-three of the group members were in fact infected. The rest were coming to the centre so they could collect the 80-cent transport allowance for the meetings. Told the news that they were HIV-negative and could not stay in the group, many were distraught. They were walking great distances to attend because the allowance was the only thing feeding their families. One day when Winstone gave a young woman named

Jennifer the happy news that her TB had been successfully treated, she
responded by bursting into tears: without TB, she would no longer qualify
for a weekly parcel of soya powder and beans, the only source of food
for her three children.

"When I went home I couldn't sleep," Winstone wrote about those
days. "I felt terrible. What was the use of setting up Kara Counselling in
Kabwe if the people wished they had AIDS so they could get a few cents?
How could we fight TB if patients felt happy to be sick so they could
get a few pounds of soya powder? What the fucking hell was I doing
here?" He thought about his most recent speaking tour in the United
States, where he was told about a cat with kidney problems on dialysis,
saw massive sport utility vehicles with built-in DVD players, heard that
the leading epidemic in the country was obesity. "And here I am stuck
with Jennifer and Joyce in my little office as they wish they had the
most serious and fatal disease to have hit the world so they can get 80
cents every week." Some days, it was hard just to go into work, knowing
what waited there for him.

While Winstone knows his decision to go public had a huge impact
on people, he sometimes regrets it—he still gets hassled nearly every
time he orders a beer. And while he's had far more than the six years he
originally hoped for, HIV still colours his life. The poems he wrote the
day he learned he had HIV were never published, but he has since had
his writing both printed and posted on AIDS sites on the internet. In
2004, he wrote of life with HIV

> Yes, I have lived positively with HIV for a dozen years.
> Yes, I have given hope, I hope, to some people.

WINSTONE ZULU

# about this epidemic is its sacredness and its meaning."

Yes, I try not to be weepy most of the time.

And yes, I am glad to be here.

But the fact remains that I will have a far shorter life than if I had stayed away from HIV. Morbidity and mortality are a permanent feature on my daily agenda.

I know what fear is. Fear of losing weight until you have no more lips to cover your teeth. Fear of being rejected by those who are closest to you. Fear of being cold and dead.

Alone in that coffin. Fear of leaving your children, your wife, your parents, friends—Lusaka. Oh yes, I love this city and I will surely miss it.

I know what anxiety is. The uncertainty of what will befall me tomorrow. Tuberculosis, herpes zoster, pneumonia, Kaposi's sarcoma, oral thrush, fungal rash, viral rash, bacterial rash, diarrhea, meningitis, cytomegalovirus, loss of weight until everyone can tell.

I know what anger is. Anger at myself for getting myself into this mess. Anger at God for not protecting me from this pestilence. Anger at the scientific world for not discovering a cure within my lifetime. Anger for still being alive.

I know what discrimination is. Being pushed off a bus by ignorant people who thought I was infectious by merely touching them. Being denied a chance to study in Russia, the USA, Canada or Australia. No red meat, alcohol, sugar, Coca-Cola, sex. Having special laws made for me. Being denied employment, promotion, insurance, God's blessing when marrying. Written off.

Beyond the personal cost, he mourns what the disease has cost Zambia as a nation. No one thinks it shocking that he lost five siblings, that his elderly parents have eighteen orphaned grandchildren. "One of the horrible things about this epidemic is that death has totally lost its sacredness and its meaning," he said. "I go to Mandla Hill"—Lusaka's posh shopping area—"and all these people are out shopping and it looks so normal. Walk five streets from there to the graveyard and all these people are being buried. How are we still functioning? When this whole thing is over, everyone will stop and cry. But at this point we are numb."

Winstone and Vivian have made their stand in the face of numbness by building a family. By 2000, it was clear that the interventions for pregnant women with HIV could effectively prevent them from passing on the virus, and they could get nevirapine and Caesarean delivery in Lusaka. They had a son, Mtunduwazanso, whose name means "the clan has come back again," in honour of Winstone's lost brothers, and a daughter, Mwenda; both were successfully delivered HIV-negative. Michael, their adopted son, was not so fortunate. He has twice had tuberculosis and is on ARVs.

In 2004, Winstone made another public appearance to advocate for better treatment of TB, at the International AIDS Conference in Bangkok. This time he shared a stage with the one TB survivor better known than he: Nelson Mandela, who had the disease while a prisoner on Robben Island. Mandela pleaded for more attention to the disease, more resources for treatment and faster diagnoses. And he singled out the young man on the stage next to him: "I want to acknowledge and thank Winstone Zulu, who will share his experience fighting HIV and TB with you," Mandela said. "We need more advocates like Winstone to tell the world about TB and the effect it has on so many millions of people."

A few minutes later Mandela stood to make his way out of the room, surrounded by bodyguards and photographers and breathless admirers. Winstone leaned on his crutches and watched them go. I nudged him with an elbow. "Not every day Nelson Mandela talks you up," I said. Winstone laughed and shook his head. "I can't believe that," he said.

And then he turned so that he could just see Mandela's retreating back, and spoke again.

"I want to live that long," he said. "Long enough to have so many lines on my face."

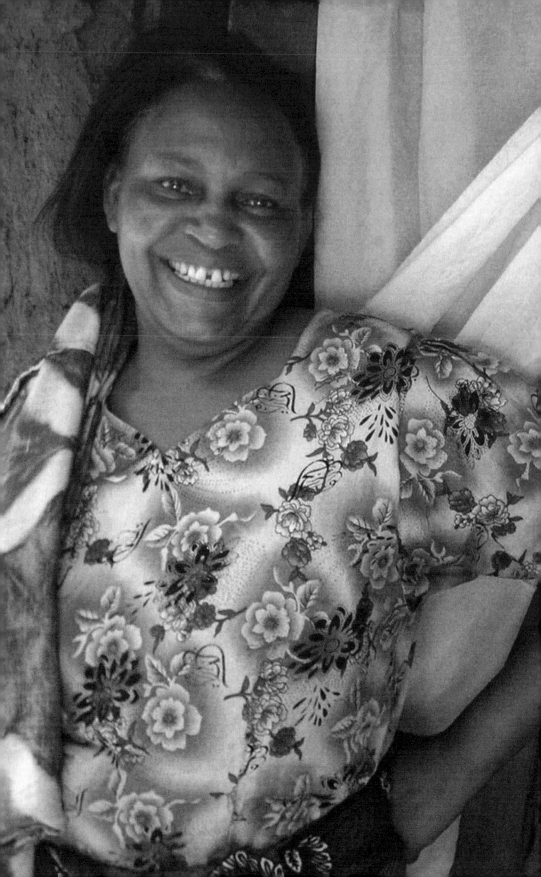

# EIGHTEEN

# AgnesMunyiva

I lay down to test the mattress: it was lumpy and totally unyielding, not the sort of place one would want to spend much time, which seemed a little odd, given the purpose of this room. Agnes Munyiva saw my wince, laughed and patted the bed. "You need it to be hard, because otherwise you could get hurt when the men are pushing on you," she explained.

The mattress, stuffed with lumpy cotton and resting on a plain metal frame, fills most of her room, just one metre by two. The walls are made of mud, the roof of scraps of tin. The air has a tang from the raw sewage and rotting food scraps in the alley outside, and Agnes tries to keep the clouds of flies at bay with a crisp white muslin curtain in the doorway. Remnants of linoleum, pieced together like a quilt, cover most of the dirt floor. She has a kerosene burner, for making tea, and a gas lantern. Two mouldy calendars, giveaways from insurance companies many years back, are tacked to the walls, the only decoration. A collection of worn facecloths hangs drying on a small clothesline. Beside the bed she keeps a large white box, containing the best part of a gross of condoms.

Agnes rents this room for 900 Kenyan shillings, or $12, a month, bed included. She doesn't live here—she also rents another room, a bit bigger than this one, on the other side of Majengo, a slum neighbourhood on the edge of Nairobi. She shares that room with the three youngest of her five children. They have never seen this one. This room is just for work.

Agnes arrives here around six o'clock each morning, when the sun is climbing in the sky, and she makes sure she is on the way home before the sun sinks again twelve hours later—she is a lady of the evening who works only in the daylight hours. There is plenty of rape and theft and murder in Majengo in the daytime, but at night the streets are completely lawless. When Agnes arrives in the morning, she sweeps the patch of floor and the narrow alley outside. She makes a cup of tea, sips it from a battered tin mug, stacks the cloths by the bed. Then she takes a low three-legged wooden stool into the alley, sits down and waits for business. "*Karibu*," she says as men pass—Kiswahili for welcome. She gives them a wink and her slow smile that unfurls like honey off a spoon. "We all try our luck each time a person passes," she explained. "If he stops to look at me maybe he is interested, but if not, maybe he is used to someone else." In front of every third or fourth shack in the streets, a woman sits on a stool, modestly dressed like Agnes, who wore a bright wrapper printed with blue and yellow chickens on the day she introduced me to a working woman's life in Majengo.

Most days, a man stops before she has been in the alley for half an hour. "They are people on their way to work. Or men on the road who spent the night away from their wives—they pass here for breakfast." When a man stops at Agnes's soft *karibu,* she invites him to step into her room. "Most men are discreet—the ones with wives want to get in the door very quickly." Inside, they negotiate. The price is set at between 50 and 100 shillings—75 cents to $1.50. She slides the door closed, but the scratchy sounds of a neighbour's transistor radio drift through the screened window; her customer knows he must be silent. "We even tell them not to make a lot of noise," Agnes said, sounding very prim, "because there could be a family in the next house." She removes her wrapper, lies back on the bed, her arms above her head. She does not embrace the client, whispers no encouragement. This is a brisk transaction. "If your five minutes are over and you are still there"—she pointed at her chest—"you have to pay another 50 shillings," she said firmly. Business concluded, her client steps over the curious chickens in the doorway and back out into the alley, and

Agnes cleans up with the cloths and a pitcher of water from the standpipe at the end of the alley. Then she returns to the stool.

This interaction is repeated a dozen times each day. A fair portion of the men who stop have spent time with Agnes before: "The service must have been good, so they come back," she told me with a giggle. At the end of the day, she padlocks the door and takes home perhaps 500 shillings, enough for some food bought at the market stalls on the way, and a bit put aside for the next installment of the children's school fees, or some kerosene or soap.

Agnes came to Nairobi from Machakos, two hours to the east by bus, in 1971. She was twenty years old. There was only the exhausting work of farming at home, and she hoped to find a job in the city. Before long she was hired as a maid in a middle-class house. That lasted a year, and then she found more work mending clothes, and then casual labour in the indus- trial area on the edge of the booming city. That led to a job making paper bags in a factory—but she injured a finger in the machinery after a couple of years and was fired. By then she had had three small children, fathered by a couple of boyfriends who hadn't stuck around. Her mother had died back home, her father was unwell, and she felt there was no one in Machakos to whom she could turn.

Agnes had only one room, then, in Majengo, the sort of chaotic com- munity at the edge of the city where so many of Africa's rural poor end up. Majengo is built around a vast market for *mitumba*—second-hand clothes given by North Americans and Europeans to charity shops that end up shipped to Africa in giant bales. Traders from all over East Africa come to hunt for bargains in First World cast-offs. The market also sells everything from plastic washbasins to jerry-rigged scrap-metal satellite dishes. There are food stalls and tearooms and hostels for the travellers. Thousands of people move through here every day, many with a little disposable income suddenly in their pocket: like similar communities the world over, it is a natural centre for sex work. In addition to the travellers from out of town, men from all over Nairobi—police officers, civil servants, welders, street sweepers, teachers and taxi drivers—seek out the anonymity of the vast market for their occasional sexual encounters.

# "In the neighbourhood who were doing it, and try it. I had children

When Agnes was despairing about how to make money, how she would survive in the city, her neighbours suggested she try *umalaya,* sex for money. "In the neighbourhood there were other women who were doing it, and they encouraged me to try it. I had children who needed food." And so, with great reluctance, she began to sit on a wood stool outside her home and try to catch the eye of men who passed by. She never imagined, in those first few weeks, that she would be earning a living this way thirty years later.

Today thousands of women work in the alleys of Majengo and the other sprawling slums of Nairobi, but only one or two of Agnes's friends from her first days in the business are still around. "The ones I started with are no longer here—they have died," she said simply. "Most of the people I have worked with have died." Beginning in the early 1980s, women started to get thin, with sharp coughs and white fur that coated their mouths and throats; back then they called the illness Plastic, Agnes said, because city workers hastily wrapped up the bodies of people who died that way in plastic sheeting. Some of the women died there in Majengo, and others went back to the village when they grew too sick to work. But Agnes remained healthy, year after year.

What happened to her—or, more accurately, what didn't happen to her—would prove to be one of the greatest discoveries in the twenty-five-year battle with AIDS. She would acquire, over the next two decades, a certain fame, in the world of virology and infectious disease, as one of *those* Nairobi prostitutes. But Agnes's body would be slower to give up its secrets than anyone imagined.

This story starts with chancroid, a venereal disease that causes suppurating ulcers on the genitals. On the other side of the world from Nairobi, in the Canadian prairie city of Winnipeg, there was an outbreak

# there were other women they encouraged me to who needed food."

of chancroid in the late 1970s, and infectious disease experts at the University of Manitoba began to investigate. Before long they had figured out how to grow the bacteria in the lab—but the outbreak had quickly been brought under control by public health officials, and the researchers were left without patients. That might have been the end of it, had a Winnipeg microbiologist not got talking to a colleague from the University of Nairobi at a conference a few months later. "You want chancroid?" the Kenyan asked. "We've got chancroid."

And so Allan Ronald flew to Nairobi in 1980. He soon noticed that sexually transmitted infections, or STIs, such as chlamydia and gonorrhea were rampant. He also noticed that most of the people seeking help at government clinics for these infections had in common the fact that they frequented prostitutes in an industrial slum. He and a couple of colleagues set up a shopfront clinic in Nairobi, offering free treatment to anyone in return for participation in medical research. Before long the operation expanded into slums around the city. They were candy-store settings for young Western researchers, with more weird microbes coming through the door in a single morning than they might see in a year back home. And their patients were more than happy to participate, in exchange for the top-notch health care they could never have afforded to purchase in Nairobi. "Here we got treatment if we were diagnosed—the city clinic never had any drugs," said Agnes, who first attended a clinic in 1983 and soon became a regular. And, she said, she and the other women felt less judged in the research clinic; no one gossiped about the way they earned their living.

In those first few years, the Manitobans and colleagues from other universities in the West who joined them did some important research on sexually transmitted diseases, and the impact on children whose mothers were infected with gonorrhea or chlamydia. But the discovery that would rock the scientific world came from the whim of a graduate student. In 1985, Joan Kreiss, a student researcher from the University of Washington, decided to test the sex workers, including Agnes, for HIV. The virus had been identified in New York four years earlier, and Kreiss wanted to use the new test for antibodies to HIV. Her older colleagues were dubious. They suspected, from post-mortems on patients who had symptoms similar to those being reported in New York, that HIV was present in the city—and years later, tests of stored blood from East Africa would show that in fact some communities in the region at that point had infection rates as high as 20 per cent. But there was not a single documented case of AIDS in Kenya at the time, and many scientists were doubtful that women could even catch the disease through sex. So no one was prepared for what Joan Kreiss found. Two-thirds of the women she tested were HIV-positive.

Her findings—one of the earliest recorded signs of the African epidemic—did not go over well. The government of Kenya threatened to deport the foreign researchers and shut the whole project down. "The government said, 'It's not true what you are saying! You're going to drive the tourists out of Kenya!'" recalled a rueful Elizabeth Ngugi, a community health professor at the University of Nairobi. She was working ("in the mud and in the sun and in the rain and in the dust") to get to know Agnes and the Majengo women, building relationships that would be the core of research through the decades. She soon organized six hundred women into support groups, brought them into the clinic for classes on sexually transmitted diseases, gave them condoms and encouraged them to present a united front to clients, insisting on protected sex.

Over the next few years, research involving the women yielded two big discoveries. The first was that mothers passed HIV to their babies in breast milk. Researchers already knew there was some transmission of the virus this way, but a study in the slum showed that the longer a mother breastfed, the higher was the risk of transmission—and that far from being negligible, this was in fact a major source of infection. The second major finding was that a person with a conventional STI such as gonorrhea has a much higher chance of contracting HIV—as much as 70 per cent higher—than a person not infected. All of this, however, paled beside a discovery that emerged in the late 1980s.

Frank Plummer, now the director of Canada's Centre for Infectious Disease Prevention and Control, in Ottawa, worked in the Nairobi project from its early days. He was intrigued by these HIV-positive women, who gave the lie to so much of the predominant thinking about AIDS at the time—that it didn't exist in Africa, that women couldn't get it, that hetero-sexual sex was no real risk. By 1988, he had noticed something bizarre: over time, more and more of the women were testing positive for HIV—but not all of them. Some, including Agnes, were still around, three and four and five years later, and in their biannual HIV tests, they were still negative. Plummer began to track them closely, and concluded that a small number of the women—perhaps 5 per cent—were simply not getting infected. "They're basically immune to HIV," he told me. "Their immune systems for whatever reason are able to recognize and kill HIV." In the study of a particularly impenetrable virus, this was a massive discovery.

Keith Fowke, a professor of medical microbiology at the University of Manitoba who was then a student working under Frank Plummer in Nairobi, explained it like this. "We did the models and found that these women were not just really, really, really lucky—it was beyond the statistical chance of luck playing a role. We estimated that many of these women have had five hundred to two thousand sexual exposures to infected men when they weren't using a condom." Surveys found that a quarter of the men who frequented sex workers in the area were HIV-positive. And while Elizabeth Ngugi's shack-to-shack education efforts had early success getting Agnes and the other women to use condoms with some of their one-off clients, there were still many exceptions: men would pay extra not to use condoms—money that women hard up for cash were reluctant to forgo—and sex workers didn't use them with their "regulars," men they saw every week or two. Ngugi's surveys found that the women used condoms, at best, only 75 per cent of the time, so there could be no question that Agnes and a handful of others had been routinely exposed to HIV over a decade or more.

# "I just thank God," as she does now. she wasn't sick. thanks for it at Mass

Yet they weren't infected. It wasn't good nutrition—the women did not earn enough to eat well—and it wasn't that they somehow took better care of themselves, because they had had other STIs and ailments. Something else was happening to make these women immune.

Then Frank Plummer and his team noticed something even more peculiar. The women's likelihood of being infected with HIV/AIDS was related to the length of time they had been doing sex work: the longer a woman had been selling sex in Majengo, the *less* likely she was to be infected. If she'd been doing it for five years and was still HIV-negative, the data suggested, then the odds were she was going to stay that way. These findings were so counterintuitive that Plummer and his team struggled to find any-one who would publish them. The phenomenon didn't get major attention until two years later, when he described the resistant women at the International AIDS Conference in Amsterdam in 1992.

Once the public really began to understand that there were people who were immune to AIDS—and the dark irony that it was the sex workers vilified for spreading the disease—Majengo became a focus of attention. Television news teams poured into the slum, clamouring to meet the women. The attention left Agnes baffled. "I just thank God," she said then, as she does now. She couldn't explain why she wasn't sick. She could just give thanks for it at Mass every Sunday morning.

The researchers, however, were frantically trying to decode what was going on in the bodies of Agnes and the other women. "Either the virus couldn't infect their cells at all or the virus could but their bodies were clearing the infection in some way," explained Keith Fowke. "But when we isolated the blood cells of some women in the lab and exposed their cells to HIV, it could get inside their cells and was able to replicate and able to grow just fine. So we started looking at their immune system—HIV was able to establish initial infection and the immune system was able to clear it," Fowke said. "We've really found cells that can kill HIV in these women."

Agnes has, in effect, a callus: the first time she was exposed to the virus, her body produced enough killer T cells to fight it off. This part isn't unique—the body of every person who is exposed to HIV mounts some level of response, and sometimes manages to fight it off; a single exposure does not guarantee infection. But Agnes's body, it seems, not only produced sufficient and strong enough cells to fight the virus off the first time, it then produced a whole raft of those killer Ts, flooding her system with guardians whose sole brief was to keep an eye out for cells infected with HIV. The infected cells have a distinct pattern of little bumps on them, called epitopes, which act like a red rose in the lapel as far as the killer Ts are concerned, letting them know just which cells they want to hunt down. Then every subsequent time—probably thousands of times—that HIV got into Agnes's body, her killer T cells drove it back. A person does not normally maintain a large number of killer T cells for a long period—just long enough to kill something off, then production drops. But in Agnes, fairly constant exposure to HIV kept her killer T cell count high.

This conclusion was reinforced when Frank Plummer and his team noticed that women who take a "sex break"—who make a trip home to the village for a few weeks, or save up a little money and leave sex work for a while to try selling shoes instead, or hook up with a regular who keeps them in cash for a year or two—were far more likely to get infected, almost immediately, if they returned to sex work, even though previously they had had years of apparent immunity. On the break, their bodies stopped making the killer T cells, leaving them vulnerable again.

The Nairobi women aren't the only people in the world immune to HIV. Some Caucasian men have been found to have a genetic mutation that means their cells lack one of the molecular "hooks" that HIV latches on to, and so they cannot be infected. And no doubt there are other groups of people who, like these women, are able to kill off the virus—but it is much easier to see, and monitor, in this community of women who are repeatedly exposed to the virus than it would be in, say, a group of nuns in a convent in Europe. They might be immune to HIV too, but how would anyone ever tell?

From the moment it became clear that Agnes and a handful of other women in Majengo—about a hundred to date—really could fight off the virus, the researchers in Nairobi hoped that their biology would hold the secret of an HIV vaccine. Soon a team from Oxford University was at work on a vaccine that used the epitopes (the tell-tale bumps on infected cells) that triggered Agnes's killer Ts. They hoped it would provoke other people's bodies to produce killer T cells in the same way that the real virus appeared to trigger production in the sex workers. Trials began in Nairobi in 2001, and a second trial was mounted by Pontiano Kaleebu and his colleagues in Entebbe a couple of years later. But despite high hopes, the Oxford vaccine didn't cause that explosion of killer T cells. And so it was back to the painstaking work of trying to figure out the secret of Agnes's immunity. "Sometimes a vaccine feels impossibly far away," sighed Keith Fowke. "All our knowledge about these HIV-resistant people is interesting and I feel it's important . . . but it is frustrating."

For Elizabeth Ngugi, watching as AIDS decimates ever more of this community where she has built such strong ties, the gains are hollow. "Yes, it's fascinating," she told me. "But sometimes I feel very sad. Sometimes you are not a scientist but a friend, and you feel the emptiness inside."

There was a certain sense of breath-holding among the Nairobi researchers when Frank Plummer and his team first proved the women's bodies were able to kill off HIV, but that breath has long since been let out. Today the research strategy in Majengo revolves around intense study of Agnes and the other resistant women (who make up about 5 per cent of the cohort at any one time), from analyzing their genome to breaking down the chemical components of the mucosal membranes in their vaginas, in an effort to figure out what may be protecting them. So far researchers have not found anything present in 100 per cent of the women, so it may be that the protection comes from multiple overlapping factors, including some that are genetic. There is a strong family correlation—people related to an HIV-resistant woman seem to be half as likely to get infected as people who are not related.

Agnes is aware that she is a fascinating specimen. "Most of the people have been very interested in me," she said matter-of-factly. But she has no understanding of the biological basis for her HIV resistance. "No one has told me," she said with a shrug. She gets good, free health care at the clinic, for the occasional sexually transmitted infection and also for respiratory infections which plague residents of the polluted slum. So she is happy to give them her blood a couple of times a year, and to enjoy a sense of contributing something to her community.

But Agnes's survival has served to highlight a disquieting aspect of this research. She has come to the clinic for more than twenty years. In that time, more than $22 million in scientific grant money has flowed through the project, and many of the researchers have earned reputations as the top experts in their fields. Yet Agnes and a handful of other women are still selling sex, to an average of eight clients a day, still for a dollar or two each time—although they say they would like nothing more than to get out of sex work. When I asked her what she would like to do instead, Agnes's broad face lit up. "Any kind of job I could do. I could be a cleaner or anything. But it's very difficult to get a job—you have to know somebody to get a job." And Agnes said she doesn't know anybody who could help. With only limited literacy after three years of primary school, and no other skills, Agnes said she sees no other options. "It's embarrassing, this profession," she said. She refuses to discuss what she does for a living with her children, although she is sure they know. "I've never told them what I do, but I think they can see it. I think they know what I'm doing is not good but they know I do it to provide for them."

Agnes's frustration with her life in sex work raises troubling ethical questions about research, the kind that bedevil investigations into AIDS vaccines, prevention technologies and treatment, all of which, by definition, involve large groups of poor Africans, the people most at risk. What obligation does a researcher such as Frank Plummer have to the women who have given him their blood for twenty years? What does this project owe Agnes?

"Those are difficult questions," Plummer told me. "My philosophy has been: try to help as many people as we can with what resources we have so we can ultimately solve it. We provide treatment for a lot of medical conditions and counselling for safer sexual behaviour and free condoms and referral to other medical services—which prevents about ten thousand infections each year. We do have an obligation to provide some basic level of care, and since 2004 we have provided ARV treatment, which is an important step. But ARV drugs are not going to solve this problem." Plummer doesn't disagree that women like Agnes need a route out of prostitution. "I don't know what those ways out are, though, and anything we could do is just working on the margins—it's unlikely we'll be able to do anything to get them to the point that they're not partially dependent on sex work: you can only make so much money selling tomatoes or weaving baskets."

His Kenyan colleague Elizabeth Ngugi is unconvinced by this line of argument. "These women have given the world such a huge body of knowledge, but what has the world done to help them change? The research findings have given us so much, but what have we given back? There is more research money coming all the time—quite clearly there is an imbalance." In 2002, she received funds from a donor agency to train 120 of the women in new skills such as dressmaking and hairdressing, and she said 80 of them successfully made the transition out of sex work. She has helped a few others make their way to local benevolent agencies and out of the business, but most are stuck, and the research budget includes no funds to give them other options—a grim irony when, as she pointed out, they have educated all the women about what a huge risk sex work is to their lives.

Frank Plummer agreed that the women need basic education in numeracy and savings and small-business skills. "But you can't get a research grant for that," he said. The ethics of science today require that the women get counselling and condoms, but ethics approval boards make no demands about math classes or instruction in how to set up an alleyway beauty salon.

There is a small patch of grey at Agnes's hairline these days, and her body has thickened to that of a woman of a certain age. "I'm getting old," she said. "There will be a time that I'm too old—at around sixty. Maybe ten years from now clients will not even look for me. It will be difficult." Now she feels lucky to get 100 shillings from a client, when a young woman newly arrived in Majengo might get as much as 300—although in any case trade is not what it once was. "Ever since we got this disease, business has dropped. Most men go home to their wives on the weekend." Of the men who still buy sex (and she manages to find nine or ten each day), most now agree to use condoms—but not all, and Agnes worries. She would like to start a small business that would keep her family when men no longer stop outside her room, but she used all the few thousand shillings she had saved to put up a single-room house on the land her father left her back in the village: insurance in case her luck runs out and she needs to go home.

Agnes's mysterious immune system has garnered her considerable fame in the world of AIDS, but little else. She lives a life almost totally unchanged from her first days in *umalaya* thirty years ago. "I can buy our daily food out of what I earn, and that's all," she told me as we sat in the shade of her bustling alley. "I don't feel famous. It's only that my problems push me to do sex work. If I could find something else, I would."

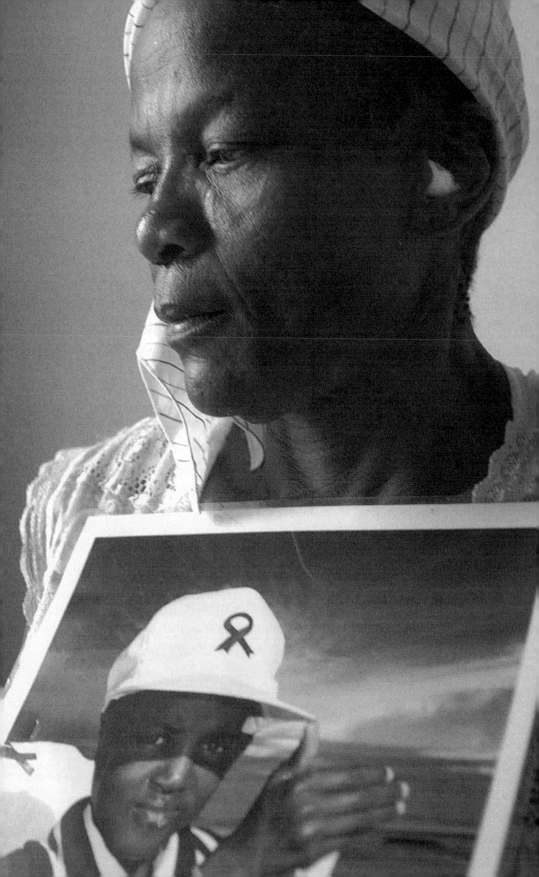

# NINETEEN

# MphoSegomela

his is my favourite story about Mpho.

Her mother had died of AIDS when Mpho was a baby, and her granny, Magdeline Segomela, was raising her. They lived in the township of Alexandra in Johannesburg, where Magdeline belonged to a support group for grandmothers looking after orphans. The group helps the women out in different ways—emotional support, and perhaps a food parcel every month, and a small bus to take the children to school because many are too sick to walk. Magdeline was supposed to collect money from the group to pay the bus driver, but one day in 2003 she was feeling sick, so she sent Mpho to collect the 100 rand—about $15.

Mpho (pronounced *Mmpoh*) picked up the money as she was supposed to, but she didn't give it to her granny. Instead she spent the whole 100 rand—a small fortune for a child in Alexandra—on a bag of candy at the corner store. The next day she gave sweets to every kid at school, and basked in her sudden popularity.

When Mpho was naughty, she was naughty with style.

I got to know ten-year-old Mpho and her family not long after I moved to Jo'burg, through Rosina Letwaba, the indefatigable nurse who had founded the support group. Every week, it seemed, she had another tale about Mpho. "That girl!" Rosina would say, throwing up her hands in mock

# When Mpho was naughty,

horror. I loved the stories, and in early 2005 I asked Magdeline if I could start writing regularly about her family. Mpho, then twelve, her grand-mother and her aunt Ellen were all living with HIV. I thought that telling their story, as they struggled to keep their family together in a community with one of the highest HIV infection rates in the world, might get news-paper readers interested in AIDS. Who could help but be seduced by the misadventures of Mpho? Even when her legs were almost too thin to hold her up, she had a plan to scheme her way into another 100 rand or bag of sweets. She was going to take trips, to get famous. She was wiry and feisty and she had inherited her grandmother's scrappy survival instinct.

But I spent much of that year on the road elsewhere in Africa, and somehow I didn't get around to sitting down with Mpho and her family. And then suddenly it was Thanksgiving, and Rosina and her sons came to my annual dinner. She and I were rolling out the crust for pumpkin pie when she told me quietly that Mpho was sick, that she was "coming to the end of her journey."

I heard her, but I didn't take the news too seriously: Mpho was tak-ing ARVs, which Rosina had helped her get through a local clinic six months before. I was sure—I convinced myself—that she would thrive. I knew Mpho had survived far, far past the life expectancy for a child born with HIV, and that most likely her organs were irreparably damaged before she got the drugs. But I let her bravado persuade me she would be fine. I made a mental note to go out to Alexandra that week and see her. But I got busy.

Rosina called late the next Friday night. Mpho was gone. And her aunt Ellen had been taken to a hospice for palliative care, by then too sick to stand.

# she was naughty with style.

A few days after that, the neighbours put up a tent in the street outside Magdeline's cement-brick shack, and the women started chopping vegetables for the community feast that accompanies a funeral here. A strong gust of wind swept through the township and nearly blew the tent away. As the canvas walls billowed and snapped, Rosina gave a bittersweet laugh. "That's Mpho," she said about the tearing wind. "She's so angry."

The next day we came for the funeral. Magdeline—who had buried one daughter, and now a granddaughter, and saw still another funeral coming—looked at us and said simply, "I'm lost. I'm lost."

At the graveyard, there was a struggle: there was no space left for new graves, no space for the coffin of even a frail and wasted twelve-year-old. And so in the end, they reopened the grave of Mpho's mother, dug down, and buried her daughter on top.

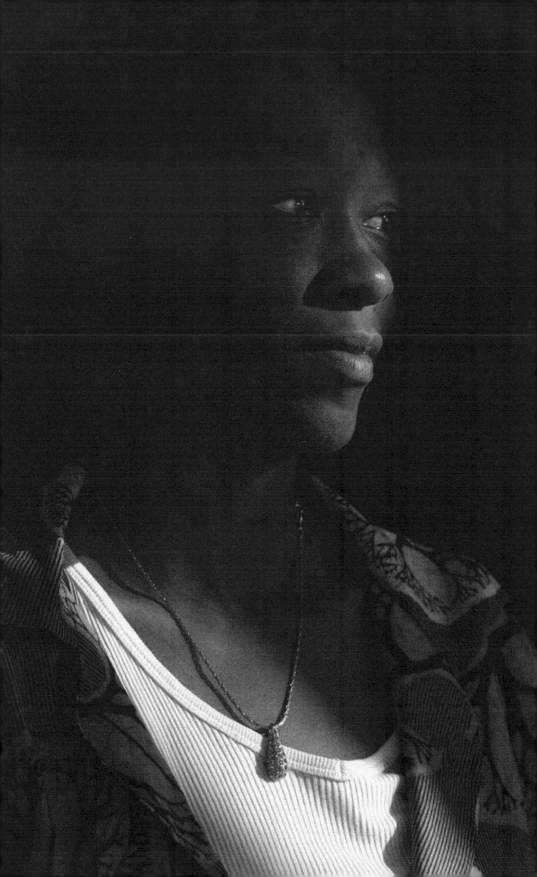

# TWENTY

# AnneMumbi

**T**he first time Anne Mumbi saw a classroom beneath a tree—a teacher with chalk and slate, and rows of children crammed together in the shade—she could hardly believe it. How could this most cliché of images of Africa be here in her own town, in the 1990s? "I said, 'My God, is there no government in Zambia?'"

There was, of course, a government—but it wasn't doing much to help. Anne was then a project officer for the international development agency Oxfam. She was working on income projects—things like teaching people how to grow hydroponic vegetables for sale in city markets—in the poorest neighbourhoods around Kitwe, a copper-mining town in the north. And the children beneath the tree had just joined her caseload. Their parents had been thrown out of their jobs and lost their homes in the privatization of Zambia's mines. They had come back to the villages outside the city, where there were no schools—and the Ministry of Education said it couldn't build them because its budget was frozen by the World Bank as part of the same economic restructuring program that privatized the mines. (The bank, on the other hand, said the government was so bloated and corrupt that it could borrow no more money, and would have to pay teachers with what it had.)

Anne did what she could. But before long her income-security work started to be undermined by something else. As fast as she trained people in new skills, they died. "Everything we were doing was amounting to nothing because we were losing people—we would have a person who is very good with volunteers, a leader in the community, and then they would die and you lose the skills and the knowledge. You see fields grown over because the parents died and the children don't know how to grow there." The problem, of course, was AIDS. One in four adults in the Kitwe area was infected.

She saw it at work, and she felt the impact of the disease at home as well, as she and her husband, Alex, took in their siblings' orphans. Soon there were nine of them living with Anne, Alex and their three children. "You just say, 'Here we are—come!'" she said. "But twelve kids . . . it's expensive. We were extending our house, planning to rent it out. Little did we know that we were extending it to fill it up with children."

Anne decided that it was time to tackle the big problem head on, and she left her aid work for AIDS work. Today she runs an organization called Children in Distress. CINDI, as it is known, was founded in 1994 by women alarmed by the growing number of grimy, barefoot children living in the streets in Kitwe. They started to register the orphans—no state agency was doing it—and to organize "community caregivers" in the slums and villages to keep an eye on the kids and let CINDI know what they needed. They started free "community schools" to teach the basics of literacy, and arranged food parcels. When I visited, there were twelve thousand orphans on their books, and twenty thousand had been assisted since the group began. One CINDI orphan, Anne told me with pride, has grown up to serve as Kitwe's deputy mayor.

I met Anne, a slim woman whose quiet and calm demeanour masks a fierce sense of social justice, in the southern African winter of 2006, when I was writing about the impact of AIDS on Zambia. Over the course of the few days we spent together, she showed me the many ways the disease has hit Kitwe. In shelters run by CINDI, I met orphans with no one to pay their school fees, and sick kids the staff was trying to get on ARVS. She whisked me through Kitwe Central Hospital, where the director showed me his staffing charts—more than half his jobs for nurses were vacant. Sixteen patients had died in the past twenty-four hours, all but one of AIDS. I saw a small workshop where a CINDI instructor was training a dozen grandmothers and teenage girls—each of them raising three or four orphans—how to use ancient Chinese treadle sewing machines: Anne has a vision of employing the women in a garment company to supply overalls to the mines. She took me to a village called Kamfisa, forty-five minutes' drive outside of town, where we met women too old and too tired to work their family plot and wondering how to feed the grandchildren they'd been left with. We stopped outside the Home Affairs office, and Anne pointed out the people with bedrolls, planning to sleep out overnight so that they could be first in line in the morning—with only one or two clerks left to work in the office, it can take months to get a passport or a death certificate.

All of that was bad, but Anne wanted me to understand that there was more to it than just the disease. A 25 per cent HIV prevalence rate would be devastating anywhere. But a complex mix of factors has made the impact of AIDS on Zambia far worse than it might have been—factors that have made people poor, and thus at greater risk of exposure to the disease (because they are migrants, or sell sex, or because they can't buy condoms or pay to go to school and learn how to protect themselves), but also factors that have undermined the ability of their country to respond. This part of the picture is much harder to see; it takes a thoughtful observer such as Anne, someone who works in the eye of the pandemic but retains the ability to step back and assess the larger picture.

Zambia has never had a war. It has fertile land, plenty of water and vast mineral riches. And yet its people are as poor today as they were at independence, nearly fifty years ago—and when AIDS came, they had nothing with which to cushion the blow. Anne was quick to stress that African governments have played a key role in all of this: Zambia is one of the poorest countries in the world today due in no small part to poor economic planning, bad governance and corruption. But just as important are forces beyond its control.

# "It's so heartbreaking, with all its rich resources, and good rain. a peaceful country

As Anne explained it, there are three main external variables in the AIDS equation: debt, aid and trade. Zambia, and indeed most of the countries of sub-Saharan Africa have for decades been crippled by debts their government couldn't possibly repay; they have received aid that was insufficient and poorly targeted and often took as much money out of the country as it brought in; and they have been foiled by trade barriers that shut their products out of rich-country markets even as they were forced to open up their own natural resources to foreign exploitation.

Before I met Anne, I had seen this pernicious mix of factors at work in other parts of Africa. Lesotho, where the prevalence rate is 29 per cent, had, a few years ago, a healthy garment industry, the result of a piece of U.S. legislation passed in 2000 that gave a handful of African countries tariff-and-quota-free access to the American market for textiles and a few other products. It was a big boost for Lesotho: soon nearly half of the country's employed workers, almost all of them women, stitched sweat-shirts for the Gap and other U.S. firms. Those workers didn't earn much—an average of about $5 a day—but they had jobs. They could pay school and medical fees, and the factories provided Lesotho's struggling government with a tax base to try to build its health-care system.

Then, on 1 January 2005, a World Trade Organization deal called the Multi-Fiber Agreement expired. Most people had never heard of it—certainly the women stitching T-shirts in Lesotho never had. The deal gave the poorest nations preferential access to major markets, including the United States and the European Union, by limiting the amount that giants such as China were allowed to export. Without the cap,

# this beautiful country
# its good land
# It's a beautiful country,
# —with a terrible policy."

Lesotho couldn't compete and the factory owners, most of them Taiwanese, packed up and headed for China and Bangladesh, where a better-developed industry would allow them to make their T-shirts more cheaply. Overnight, half of Lesotho's garment industry disappeared, because no regulations were in place to protect a vital industry in one of the world's poorest countries.

I have seen it in Kenya, too, where the health system is desperately short of staff, and in need of nurses in particular to mount a full response to AIDS. The International Monetary Fund, as a condition of its loans to the Kenyan government (and a condition of the lending recommendations it issues to other donors), sets economic targets which restrict the number of civil servants Kenya can employ, on the grounds that public sector spending must be checked. And so the government can't hire new nurses even though there are thousands of out-of-work nursing graduates in the country.

But in a couple of days spent with Anne around Kitwe, I could see the intersection of all these things—the impact of international trade policy, of external debt, of aid and the lack thereof—in one grim package. "In this country, only people with a bit of money have life," she said as we left the hungry children in Kamfisa. "We're just in a terrible state. People die in their houses because they know that if they go to the hospital there is no one there—they die without even a little Tylenol to relieve the pain because they can't even afford that. It's so heartbreaking, this beautiful country with all its rich resources, its good land and good rain. It's a beautiful country, a peaceful country—with a terrible policy."

Anne was born in Kitwe in November 1966; when she was a young girl her father retired from the national police force and the family moved up north to farm. She always wanted to go back to the city: "I knew the only thing that could take me out of the village was education. So I read and read and read—I never let a book pass without reading it." Her escape plan worked, and she graduated from the University of Lusaka. There she met and married Alex Mumbi, who was entering the new field of computer engineering, and they moved back to Kitwe when he got a job with the national copper-mining company there.

Zambia, she explained as we drove past the mountains of slate-grey mine tailing dumps that surround Kitwe, is all about copper. That was true at independence in 1964, and despite years of discussion of economic diversification, it is still true today. At independence, the government bought a 51 per cent interest in most major mines, taking back mineral rights that had been held by British mining companies. In the early 1970s, that meant plenty of state revenue: the mines, then at peak production, produced 12 per cent of the world's copper. Kitwe, when Anne moved there as an adult, was a company town: the state-controlled monopoly eventually employed thousands of people, who were members of strong unions, and housed them in tracts of small, bright-coloured houses all around the city.

But the state-run mines became overstaffed, inefficient and unproductive; managers let the infrastructure rot. Then the price of copper slumped, and Zambia's export earnings were cut in half. By 1976 the government had a cash crisis and began to borrow more and more money from the IMF. A mere decade later, Zambia was one of the most indebted nations in the world.

The IMF was happy to lend, but the bailout came with conditions: the financial agency ordered President Kenneth Kaunda to liberalize the economy. That meant lifting price controls, devaluing the kwacha, cutting government spending and ending costly state subsidies that kept the price of food and fertilizer artificially low. Those moves, Anne recalled, hit poor people hard—the price of food shot out of reach overnight; the 85 per cent of people dependent on agriculture could no longer afford fertilizer and saw their small crops shrink. At the same time, the international lenders imposed user fees on social services, saying every citizen, no matter how poor, should pay something for health care and education. "The policies of these giant institutions, the World Bank and the IMF—they devastated us," Anne said. "The subsidies had helped tremendously in food security. At the same moment that they put fees on education, all kinds of people were being thrown out of work. So many kids were out in the street."

Other international donors were pouring money into Zambia, but that funding came with the caveat that the country had to follow the whole IMF prescription. There were other strings attached, too: some 40 per cent of aid for Zambia was earmarked either to pay expensive consultants (who come from G8 countries) or was "tied"—meaning it had to be spent on goods or services from the donor country. Donor governments funded projects that met their particular interests, regardless of how that fit with the Zambian government's plans; the donors made their aid pledges on one-, two- or at best five-year cycles, so a project would be in vogue for Zambia one week and cancelled the next. In Kamfisa, for example, Anne pointed out several hand-pump boreholes that are remnants of a foreign-funded clean-water project begun a decade ago. The pumps broke a few years later, but no one in the village knows how to fix them, so people in Kamfisa went back to drawing their water from a muddy, unprotected spring.

Meanwhile, the structural-adjustment program drawn up by the World Bank didn't have the anticipated effect of boosting the economy; by 1990, in fact, the economy had shrunk so much that nearly three-quarters of Zambians were living below the poverty line. President Kaunda had little choice but to privatize some of the state-controlled agencies. The public service was bloated with clerks appointed through nepotism; bureaucracy was so thick that foreign investors would have nothing to do with Zambia.

Kaunda, who had ruled a one-party state for decades, finally called multi-party elections in 1991. He lost to Frederick Chiluba, who launched a much more ambitious privatization plan under the auspices of the World Bank. In fact, Zambia was soon held up as the bank's poster country—and Chiluba's liberalization program allowed him to borrow even more, so that total debt stood at more than $7 billion by the end of the decade. Now, Anne explained, a huge portion of Zambia's earnings, and donor assistance, were flowing right back out of the country as debt repayments. The primary demand the bank placed on Chiluba was that he privatize the copper monopoly; by 2000, foreign firms had purchased most of the mines. No question, Anne said, those mines had become inefficient and absurdly overstaffed. But with privatization, hundreds of thousands of workers were left unemployed overnight. They included her husband, Alex, who had been a hardware engineer for the state mining company. All the rows of mine houses emptied out, and people crammed into shacks in the slums or headed back to their villages. And a few weeks later she came across the children sitting crammed together at "school" beneath a tree.

"Of course we blame the international financial institutions, which pushed through the privatization without thinking about the poor," she said. But Anne also laid much of the blame on Zambia's own government. The global anti-corruption agency Transparency International has called Zambia's privatization program a "looting exercise." The process was finagled so that members of the ruling elite, who partnered with firms from South Africa, North America and Europe, got a cheap deal on national assets. A parliamentary investigation later found that untold millions of dollars of proceeds from the sales never made it to the national treasury. Some of the cash wound up in the foreign bank accounts of cabinet ministers; some was used to shore up Chiluba's political fortunes.

No one in Zambia was insulated from the corruption, and in 1994 it worked its way right into Anne's office. The cabinet minister representing the Copperbelt was awarded 96 million kwacha (then worth $100,000) to repair a bridge near Kitwe—but spent only 5 million ($4,800) of it, leaving the bridge a shambles; the rest of the cash "disappeared." Local residents were furious, and Anne lent a group of them her fax machine to mount a campaign. The Zambia Broadcast Company sent a reporter, who put pictures of the crumbling bridge on TV—and was promptly fired. The minister showed up in Anne's office a few days later, threatening to "destroy" her. Anne was unshaken. "I said, 'Bring the books. If you say you are the father of the Copperbelt, you cannot steal from your children.' He said, 'No one talks to me like this!'" The community activists raised such a ruckus that President Chiluba was obliged to investigate where the money went. A tribunal found the minister responsible—so he was removed from his job. Within months, however, he had been appointed to the protocol team in the president's office and nothing further was said about the bridge (nor was it fixed). Anne was disgusted, if not surprised. "I realized I had touched a live wire."

As Anne told me this story, we were driving past vast tracts of unused farmland, green even in the southern African winter because Zambia has vast reserves of water. "Copper is not the only thing this country has," she said. There are opportunities in the cities for manufacturing and industry, for example. "And the government talks about small-scale mining, tourism, agriculture. But still we are depending on mining. Only tourism showed any growth, but the businesses are owned by South Africans and they take the profits out of the country. Small-scale miners and local farmers can't access loans. The ones who need help never get it."

Her country could be an agricultural powerhouse, she said—she knows, from her work in the villages, how fertile the land is, how people could grow not only food for themselves but market crops, if they had assistance for irrigation and fertilizer. Kitwe is close to the border of the Democratic Republic of Congo, a massive untapped market, but instead of local farmers growing food to sell there, trucks carrying South African and Kenyan fruit and grains rumble through town. "The land is owned by the mines or the chiefs—very little of it is available. Anyone who wants to buy land and clear it has to go through several different government ministries, and the bureaucracy is torture."

Anne has worked with farmers trying to expand into commercial coffee or flower production, but given the way global trade works, she said, there doesn't seem to be much point. "When you talk about trade, policy at the international level affects us—we're not at a level where our local farmers can participate on an equal basis," she said. "The West has a history of exports. Their agriculture industry is well developed and they export at volume. Our farmers have ten bags or forty tons—not a million tons." Africa's share of global trade dropped from approximately 4 per cent in 1970 to 1.5 per cent in 2004, in large part because international trade laws are entirely stacked against the continent. Rich countries heavily subsidize their farmers (cotton growers in the United States, or dairy and produce growers in Europe), allowing them to export into Africa at prices against which African farmers can't possibly compete. At the same time, those rich countries protect their own markets with tariffs and quotas that keep out African products. The amount that the G8 countries spend subsidizing their own farmers far exceeds the total amount the G8 sends to Africa in aid money.

In recent years, "trade not aid" became a mantra of international donors. Frustrated that poverty in Africa remained unsolved by the influx of $500 billion in aid money since the late 1960s, they began to cut grants, and instead championed foreign investment and private-sector-driven growth in the hope that these would have a more lasting effect. It was, as Anne showed me, a good theory in the abstract but one that breaks down entirely in the face of the reality of Kitwe. "Who would invest here?" she said. "You have a workforce with high rates of HIV, no infrastructure, the only lucrative industry is extractive and it could leave at any moment."

In 2005, Zambia got the promise of new help. After a massive campaign by activists that included the anti-debt Jubilee 2000, Make Poverty History and the celebrity-heavy "One" initiative, culminating in the simultaneous Live8 rock concerts around the world, the leaders of the G8 countries met in Gleneagles, Scotland, to draft what was touted as a new deal for Africa. They promised 100 per cent debt cancellation for qualified countries (those, that is, who had the World Bank stamp of approval on their economic policy); trade reforms that would end subsidies and quotas on poor-country exports; universal access to AIDS treatment within five years; and an additional $50 billion in aid for poor countries, double the current level, by 2010, with half of it for sub-Saharan Africa. And, they said, they would make it better aid—with fewer restrictions on how to spend it and more freedom for recipient governments to determine their own priorities.

On the debt front, this meant good things for Zambia. The country had already had some relief from its massive foreign debt a few years earlier when the international financial institutions had proposed a "heavily indebted poor countries initiative." HIPC, as it is known, recognized that no country could get out of poverty if it was spending as much as a third of its budget on debt repayment—which many countries in Africa were (vastly more than they were spending on health and education). Often, these countries were paying debts that grew out of Cold War spending sprees or the whims of corrupt dictators. South Africa, for example, is still paying off the loans that bankrolled apartheid. Under HIPC, borrowers who followed a plan of economic and governance reforms had their debt payments partially suspended, and if they stayed "clean" for a few more years, some of their debt was cancelled outright. The process was painfully slow, but finally in 2000, Zambia qualified for the cancellation of $3.8 billion. That figure was a bit less than half its external debt, and it left billions more. So few countries received real relief that debt became the focus of the grassroots Jubilee 2000 campaign, which finally won the G8 promise of total debt eradication. On January 6, 2006, the IMF cancelled debts from nineteen of the world's poorest countries, including $6.5 billion from Zambia.

Then Zambia, like many other countries, channelled the freed-up money into social spending, making basic health care free in rural areas and for all people over fifty-five and under five. It pledged to hire 4,500 teachers and build dozens of new schools, to hire health-care staff and to buy more drugs, including ARVs. This, Anne said, held some promise.

But within months of the G8 summit, there were ominous signs that the pledge on aid would not be kept. In order to make it to the promised

Some evenings, when she
light and goes to lock the
more child, in dirt-stained,
waiting at the door,

$50 billion by 2010 through the proposed graduated increases, the G8 countries would have had to increase their aid spending by $3.5 billion that first year. In fact, spending increased by only $1.6 billion. A key part of the promise to Africa was more money for AIDS. But when the Global Fund held a pledging conference three months after the G8 summit, rich countries met less than half the fund's estimated needs, leaving a $3.4-billion shortfall. The United States is the single largest donor to the fund to date, accounting for nearly a third of its budget, but AIDS activists calculate, based on the size of the American economy, that the U.S. share should be three times the amount it gives now, while Canada is giving only a quarter of its share, and Australia an eighth.

On trade, the picture was even more grim. Five months after the G8 summit, negotiators gathered in Hong Kong for a key round of talks meant to level the playing field for the developing world. But the meeting produced no end to subsidies—the United States refused to stop payments to its cotton growers (which would have been a boon for Africa, boosting prices of this key crop by at least 10 per cent), while France and Italy wouldn't give up subsidies for their farmers. Rich nations also refused to remove tariffs on value-added products, thereby locking poor countries into continuing to export low-value raw materials rather than building up their processing industries. The G8 had agreed that 97 per cent of exports from Least Developed Countries would be free of duty or quotas, but because those countries export such a small range of products, the 3 per cent loophole allows rich countries to exclude the handful of key sectors, such as textiles like those Lesotho T-shirts, which they view as finally switches off the office, she finds one too-small clothes, or curled up at the gate.

threatening to their own economies. And, in return for the 97 per cent, the G8 demanded that developing countries make radical cuts in tariffs on industrial goods—opening up their own markets to businesses from abroad that are better developed and difficult to rival.

Meanwhile, many of the policies from the structural-adjustment era remain in place: the Zambian government is restricted by the World Bank from spending any more than 5 per cent of GDP on salaries for civil servants—so unless growth takes off, that means no more nurses at Kitwe Central Hospital.

Many evenings, Anne is still at her desk long after sunset, a mountain of files and paperwork held in a pile by the strategic placement of her well-worn Bible. The demand for CINDI's services seems to grow all the time, she said—while more people with AIDS are on ARVs in the area, it is not enough to have any visible impact on the death rate. The government has made primary education nominally free, but because schools are so under-resourced, they demand "development fees" or other add-on charges that continue to keep children out of class. Every week, her staff registers more orphans who need a place in CINDI's community schools, or food parcels, or someone to take them to the clinic and buy them medication. Some evenings, when she finally switches off the light and goes to lock the office, she finds one more child, in dirt-stained, too-small clothes, waiting at the door, or curled up at the gate.

She worries that CINDI's funding—which currently comes from private European and Canadian charities—may not be any more sustainable than the aid on which the Zambian government relies. "Our partners may not always want to help," she said. So she is trying to expand CINDI's work away from the food parcels and fee-paying and into enterprises such as the garment factory for miner's uniforms.

After long days at the office, Anne goes home to her overflowing house. She is determined to try to stanch the impact AIDS has had on her family. She gathers all the kids around the kitchen table on Saturday nights, twice each month, for discussions about sex. "We have stopped using traditional modes in our culture, where a grandmother or an aunty would have been the one to talk openly about those things—we're not living in those communities any more, that role is totally broken." So she and Alex take a deep breath and talk frankly to all their kids. It has paid off; the children announced that they all wanted to be tested for HIV. "I said, 'What if you are found positive?' They said, 'It's okay, it's better I know and if I get sick I can take medicines.'" She has other, more subtle, strategies at work as well: for example, the household runs on a rota where everyone, even the boys, has to make a meal each week. "You must put every effort in place to import a different culture. We need a culture that teaches girls assertiveness, and one that values life."

If Zambia can raise a generation that remains HIV-negative, she said, then there is much to be hopeful about. And yet she looks at her kids—the twelve at the kitchen table, the hundreds and hundreds who come to CINDI centres each week—and she wonders what kind of a country they are going to inherit. "Zambia without HIV would be very different—we've lost a lot of the brilliant young people I knew at university. Teachers, public servants. Your development depends on the human capacity you have." And despite their best efforts at CINDI, there is a limit to what they can give these kids. "It's no longer a matter of school fees, it's the *care*. The children are not growing up in a stable household— they don't experience family care. What kind of leaders will we have in twenty years if these are the children we are growing? They are the next generation of doctors, but is this the kind of education to make them into doctors? Or leaders?"

Through CINDI she does her best to keep that next generation off the street, and she and Alex do what they can for the children they inherited. But for things to change, Zambia needs leaders who will govern honestly, and win its battles on the world stage. "And that," she said, "is a lot to ask of these children."

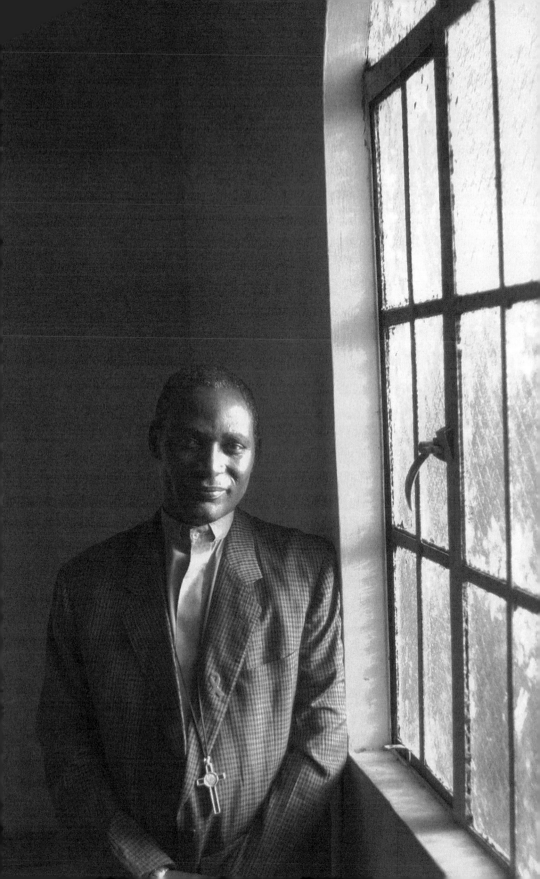

# TWENTY-ONE

# Gideon Byamugisha

"God," the priest said, striding out of his little chapel, "should be left out of this." Late-afternoon sunlight was streaming through the blue and yellow stained-glass windows, and he was warming to the topic. People are forever dragging God into discussions about AIDS in Africa—they talk about God's curse, God's vengeance on sinners, God's great test of humanity—but in the learned opinion of the Reverend Canon Gideon Byamugisha, God doesn't belong there at all.

"God did his part the day he showed how HIV is transmitted. If God wanted to punish us, we would still be searching. But in the first ten years we knew the roots of the cause, and of prevention. In the next five years we knew the roots of prolonging life. God gave us wisdom." That was God's job.

Now it is an issue of politics, economics, gender and access to resources. Big, messy, complicated issues—human issues. It's so much easier to invoke God than to deal with any of those.

Gideon has given these matters considerable thought, as I quickly discovered when I travelled to Uganda to visit his parish outside Kampala in 2006. I had seen him speak a few times, and heard him quoted often, and I was curious about the unconventional ideas on AIDS that came from this slight man in a clerical collar and sober grey garb. He invited me to visit his small congregational centre, where he was in the process of constructing a shelter for AIDS orphans.

Gideon is from Kigezi in the southwest, near Uganda's border with Rwanda. Born in 1959, he is the eldest of fourteen children. He qualified as a history and geography teacher, and worked as deputy headmaster at a secondary school, before deciding in his twenties to study theology and become an Anglican priest. At the seminary, and later when he began to teach at the theological college, his interest lay in esoteric questions about the philosophy of religion. These more temporal matters, of HIV and the power and equity issues that underlie its spread, were thrust upon him only later, more of an assault than a vocation.

Back in 1990, Gideon and his wife, Kellen, had a new baby daughter, Patience, and they were making plans to go abroad. Both were accepted to graduate programs at a British university, and they were, Gideon said, eager to study, to travel and to grow together into a life in the church. And then one day in April 1991 his vibrant wife—his twenty-five-year-old wife— woke up with chest pains. A week later, she was dead.

Gideon barely remembers the next few months, left suddenly alone with a baby daughter and a demanding ministry, his dreams of life in England abandoned. He does remember a visit from his sister-in-law, Eunice. Eunice is a nurse, and she was with Kellen in the hospital for the last few days of her life. She alone knew that Kellen was tested for HIV, and for six months she had been living with a secret: Kellen was positive. Finally Eunice worked up the courage to tell Gideon.

He was stunned, and scared—could AIDS have killed Kellen that quickly? Could it kill him? Could it kill his tiny daughter? He went immediately to be tested, then waited an agonizing two weeks for the results. He, too, was HIV-positive. (Their daughter, to his relief, was negative.)

Then Gideon faced a huge dilemma. He could not imagine keeping this a secret. "I didn't think I could live a double life—put on a smiling face, have my students asking, 'How are you, teacher?' 'I'm fine,' when I'm not fine. The preacher would say, 'Is there anyone with prayer requests?' and could I say no when actually I need all the prayers in the world?

Would this be a person of integrity?" Yet there was not a single member of his church living openly with HIV. Not just in his diocese, or his country, but anywhere in Africa. If people knew he was infected, he stood to lose his job, his ministry, his whole community.

Nevertheless, he told. First the principal of the college and then other staff members. "At the college they said they would support me, but they told me not to tell anyone else." Gideon rejected that idea. "I said, 'I am not going to accept for you to be comfortable at my expense.'" He told his students, who were, for the most part, encouraging, and then began to tell—and warn—the wider church community. "It was very risky," he said. "It's still risky. There are still people who are uneasy about my message—'Why is he talking all these stories? Doesn't he care about the image of the church?'"

But Gideon did not see HIV infection as something that undermined either the church or his moral authority as a priest. "There is not one time I ever felt guilty about my status," he said. "The only regret I have is that I lacked information. I have all this education—two degrees, one first class—but I failed an HIV test."

As word spread, there was one thing everyone wanted to know: how he got infected. "I always say, I am a priest who did some good things like some of you, and failed in some, like others. But because I lacked information, I got infected." He doesn't know when it happened: he and Kellen did not test before their marriage, so either of them might already have had the virus. Plus, in 1988, Gideon was in a serious cycling accident and needed a blood transfusion (at a time when few blood supplies in Africa were screened for HIV) and many injections. "I never asked if the syringe was clean."

Over the next couple of years, Gideon adjusted to a public existence. In 1995 he agreed to speak at the pan-African AIDS conference, held that year in Uganda. There, the sight of him in his collar caused a stir: it was nearly unthinkable, a priest saying he had HIV.

Gideon's parish is located about twenty-five kilometres outside Kampala. To travel in and out of the city he takes mini-bus taxis, which

# It was nearly unthinkable,

often have logos emblazoned on their rear windows: "God Protect Me" and "Safe in the Arms of Jesus." In the streets, he passes the Allah's Mercy Halal Butchery and Trading Store and the Jesus Saves Pharmacy. Two of the four television channels in the country show religious programming all day long. President Museveni is a born-again Christian, and the first lady likes to lead prayer vigils in the streets of Kampala. Uganda is a country soaked in religious faith, and it is not unusual on the continent: Africa is the site of the most rapid growth in followers of both Christianity and Islam.

Christianity came to Africa some fifty years after the death of Jesus, spread by disciples down through North Africa as far as Ethiopia. The next Christians in Africa were Portuguese and Spanish explorers who came ashore to plant crosses in the sand and claim the Cape of Good Hope for God and king. In the 1800s, missionary societies mounted efforts to convert the African heathen, and began constructing the networks of mission schools and hospitals that still operate today. There were 8.7 million Christians in Africa in 1900; there are 390 million today. The Centre for the Study of Global Christianity, in Massachusetts, says that the technical centre of the Christian world—the point where there are equal numbers of Christians to the north, south, east and west—is Timbuktu, in mostly Muslim Mali, and predicts that that point will shift west to Nigeria in the next hundred years.

About half of African Christians belong to either the Roman Catholic or Anglican churches, traditionally the strongest faiths here. (More than half of the world's eighty million Anglicans live in Africa.) But many Africans are leaving the once-dominant churches that originated in Europe for the new evangelical and Pentecostal churches that have adapted more deftly to African societies. These new churches work

# a priest saying he had HIV.

in local languages, employ local music and worship practices, and emphasize a healing and deliverance approach: the faithful ask God for specific protection—from unemployment, or burglary, or HIV infection by a philandering spouse—and the strategy appeals in societies where most people have real questions about their day-to-day survival. The evangelical religions emphasize tithing (paying 10 per cent of one's income to the church), a practice that resonates with many indigenous animist African religions that require sacrifices of food or livestock.

Islam came to Africa in the seventh century, first with invading armies from the north that swept down through the powerful kingdoms of the Sahel and into West Africa, and later with the Arabs trading in slaves and minerals who colonized East Africa. Today some of the ancient Muslim societies endure, such as the centre of Islamic learning founded in Timbuktu in the twelfth century, while many converts are being drawn to the faith through social agencies funded by the Persian Gulf states, which bring education and clean water to long-neglected areas, and through "missionaries" much like those used by Christians a century ago.

The strength of the churches and mosques, and the depth of faith of their followers, means that religious organizations have a social and political power in Africa that is barely conceivable in the West. Only Sudan and Somalia have governments that explicitly try to govern under religious law (in their cases, sharia), but in almost every country religious organizations are the core of civil society and a main provider of social services. Thus they have played a central role in the response to AIDS—and in most cases, their record is grim.

Religious organizations, Gideon said, have both inadvertently and deliberately contributed to the spread of the disease and to the shame and fear that surrounds it. Most churches say that abstinence and fidelity within marriage are the only permissible ways to protect oneself from AIDS. The Catholic Church, with 116 million followers in Africa, still forbids the use of condoms; the Southern African Catholic Bishops' Conference, whose faithful live in the most infected nations in the world, warned in 2001 that "condoms may contribute to the spread of AIDS," creating baseless fears that the virus could somehow pass through latex; the Catholic prohibition on condoms extends even to couples in discordant marriages. The new churches are no better: evangelical sects in Nigeria fill converted airplane hangars for services where they promise to cure AIDS through prayer. Many churches condemn those who are infected as sinners who have received the punishment they deserved, and the same message has been spread in Islamic mosques and Hindu temples as well.

Yet Gideon said he can understand this response. "You can't blame religious leaders," he told me gently. "The first people to talk about AIDS in Africa communicated it wrongly: they said, 'This is a new disease, there is no cure, there is no vaccine, it's coming through homosexuals.' And then in East Africa we added prostitutes and truck drivers." No one anticipated the scale of the epidemic, or that it would sweep through the population as a whole; priests and imams thought that it would be enough to encourage moral behaviour. "They did not expect even religious leaders and their children to be affected."

From the moment Gideon made his HIV infection public, he found himself in heavy demand for public meetings and conferences, expected—as the only openly HIV-positive priest—to speak for all faiths, for all religious leaders. "By 1998 I was feeling my energy going down. I wondered, 'This ministry is so big: why am I alone?' Whenever someone introduced me, they would say, 'This is the first religious leader publicly living with HIV in Africa'—and I would think, Where is the *second*? I knew I could not possibly be the only one."

In fact, in his travels he had been collecting business cards from other clergy who approached him privately to disclose that they, too, were infected.

And it occurred to him that if he could get them all together, they might feel a comfort in numbers that would allow them to speak more freely. In 2002 he secured funds from a Christian aid agency to host a meeting in Harare. Forty-two religious leaders, ordained and lay, attended, and Gideon said it took them only a day to decide that they wanted to organize into a continent-wide network—both to support and care for each other and to try to have more influence on the policies of their churches. "I thought," Gideon said, "that if we are many, the positive change would come quicker."

Only Christians attended that first meeting, but they quickly moved to open up the group to other faiths. "It's the same stigma if you're Muslim, Hindu or Baha'i," he explained. However, it is also true that those African countries that are predominantly Muslim have, on the whole, much lower prevalence rates than predominantly Christian ones. This is due to a combination of geography—in West Africa, home to substantial Muslim populations, the far less infectious strain HIV-2 predominates—and to differing cultural mores that lead to lower rates of sexual transmission. Muslim societies, for example, often put much stronger prohibitions on premarital sex and infidelity than do Christian ones, while traditional values such as polygamy or a girl proving fertility by bearing a child before she weds coexist with Christian custom. And while Muslim marriages are more often polygamous, those marriages in conservative societies are usually faithful, and as such offer little risk of HIV infection.

Gideon's recruits decided to call themselves ANERELA—the African Network of Religious Leaders Living with or Personally Affected by HIV/AIDS—and gave themselves the tasks of offering "a network of support without judgment" and acting "as witnesses to hope and forces for change" in their congregations and communities. At first only a handful of them had the courage to join Gideon and publicly declare their HIV-positive status. But they all recognized that they occupied a unique position: their institutions are often the most powerful force in a community, and they had innate authority and credibility, plus a ready-made audience and access to resources and infrastructure far greater than that of most groups dealing with HIV/AIDS.

Today ANERELA has 1,300 members from eleven countries, although not all those members are open about belonging. Three-quarters of the members are male, reflecting the predominance of men in positions of religious authority on the continent. "Not all are positive or know their status, but they are personally affected," Gideon said. "Perhaps they have lost a spouse or a parent or are nursing a child. You see, a person with a positive daughter gets the same amount of stigma as a person infected. People say, 'This disease is for promiscuous people so this pastor does not control his children.'"

As the response to AIDS has accelerated in recent years, the engagement of religious organizations has grown too, and Gideon is ever more in demand. President Bill Clinton invited him to the White House in December 2002 for a meeting on faith-based responses to the pandemic. The international aid agency World Vision asked him to head its church partnerships program on AIDS. He has written widely on HIV stigma, and his own experience, "not dying from AIDS, but living through it." He began his own care program, which includes the orphan centre to house, educate and entertain children from the congregation.

In the years since his diagnosis, he has come to see religious leaders as being in one of two camps. "Some are using their authority to control AIDS—they gather children, adults, and give them information about prevention. On the other end of the spectrum you have leaders who are using AIDS to control their congregations. The first group will do everything possible to destigmatize AIDS: those who are positive are welcomed, supported and prayed for. When they reach their deathbed they will be escorted well, given all possible care for their journey to the other world. The others are intolerant people who say, 'Stop sinning,' or 'The wages of sin is death.' They quote Deuteronomy 28: 'The Lord shall make the pestilence cleave unto thee'—they say repent or you will die of AIDS. And they don't like us people with long-term survival." At this, the impish priest gestured to himself, shiny with health fourteen years after his diagnosis, and had a good chuckle, before turning serious again. "They use the disease to justify their failed sermons and their theologies of damnation."

But, he said, as we sat in the shadow of his chapel, their logic is weak. "If this is a disease come to punish sexual sinners, why are there sexual offenders who are not infected? If this is God's punishment, why are virgins getting infected after they waited thirty-four years for their marriage night?" The pastors who talk of punishment like to quote the Bible, he noted, and indeed Christian scripture says, for example, that the family of a sinner will be punished up to the fifth generation. But then, Gideon observed, the Bible has been used to justify all manner of things—apartheid, Jim Crow laws, the slave trade.

As angry as the moralizing makes him, he also believes that credit is due: over the years that he has lived publicly with HIV, he said, many religious organizations have made considerable progress on the issue. In some of the worst-affected communities, churches have taken the lead in the response. In Uganda, Catholic Relief Services is a major supplier of testing and counselling, and has put thousands of people on ARVs through the clinics it supports. In Zambia and South Africa, individual priests and nuns have defied the Vatican to distribute condoms. Church hospices have nursed the dying, and congregations have organized teams to tend the sick and raise the orphans. Gideon was heartened when, in 2006, the Catholic Church announced that it would reconsider whether it might be a "lesser evil" for people in marriages where one person has HIV and the other does not to use a condom rather than spread the infection. (The Anglican Church has permitted the use of condoms in marriage since 1991.)

In March 2006, Kenya's Anglican Church issued a public apology for having shunned people with HIV/AIDS. "Our earlier approach in fighting AIDS was misplaced, since we likened it to a disease for sinners and a curse from God," Archbishop Benjamin Nzimbi said at an ANERELA gathering. "We apologize for earlier abandoning our flock, which was as a result of our ignorance of the disease, but today we are more informed." Islamic institutions, which have come later to the game because their faithful were less affected, have also recently launched education, orphan and anti-stigma projects.

"It is not God's plan that
old. Or twelve. Or thirty.
knowledge and skills to
death. Now it's about

But at the same time, more and more religious communities are
requiring mandatory HIV testing for any couple seeking to be married in
the church or mosque; some deny marriage to those who test positive. And
many institutions continue to promise cures for AIDS at healing services.
Pastors still do not understand the mechanics of infection, Gideon said,
believing that people are cavalier or stupid, instead of weak and ill-
informed. "Their message of 'choose life'—well, who would choose death?"

In those first years after Kellen died, Gideon, missing her terribly, tried
his best to raise their daughter, Patience, on his own, and considered the
conundrum of his celibate life. He had a fatal illness on the one hand, and
on the other, he was still very much alive. He did not believe God meant
him to be celibate, but as a devout priest, he also had no intention of
seeking physical or romantic comfort outside the vows of a marriage. Yet
how could a person whose days were numbered get married? He concluded that the best solution might be a wife who was also living with
HIV—who would have no illusions about what his infection might mean
for their future together. He began asking around among friends, and he
was introduced to Pamela, then twenty-one, a capable and congenial
woman whose husband had died of AIDS not long before. Yet when they
announced their engagement in 1995, church leaders were appalled and
tried to dissuade them from marrying. Their reaction left Gideon baffled,
and frustrated that they could not understand the immense loneliness
that comes with living with HIV, or the care with which he and Pamela
had made this choice.

people die at eight years
God gives us the
prevent or postpone
what people do."

The next year, he fell ill. He lost 20 kilograms in a matter of months, and his CD4 count plummeted below 100. His doctor said Gideon would be lucky to live six more months without antiretrovirals—but the drugs were not available in Uganda to anyone but the wealthy elite. The bishop of Kampala launched a crusade to keep Gideon alive, mobilizing the church network, and found support from two individuals Gideon called "Good Samaritans" (one in the United States and one in Singapore) who began to send him ARVs in 1997. He has enjoyed excellent health ever since, and Pamela remains healthy without treatment, working long hours in the hardware store she owns.

When they were married, they agreed they would not have unprotected sex because of the risk of cross-infecting each other with a different strain of the virus or of giving birth to infected children. But Pamela hankered for babies. Gideon pleaded with his new wife to be patient: "I said, 'Let's postpone until God gives us a miracle." The miracle came in 2000, in the form of public access to drugs to prevent mother-to-child transmission. They had a daughter, Love, and another two years later, Gift. Both girls are HIV-negative.

The couple nevertheless faced criticism for this decision, too. "People said, 'Don't you feel guilty that you're producing children who will be orphans?'" The answer is no. When his girls are old enough to ask about their parents' HIV status, Gideon plans to tell them, "Your parents waited seven years to have you so as not to infect you. If we die it will be because society is so unjust that we could not get access to the resources to keep ourselves alive." And then, he said, "it's up to the kids whether they blame their dad who took the risk, or the world, which is not a fairer place. If I die now it will not be of AIDS. It will be of the structure of society."

Gideon has been radicalized by his struggles and the deaths of people he loved, and he speaks most often of AIDS not as a medical or spiritual issue but as a political one. "We know AIDS needs a clinical approach, but that won't succeed if poverty stays the same, literacy stays the same, inequality stays the same. HIV shows us the holes in our relations: how we trade with one another, how we relate as genders, how we deal with one another on governance and politics. Those are the things we have to fix."

In his own country, he saw George Bush's President's Emergency Plan for AIDS Relief (PEPFAR), the biggest donor, insist on abstinence-only education as the pillar of prevention programs; the driving force, he said, is not an understanding of what's best for Ugandans but rather the influence of the evangelical Christian lobby in the U.S. on the Bush administration. He watched PEPFAR insist for its first crucial years of operations that Uganda use its funds to buy only brand-name drugs, not the generic drugs that cost five times less and so might have treated five times as many people—not, he said, because those branded drugs were any better, but because of the lobbying strength of the U.S. pharmaceutical industry, which was determined to keep the generics from gaining ground in the AIDS field. These are the kind of inequities he will help his three daughters understand.

Life with AIDS has also reshaped Gideon's faith. He remembers, more than a decade ago, when he gave sermons about "God's will" or spoke at funerals about God giving and taking away. He doesn't do that any longer. "It is not God's plan that people die at eight years old. Or twelve. Or thirty. God gives us the knowledge and skills to prevent or postpone death. Now it's about what people do. We've never seen a disease so vulnerable to the right policies. HIV is not like cancer. If we adopt a combination of prevention approaches, and protect the blood supply, the disease will retreat like it did in the U.S. We know what works. We can defeat AIDS if we do the right things. And we *know* what those are."

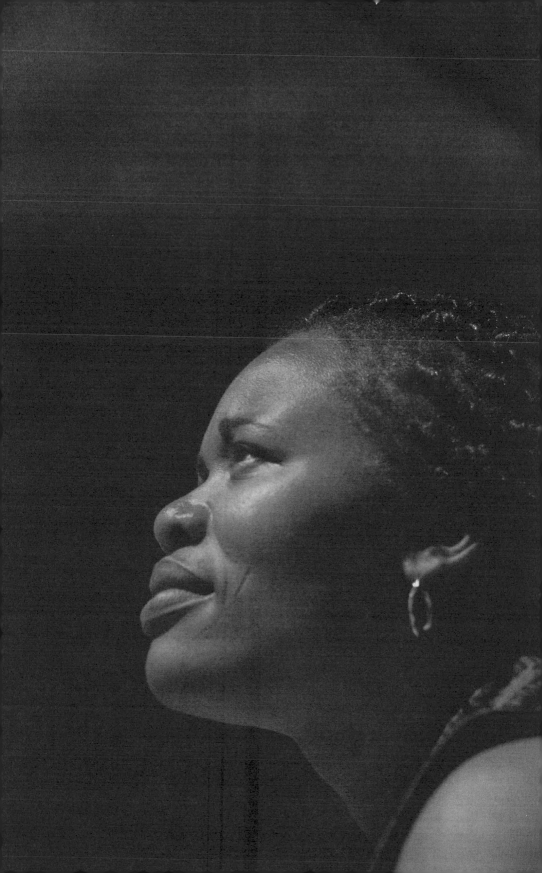

# TWENTY-TWO

# IdaMukuka

A t the clinic, they said she could work magic. There was no case too difficult—no fuming husband, no terrified wife, no cavalier playboy, no churchgoing matron—whom Ida Mukuka could not persuade to test for HIV. A man would arrive at the red-brick Chelstone Clinic in Lusaka sputtering about his cheating wife and the scourge she had brought into their home, and in a couple of hours Ida would have him signing up for training to lead a support group for other men with HIV. She could sweet-talk those who tested HIV-negative into using condoms (or at least promising that they would); she could persuade those who tested positive to repair their marriages and join a class on positive living. She strode into teeming markets with a bull-horn, exhorting people to get informed about HIV; she toted her metaphoric soapbox into every kind of public gathering, explaining how people could protect themselves.

Ida is warm and comfortable talking to people, quick to squeeze a hand or give a shoulder a comforting pat, and it is easy to see why she makes a good counsellor. But those attributes mask her real weapons: acting skills worthy of Broadway and the mind of a military strategist. Each time a weeping woman turned up in her office, telling Ida she had tested positive and that her husband had beaten her or chased her from their home, Ida leaned across the desk, eyes narrowed, and started to scheme.

"I'd ask, 'What does your husband respect? Law? Government? The clinic?'" If the wife thought he respected authority, Ida drafted a formal letter on clinic stationery requesting his presence at an appointment. If, when he showed up, he was the bustling, self-important type reluctant to put down his cellphone, Ida would assume a lofty manner, then glance at her watch and mention in her best BBC English that she was terribly busy and fitting him in specially. "I could become a professional person. I behaved like a person with many degrees, although I have only a certificate. I convinced the men that they must pay attention."

If, on the other hand, the husband was an unemployed fellow from the slums who had never set foot in a government office, then Ida might just happen to bump into him in the street outside his house (after quizzing his wife about the address and his comings and goings), then lean on his Zambian hospitality for a cup of water. Ensconced in the kitchen, she would talk, in a roundabout way, of the clinic and the services available to people with HIV.

She eased the shame, pointed out the futility of blame, made clear that life could go on. She mended so many marriages in the years she spent as chief counsellor that she lost count. "When it was a very tough case, they would say, 'This one needs Ida.'"

She brought more than savvy and empathy to the job: she was also filled with a messianic devotion to the cause. Her brother Boyd—the protective big brother who walked her to school every day when they were kids—had died of AIDS. He had a good job as an accountant at the Ministry of Finance before he fell ill. In 1996 he caught tuberculosis and couldn't shake it, and finally Ida made him test for HIV. There was no treatment for AIDS in Zambia then. "He said, 'Ida, do you know there are no medicines?' I said, 'But it's better to know.'" She pumped him full of every immune booster on the market, but they did not stop his decline. Four years after he first got sick, she took him home to their parents. He raved with dementia, or sat in a corner "like a potted plant," she said, barely aware of his family. His mother and sisters changed the diapers he wore for constant diarrhea, and carried his once-powerful body from room to room.

Before Boyd lost his hold on reality, he and Ida had long, thoughtful conversations about AIDS. He didn't want to tell people what he had, but he told Ida she should, after he died: "He said, 'I used to change partners and if you don't say the truth, people won't learn. So don't hide it. This disease is nasty. It could destroy the whole family.'" When she told me this story six years after Boyd's death, tears streamed down her face, soaking all of her tissues, then all of mine. "He said, 'When I'm not there, join the fight.'"

Soon after he died, she saw a job opening for an HIV counsellor at the government clinic in the Chelstone neighbourhood of Lusaka. This, she thought, was just what Boyd was talking about. "I was very excited. I wanted to do it for my brother." And she figured her experience with Boyd would give her insight. "That's where my strength for advocacy lies—I've seen it first-hand." It was a pleasure, if not a surprise, to find she was good at it. Zambia introduced a program to prevent mother-to-child transmission of the virus, and she took on the job of persuading pregnant women and their partners to test. Soon she had a cohort of HIV-negative babies whose lives she knew she'd helped to save.

And then one day in 2003 she found herself on the other side of the table, sitting across from a counsellor with test results in his hand: her results. Ida Mukuka, well-known and widely respected AIDS counsellor, had HIV.

Ida likes to move quickly through this part of her story. The way she tells it now, she barely paused over the results. "Testing and knowing my status put me in a better position as an activist," she says briskly.

But I knew Ida then, and I remember how she kept the news secret from most people, except those closest to her and some colleagues who worked in the field of HIV. Mutual friends have told me how she couldn't tell her parents, didn't know how to tell her boyfriend, how she grew paranoid that she had swollen lymph glands in her neck and was convinced everyone was looking at her, seeing AIDS in her face.

In fact, she was quite well. She took the test not because of a persistent health problem but because of her counselling clients, who, when she urged them to test, would quite often ask, "What about you?" It was hypocritical, she thought, not to have tested herself. But she never thought she might be positive. "I was *shocked.*"

And yet, she said, she shouldn't have been.

Ida is from Kabwe, the copper mine town where Winstone Zulu opened the Kara Counselling outpost. When she was growing up, the mines and the national railway headquarters drew people like her parents from all the surrounding villages. Her father was a mechanic, her mother cared for their eight children, of whom Ida was fifth. They lived in what's called a "compound" in Zambia, an urban slum. Ida's father, who had only a year or two of school himself, wanted more for his children. "He would sit down and tell us, 'If you get education, you will live on your own, you will not need to depend on someone.'" Ida dreamed of going to the university in Lusaka. But she was in Grade 8 when, in 1986, the World Bank forced Zambia into the structural-adjustment program that privatized many industries. Her father was among the thousands of people who lost their jobs. Her family struggled to cover the fees, but she graduated from secondary school, shelved her dreams of further study and took her hard-won high-school certificate to Lusaka. She found a job at Chilenje Orphanage, washing diapers—but that didn't last long. Ida is a natural leader, and soon she was promoted to supervisor of the caregivers.

Around that time she began to hear about HIV. Women were abandoning babies at the home, skinny babies who were either fussy all the time or silent; staff suspected that more and more of the children they took in were infected, their parents dead of AIDS. The orphanage sent Ida to Kara Counselling, where Winstone supervised training in the basics of HIV and in how caregivers could protect themselves.

In the summer of 1994, the University of Zambia sent a researcher to evaluate the services at the orphanage, and Felix Mukuka took a quick shine to Ida the matron. He was ten years older than Ida, and she wasn't sure she wanted to marry him. "But then my heart went because he said he would pay for me to go and get my degree. Three months after we began courting I was pregnant." Felix didn't want to deal with her family, and instead arranged a hasty marriage by a judge; one of his friends pretended to be Ida's uncle and gave her away. Sometimes, she told me, life with Felix wasn't bad. He landed a job as an intelligence officer in the president's office, and they had a nice two-bedroom government flat in town. They had two daughters, Theba, a thoughtful, quiet child, and Mwamba, the stroppy image of her mother. Ida took an eighteen-month psychology and counselling course—not a university degree, but all she could manage with the girls at home. Felix, however, drank heavily; sometimes he and Ida fought viciously, and sometimes he hit her. He would disappear for days when he was drinking, and she suspected he had lovers. Then, six months after Boyd died, Felix left for a course in Germany. A week later, Ida received a call saying that he had collapsed and was unconscious in hospital there. He was flown home, and died a few days later. He had bought their daughters new dresses in Germany. They wore them to his funeral.

Felix was never tested for HIV, but Ida is certain he died of AIDS: not the lingering illness that most often characterizes the disease in Africa, but a system collapse brought on by the virus. When she was pregnant three years earlier, she had been offered an HIV test (purely for research purposes, since mother-to-child prevention was not yet available) and asked Felix take the test with her. He refused, and forbade her to test either; thinking back, she concludes he must have suspected he was positive. A quarter of adults in Lusaka had the virus by then.

The news that Ida was positive startled me when I finally heard it from a friend—I knew her as one of the savviest, most dynamic AIDS educators I'd seen anywhere in Africa. I didn't know if she had only recently acquired the virus, or now learned of an infection she'd had for years. But either way it was a lesson in the complexity of the disease, in how we are all vulnerable, even the people with the most knowledge and access to resources, because it preys on our moments of weakness, and on our least manageable emotions of shame and fear and denial. I wondered, then, if Ida would continue to work in AIDS.

On a lazy Saturday morning in June 2006, Ida and I were talking on the porch of her flat in Lusaka when I raised the subject of the irony in her positive test result. She led me into the cramped bedroom, away from the kids and the visiting relatives and the clients of the hair salon to which she rents out the back veranda. She cleared a space on her bed, wedged in beside her daughters' bunks and all their heaps of clothes and hair barrettes and skin creams. And this time, she admitted that, activist or not, the knowledge that she had HIV had left her stricken. She had spent all those years counselling people to accept their status and live positively, but she found the words were meaningless when confronted with her own infection. "I had feelings of self-loathing, that I'm no longer a human being." Rather than taking comfort in her experience and skills from Chelstone, she felt profoundly discouraged. "I'd seen the way people were treated, chased, abused. Now I realized, this is a battle that I'm going to have to fight, too."

But over that next year, Ida learned first-hand about the value of peer support. Winstone encouraged her to tell people she was infected. "He told me, 'You will be a big activist,'" and that her messages about prevention and discrimination could only be more powerful if she spoke as a person infected herself—although he was also frank about the hate and hostility he had encountered in his twelve years of living openly with the disease. Gradually, Ida acclimatized to the idea that she had the virus; in fact, the diagnosis had changed little in her life. She told her boyfriend, Cornet, a Congolese refugee she had met at church. He was unfazed. She travelled up to Kabwe to tell her parents, who took the news reasonably well, knowing there were more resources available for people with HIV compared to the time when Boyd fell sick. The only people she didn't tell were her kids. Theba asked her flat out one day, and Ida, caught off guard, dissembled, which she regrets. It took her daughters so long to find their

# 'I live with HIV. to live with HIV. I want it to end here.'"

feet in school after their father died, she said, that she couldn't bear the idea of setting them back again with the fear that they might imminently be orphaned.

Thoughts of her children redouble Ida's commitment to her job. "I always tell myself, 'I live with HIV. I don't want my children to live with HIV. I want it to end here.'" The best weapon for her daughters is a better education; she is determined that they will go to university so that they never make the sort of choice she did in marrying Felix. And she wants them to be comfortable speaking openly about the disease. "In 1991, if people had been united, I wouldn't be infected today—if people had talked about it, if there was information," she said. "This is the place where HIV should have been halted: even before the U.S.A. or Canada. People there live individualized lives; here we are a community. We go to our neighbours. Yes, we are poor, God did not give us resources. But he gave us the most powerful thing—life in a communal environment."

As Zambia geared up its response to AIDS, Ida was promoted to the job of community outreach coordinator for the Center for Infectious Disease Research in Zambia, a partnership between the government and the University of Alabama doing research and HIV treatment across the country. She swapped her bright print Zambian outfits for power suits and high heels, and, drawing on the model with which she had such success at Chelstone, she hired sixty veterans from her support groups—many of those blustering men—to run support services in all the public clinics offering ARVs. They counsel on living positively and on drug adherence. And increasingly, as more and more people get on to treatment in Zambia, Ida puts an emphasis on the importance of safer sex: too many of her clients, even her well-trained facilitators, get healthy again and return to having "live" sex, without condoms, heedless of the risk of being infected with a different strain of the virus and ending up drug-resistant. "I tell them, 'You people are going for live sex but it has consequences in the very near term—in two years we will watch you die of AIDS.'"

While Ida is supposed to be focused now on managerial issues, she still gets a call, every week or two, asking her to help with a counselling case. A few days after our Saturday-morning talk, I popped into her office and found Ida on her way out: she'd been asked to help after a husband stabbed his wife with a screwdriver when she told him she had tested positive. Ida sighed, picked up her handbag and cellphone, and called a taxi to take her to the neighbourhood where the couple lives.

"They said, 'This one needs Ida.'"

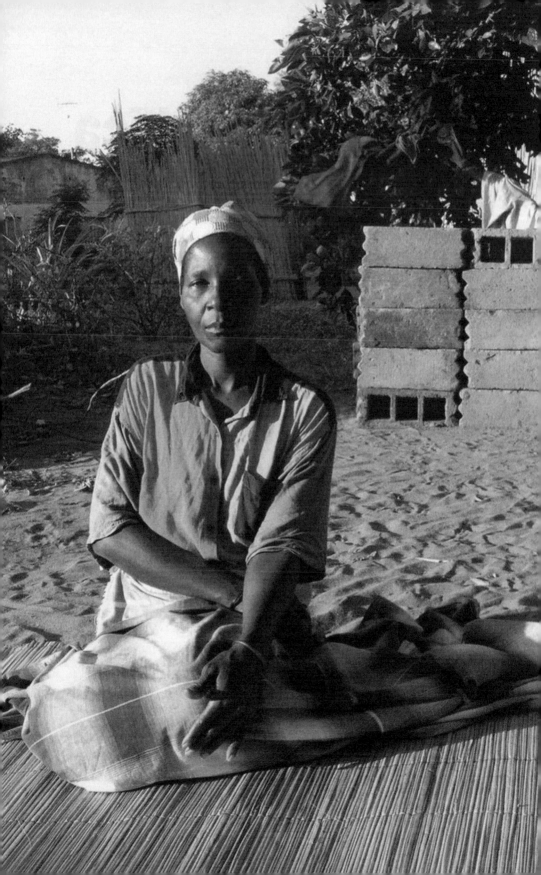

# TWENTY-THREE

# AnitaManhiça

When Anita Manhiça was in her late teens, a gold miner named Azarias Mateusse came calling: he offered her father a substantial *lobola* in blankets and grain and cash, and Anita soon found herself married. Her new husband went back to the mines in South Africa, but every year or two, when he came back to their village outside the town of Xai Xai in central Mozambique—a few miles from the home of Manuel Cossa and his family—Azarias brought Anita treasures from the city: a mattress, a sateen bedspread, new lengths of bright print *capulana,* the cotton wraps that Mozambican women wear as skirts and shawls and slings for their babies. He built a sturdy brick house with glass in the windows and a roof made of tin sheeting, the only house like it in the village.

Then, in 1985, when Anita had a couple of small children, Azarias came home with something else: a new wife, a girl of just twelve. Anita was chagrined: suddenly Azarias was putting up another brick building in the yard, and she had to share the outdoor kitchen with this girl, a child really, whose plump body her husband clearly relished. But then he went back to the mines, and she and the girl-bride, Alba Houhou, learned to live together. Alba helped with the children, and lent her strong young arms to the work in their *mashamba,* growing maize and beans.

Azarias rose through the semi-skilled jobs at the mine until he earned more than $500 a month—a fortune in Gaza province, where the average monthly income is just $25. He bought a television, a luxury almost unheard of in the village, and had an electric wire run all the way in from the main road to power it. And then in 1993 came wife number three—Graçinda Invane, twenty-three and beautiful, with high cheek bones and big gold eyes.

Once again Anita, now relegated to the position of tired oldest wife, shuffled her possessions around the homestead and made room for another family. "I couldn't say anything," she said. "He was happy having other wives, and I had to just accept it." Her husband was a Christian, like everyone else in the village, but in Xai Xai that is perceived as having little relevance to the age-old tradition of polygamy by some men prosperous enough to support more than one wife. "I was unhappy at first. But I got used to it."

Anita reckoned that it was around 1998 when women in the village started to talk about a disease from the mines in South Africa, an illness the men caught there that sent them home fevered and coughing, to waste slowly away. They began to hear about "SIDA"—the Portuguese acronym for AIDS—and how a person could catch it from having sex. Each of the wives wondered to herself if Azarias might bring this SIDA home. He was still plenty interested in sex. But they did not discuss it, not with their husband and not with each other. "I never talked to Azarias about AIDS. It would be very frightening talking to him about that," Anita told me with a shudder. What, I inquired, would have happened if you had asked him to wear a condom? "He would have beaten me," Anita replied, astonished that I even had to ask—beaten her, and almost certainly chased her from the home.

In the end, that happened anyway. In 1999, Azarias came home ill. He had all the signs of the miner's disease, but he accused Anita of infecting him, saying she had slept with other men while he was away. He told her to leave her children behind, gather her *capulanas* and get out, to go back to her family, that she was a whore not worth the price he had paid for her. "But he is the one who gave me the disease, because I never had another man,"

Anita said, still pained by Azarias's accusation, which had the whole village speculating about the morals of his prim and dignified wife. He died in 2000, at forty-two, and Anita could then return to the home they once shared. Alba and Graçinda welcomed her, the children were overjoyed— and it was a relief from the terrible shame.

By the time I met the women in 2004, Anita was forty-three, gaunt and racked by a bone-shaking cough. She was spending her days on a straw mat in the dusty yard, with barely the strength to tug a faded *capulana* around her shoulders. The stifling heat left me almost immobile, but Anita was shivering. She told me how, the year before, she was plagued by a sharp pain in her lungs. So she walked two hours to the clinic at the provincial hospital and had an HIV test. Then she endured the month-long wait for the result (the hospital didn't have a lab and had to send all its samples to the capital, Maputo). The test was positive. "I was not shocked," Anita said slowly. How could she be, when the whole village whispered about how Azarias had died?

Alba, who was then thirty-one, was also starting to feel unwell. Some days she hardly had the energy to get dressed. She sent the children to fetch water from the village standpipe—she couldn't go herself. She told me she was trying to work up the courage to go and test; her stony expression suggested she was already fairly confident of the result. Graçinda, then thirty-three, had read the signs at Azarias's house; she had taken her two children and moved to town a few months earlier. When she passed by to visit that day, she still looked healthy and strong. Unspoken, as we sat in the shade of the big mango tree, was speculation about whether she was infected as well. They were not powerless, these women—there was a hint, from each of them, that Azarias's tyranny had been countered by small acts of insubordination—but in one key way, they had been unable to protect themselves.

There was something sweet about the three of them and the warm family life they had built out of a situation they would never have chosen— it was clear that Anita had only a few weeks to live, and Alba and Graçinda were keeping close to her. But later, walking along the sand track back to

# What, I inquired, would asked him to wear a beaten me," Anita replied,

town, I thought about how many times I had heard this story, in so many other countries: from married women who had every reason to believe their husbands (miners, soldiers, truckers or simply loyal patrons of the local tavern and its bar girls) might be at risk of AIDS, might in fact be infected and getting sick. But they could not refuse those men, because they would be shamed, beaten, divorced, chased away, lose their children, be left with no money and no land and shunned by their families and neighbours, the taunt of promiscuity hanging over them. While nominally protected by law from violence and abuse in most countries, these women would rarely be judged to have property or child custody rights—not, in any case, that it would ever occur to a woman such as Anita to take a case like this to court.

When a response to AIDS was belatedly mounted in Africa in the late 1990s, it focused on high-risk groups—those truckers and bar girls. But by 2002 the statistics showed that married, monogamous women were the group at single greatest risk of infection. And no interventions at all targeted them.

Biology and the mechanics of heterosexual sex make women—who have much greater surface areas of the mucosal cells to which HIV attaches, and whose genital tissue is more likely to tear during sex—many times more likely than men to be infected with HIV in each act of intercourse. Yet a toxic mix of culture, religion and economics often leaves women unable to do anything about that risk.

What Anita needed was a way to protect herself without having to negotiate it with her husband, since using a condom, even a female condom, de facto required his consent. By 2004, I knew there was a way, at least in theory: something called a microbicide, a chemical that a woman

# have happened if you had condom? "He would have astonished that I even had to ask.

could apply in her vagina that would, quite simply, kill HIV. She would apply it hours or days in advance, and never need to tell her partner about it. The urgency was obvious: at that point nearly two-thirds of the people living with HIV/AIDS in Africa were women. In southern Africa, girls and women aged fifteen through twenty-four were two and a half times more likely to be HIV-infected than their male counterparts. And yet, for a whole host of reasons, it would still be seven or eight more years before a microbicide might reach Xai Xai. Much too late for Anita and Alba, of course, and probably too late for Graçinda, too.

To understand the history, I called Lori Heise, who heads the Global Campaign for Microbicides, a coalition of organizations pushing for HIV prevention methods controlled by women. Heise had been advocating for microbicide development since the early 1990s. Study after study shows that condom promotion can only do so much, she said. "When people are in a relationship with intimacy and expectations, they don't want to use them, for basic, human reasons. It's easy with new partners, casual partners, paying partners—many sex workers use condoms with their clients but not with their boyfriends. And that's where more and more people get infected."

When I asked Lori Heise why microbicides were still nearly a decade away, given the obvious urgency, she simmered with anger. "It's only literally within the last year or two that there has been any consensus or recognition at the higher echelons of power that this is an important component of AIDS prevention," she said. "When you talk to women, at any level, even women in the street in the United States or women in a village in Mozambique, they get it immediately, there's this instant spark of recognition: of course this is exactly what we need! But it has never ceased to amaze me how much resistance there has been among policy-makers and repro-ductive health workers, people you'd think would be the most obvious allies."

A lot of things lay behind that resistance, Heise said. First, ignorance and ill-placed optimism. In the early days of AIDS, when heterosexual women were not perceived as a risk group, a product to protect them was not a priority. Heise heard over and over again that all available resources were going into developing an HIV vaccine—no point diverting some of those resources into a microbicide, a complicated product unlike anything then available, which would be difficult to test, since women would be protected by a vaccine. Except, of course, the vaccine remained elusive, and the infection rate among women continued to climb.

Next, she said, the emphasis was placed on condoms, with the AIDS establishment convinced that with enough billboards and dis-pensers in truck stops, they would stop the spread of HIV. She called that an absurd bit of wishful thinking. "To this day so many people don't get why women can't use condoms in these marital settings—they say, 'If it were me, if I were at risk, I'd use a condom.'" Heise is a pragmatic person, not given to melodrama or overstatement, but she finally concluded that the underlying reason microbicides stayed totally off the scientific agenda, despite the ever-more apparent need, was sexism. "I resisted this analysis for a long time, but I think it has to do with the fact that it's women, vaginas and sex. There's been discomfort with and marginalization of this issue because it forces people to deal with women's bodies. People are very uncomfortable with transferring control to women and trusting them to make decisions in their own best interest."

Because of lobby efforts like hers, microbicides finally began to attract attention in the mid-1990s. But getting them on to the prevention agenda was only the first battle. Next came the research. A microbicide needs to stop HIV before it can attach its Velcro-like claws to the cells in the mucosal membranes in a woman's genital tract and thus infect her—and that is far easier said than done. Once a way is found to do it, it will take, at minimum, seven years to go from the first good idea in a lab through to animal trials, human safety trials and then a large-scale human efficacy trial, using at-risk women in a place such as Xai Xai, to see if it actually works. Once there is a working product, it will need regulatory approval, and have to be packaged, marketed and distributed in remote areas.

All of that is complicated, but the more immediate problem, even in 2004 when I met Anita, was that so few people were even looking for a microbicide. This product faces the same basic challenge that has hampered HIV vaccine development: a pharmaceutical company such as GlaxoSmithKline has to be convinced it has a reasonable chance of making money from a product before it pours millions of dollars into developing and testing it. But where's the market for a microbicide? HIV infection is still a minimal risk for women in rich countries (the major exception is black American women, who by 2005 were the fastest-growing group of new infections in the developed world). The market for a micro-bicide is Xai Xai and the villages and cities across Africa and the Asian sub-continent, where women cannot afford to pay patented prices—or pay anything at all. But sub-Saharan Africa is just one per cent of the global pharmaceutical market, and draws a correspondingly small amount of the drug industry's attention.

"There is not enough money to be made, so there is just no private interest," Lori Heise told me. "Then it falls back on to governments and foundations until it becomes a political issue." Right up to 2002, all the research on microbicides was done by non-profit and academic institutions or small biotechnology companies that were dependent on an uncertain flow of grant money. "The lack of pharmaceutical company interest in this has been a devastating blow," she said.

But a group of public health researchers in the United States decided to tackle the problem, and that year they formed the International Partnership for Microbicides, a sort of public-good venture capital fund, hoping to leverage money from governments and charitable foundations in order to bankroll the development work that pharmaceutical companies weren't interested in. The IPM and its warm and passionate director, Zeda Rosenberg, a microbiologist who headed the National Institutes of Health AIDS prevention efforts for years, had some early successes raising cash from rich-country governments—by the time I met Anita, the IPM had $100 million in its coffers. "It's not enough to get a product to market but it's a serious down payment in drug development," Rosenberg said. And then came the bigger victory: small, and then larger, pharmaceutical companies, lobbied by the IPM, began to take the highly unusual step of handing over their preliminary research and intellectual property, licensing the agency to develop drugs that showed potential as microbicides, often with an agreement for unrestricted, low-cost, large-quantity distribution in the developing world.

By late 2005, Rosenberg had new if cautious optimism in her voice when she talked about microbicide development. That year, the G8 leaders, in a communiqué after their annual summit, specifically identified microbicides as a key prevention technology. "There's clearly been a tipping point," she said. "People are starting to get it." Then both Bristol-Myers Squibb and Merck licensed new drugs to the IPM to develop them further—a new class of antiretrovirals called entry inhibitors, which worked by disabling that Velcro-like attachment through which HIV gets into a cell. The two companies were developing the drugs with an eye to using them as a treatment in people already infected with HIV, but when U.S. researchers tested them in monkeys to see if they prevented infection, they found the drugs worked better together than alone. The IPM stepped in to say it could facilitate development of the drugs used together as a microbicide, and the companies handed them over. By the time the International AIDS Conference was held in Toronto in August 2006, Bill and Melinda Gates had tapped microbicides as their big hope for stopping HIV. "We need to put the power to prevent HIV in the hands of women," the software tycoon told a crowd of tens of thousands of people at the start of the

# that it's women, vaginas and sex."

meeting, and he added that they would put hundreds of millions more dollars into the research effort through their charitable foundation. With that, microbicides became the talk of the AIDS world—a fifteen-year-old overnight sensation.

The latest microbicide candidates combine drugs that target HIV and interrupt its life cycle with a component (such as a detergent) to get in between the virus and the cells it tries to latch on to. Zeda Rosenberg hopes to use vaginal rings as a delivery method: the ring will slow-release the product so a woman could leave it in place for perhaps a month at a time. If people are going to use a microbicide, it will have to be a product that does not disrupt sexual relations or the ability to conceive a child, she explained—not if they want women to use it in a place like Xai Xai, where a woman's worth is calculated by her child-bearing abilities. This is an additional wrinkle for researchers, who need a chemical that zaps HIV but allows sperm to slip by untroubled.

People ask Zeda Rosenberg all the time why drug development can't be done any faster. To help me understand, she suggested I pay a visit to Gita Ramjee, who heads the HIV prevention unit for South Africa's Medical Research Council. She was acting as principal investigator on a half-dozen microbicide clinical trials by 2005. Ramjee works in the province of KwaZulu-Natal, where the adult HIV infection rate is about 40 per cent. When she tests a microbicide candidate, it first has to go through safety and basic efficacy studies that take a minimum of two or three years. Then, for a study to show whether a microbicide actually works she needs to recruit and screen women until she has two thousand who are not infected (that means screening up to four thousand women, because the prevalence rate is so high). She teaches the women how to use a microbicide—some, for example, are clear gels applied before intercourse by an applicator like that used for a tampon. The volunteers are also given intensive counselling about condom use and safer sex—as with vaccines, that's the basic ethical requirement for this sort of study—but Ramjee knows that many will still be exposed to HIV. In order to see if the product actually stops infection, and how well, half the women are given a placebo and half the real gel. Then Ramjee has to wait about three years, to see how many end up HIV-infected, and hope that that number is much lower (or, the eureka moment that no one in this field actually expects, that it's none at all) among those using the real microbicide.

That was the bad news. On the upside, Ramjee said, she has no trouble recruiting: the women in KwaZulu "are absolutely thrilled" by the idea of a microbicide. And while women such as Anita might need to make surreptitious use of the product (which a slow-release ring would allow), Ramjee pointed out that many men are equally enthusiastic about the idea. "Men also want a product like that. Some men say sex with a condom is not pleasurable, so if they have something that allows sex to be pleasurable, and that will prevent infection, men are also thrilled."

If one of Gita Ramjee's trials proves at least somewhat effective—say, a product that offered 30 per cent protection from HIV infection—Zeda Rosenberg and her team will swing into action to get it to Africa. First will come the regulatory hurdles: because there are no comparable products today, drug licensing agencies have many extra concerns. Rosenberg also worries about who will finance large-scale production—perhaps, she said, the Gates Foundation or the Global Fund. Then there's distribution. "In each country we have to look at, Where are women going to feel most comfortable accessing a product like this? At family planning clinics, STD clinics?" The IPM talks about teaming up with firms such as Unilever, whose beauty products are widely distributed in Africa, or Coca-Cola, the company with the widest network on the continent. "Maybe we put it on the back of Coke trucks with a health-care provider to go with them," Rosenberg mused.

That might one day get it to Xai Xai, for there was Coke for sale in the small shop at the end of Anita's road. I sat with her that day until the shadows were long and the sky streaked with orange, and thought about how a microbicide might have changed things for her. It is not a magic bullet either, of course—no small tube of gel could change the underlying inequalities that led to her infection—but it might have helped. Now Azarias's fancy television set still had pride of place in his small brick house, but the electricity was shut off long ago. The sateen bedspread was threadbare, and the small children wore worn hand-me-down clothes missing buttons and sleeves. And in the lean-to where the women cook over charcoal, there was only a small bit of maize left in the bottom of the sack. Anita lay on her straw mat, and the children brought her tin cups of water and peeled oranges from the tree in the yard. She watched them running back and forth in the sand, and smiled. "It makes me happy that all my children are healthy," she told me—they were all born before Azarias fell sick, and she is sure they are not infected—although she said calmly that her own time was running short.

I remarked, tentatively, that it all seemed rather unfair, the way things had gone in her life, and she smiled in agreement. "None of it," she said, "was up to me."

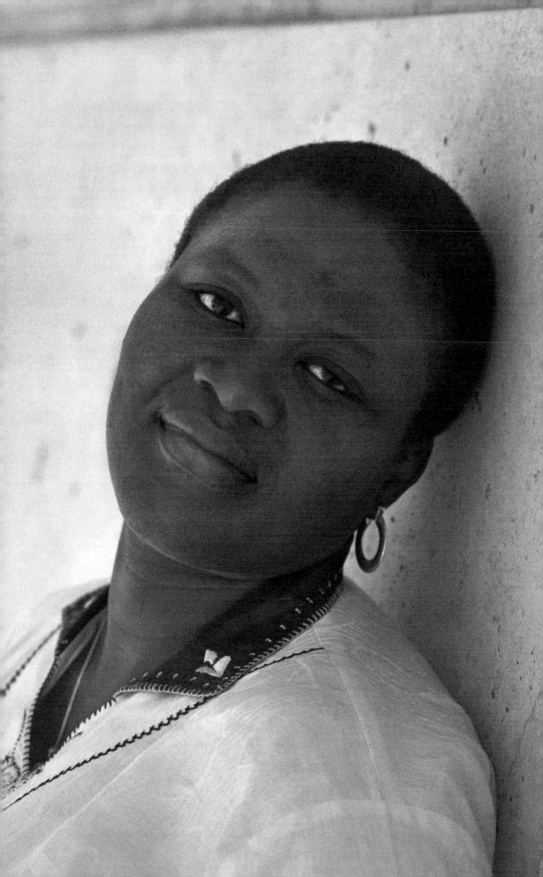

# TWENTY-FOUR

# Morolake Odetoyinbo

n that night in May 1998 when her husband came home with the news that he was infected with HIV, Morolake Odetoyinbo tugged him into their bedroom and cajoled until they made love. "He wasn't sure how I was going to take the news and I totally, totally wanted to reassure him. So that very night we did have sex. And even bringing up the subject of a condom was saying, 'Now there's a difference, things are different than before.'" She wouldn't let him say the word; she was determined to show that the diagnosis had changed nothing between them. "I promised him then that we were never going to lay blame."

Their marriage was in trouble at the time, and she feared this would be the thing that finally drove them apart. "Even though I never at any point wanted to get infected, in my heart I was really hoping, 'Let it be both of us, maybe that will bring us closer and maybe together we can fight this.'" Telling me this story seven years later, she paused, knowing that it probably sounded mad. "I say that in retrospect—it wasn't conscious at the time."

As I got to know Rolake, I learned that her two-year-old marriage had foundered because her husband was fooling around with other women—but she was determined to stay with him. Women all over Africa have told me how they could not leave their unfaithful husband, even when they feared (with, as it turned out, deadly prescience) that he might infect them with HIV. In dusty Swazi villages and bleak Mozambican country towns, I could understand—those women would be left penniless, ostracized and without options. But coming from Rolake, this argument was much harder to comprehend.

I saw her first at a pan-African AIDS conference in the Nigerian capital, Abuja, in late 2005. I was in the audience for a presentation, augmented with PowerPoint slides, on the AIDS epidemic in Nigeria, which had recently won the dubious title of the country with the third largest number of people infected, some four million. But there was a problem with the computer, the slides weren't working, and people sat patiently and fanned themselves with programs—this was, after all, chaotic Nigeria, where one doesn't really expect things to work, at least not quickly.

Then a young woman—already tall, and towering in black stiletto boots—leapt up on the stage. She wore artfully distressed jeans and a black T-shirt that proclaimed "Free HIV Treatment Now!" Silver hoops glinted in her ears; she had shiny Betty Boop lips. "As *if* it's not enough about the virus in my blood," she purred into the microphone, her Nigerian accent giving the words a rolling bounce. "Mmmm—now I'm giving them viruses in the computer too. *Sorrrry.*"

She let out a booming laugh, but only a few people in the audience joined her. The rest all looked bewildered—did someone just make a *joke* about HIV? You don't get much of that on the AIDS conference circuit.

In a minute or two the computer was fixed, and Rolake (pronounced Roe-*lah*-kay) gave a brisk, grim presentation on the state of AIDS in her country. Less than 10 per cent of those infected had access to drugs, she said. Just twenty-three of the country's thirty-six states had sites offering treatment; where it was available, the 1,000-naira ($8) fee for clinic visits kept away the people most in need.

"If Nigeria is the sixth biggest oil producer in the world, we should be able to commit to free treatment!" she snapped. "We don't have much time and all they do"—at this she gestured toward the main hall next door, where heads of government and the UN were meeting—"is talk, talk, talk." And so much of the conversation these days is about abstinence, she said;

a "remoralization" of AIDS is under way. Just when people have started to get over blaming and fearing the victims, the emphasis on abstinence, fostered both by international donors, particularly the United States, and by the strong religious lobby in her own country, is bringing the guilt back in. "I love sex with a passion," she said with another huge laugh, and a shimmy that made all of her many curves shake. "So we must have access to condoms. Some of us *need* to have sex. An abstinence-only campaign is unacceptable!" Once again, most of her audience gawked. A person with HIV insisting on her right to have sex? You don't hear that much at AIDS conferences either.

Rolake was, I soon learned, a film producer and newspaper columnist who was working as the national coordinator of the Pan-African Treatment Access Movement. As she made her way across the meeting grounds, everyone—American activists, South African doctors, Nigerian traditional leaders—wanted to talk to her. She couldn't take three steps without someone reaching for her arm; people wanted their picture taken with her. And so I struggled to understand why this tremendously smart and confident woman would go to such terrible lengths to hold on to a philandering husband.

A few weeks later, Rolake and I sat in one of several lounges in her parents' large house in a relatively peaceful neighbourhood of Lagos, and she explained it to me. It was terrifically sad, what she had to say, as she acknowledged herself. And it was also a crystalline example of how Africa— modern, bustling Africa, the Africa where Rolake lives addicted to her cellphone and Google and Belgian chocolates—is different from the West. "In this culture," she said, "divorce is your last option. Socially, culturally, religiously, everything around you screams 'No' to divorce."

A divorced woman has almost no hope of a relationship with a new man, she explained. "A single man, his family will come down hard on him: 'She's a divorcée, she's proven before that she can't keep a man at home.' Being able to keep a man and keep a home is how your womanhood is defined. Not the job you do, the head on your shoulders, it doesn't matter how intelligent you are." It was hard to believe, and yet here was Rolake, in her mid-thirties, living in her childhood bedroom in her parents' house after the shame of her broken marriage.

Rolake knows she did not have the virus when her husband was diagnosed with HIV in May 1998—three months earlier she had tested negative in a prenatal HIV screen (she lost the baby in a miscarriage a short time later). By October, when she tested again, she too was HIV-positive. Yet talking to me seven years later, long since separated and aware from friends that her ex-husband has not changed his promiscuous ways, she still assigned no blame. "It was just chance," she said. "Was this the first man I was with? No. Did I have protected sex with the others? No. It was just chance that I got this from him. Does that make him a monster? No. He did exactly what I did. He was just unfortunate, that's all. It could have been the other way round."

Her words echoed in my head for weeks afterwards. So much of the conversation about AIDS in Africa is about blame, much of that with good reason—there are a great many men who take sexual risks and infect their wives, who infect their children. There are so many women who are raped or forced into transactional sex by wars and disasters. But that's only part of the story. It is also true that many women are making conscious choices, overt or surreptitious, about lovers and sex—many of them living entirely within the parameters of what is acceptable or encouraged in their communities. And they have the misfortune to live in places where 10 or 20 or 30 per cent of people have HIV, but where few protective measures are available, perhaps none that they can afford except abstinence. And while abstinence looks logical, to some, in the face of the pandemic, it is not always, as Rolake pointed out, practical or realistic. Not everyone is going to stick to it all the time, and, as she said in a moment of gentleness, that doesn't make those people monsters, or even the authors of their own misfortune.

While Nigeria's HIV epidemic was swelling all through the 1990s, Rolake, like nearly everyone else, wasn't paying much attention. "I knew it was something that gay men, white Americans got, and some drug users. It was just not in my scope." There were a few posters touting abstinence and condoms at her university—and billboards that would come back to haunt her, big ones painted with a skull and crossbones and the message, "Beware: AIDS Kills."

Her husband was a soldier, and he was tested for HIV in a routine military screening. When he came home that night in 1998 to tell her he was positive, he made her promise she would never tell anyone. And while she was more determined than ever to keep their marriage together, she found that promise stifling: "Every single day it was in my mind but I couldn't talk about it—my husband never discussed the topic. HIV infection? Never. And if I couldn't discuss it with him then who could I discuss it with?" Four months later she confided in her father, whom she had always considered her closest friend. He persuaded her to go and get tested herself. She barely needed to read the results.

Rolake was just twenty-eight, but the doctors who tested her, and the billboards along the highway, made it clear her life was ending. "The message every single one of us got when we learned about our HIV infection—if not from the doctor, from society—was that we were going to die," she said. One thing kept her from breaking down: friends she had made when she produced a film about people with physical disabilities. "They taught me there's nothing you can't fight."

Rolake toughed it out in her marriage for four more years, keeping the secret, until she could no longer deny that her husband still had other lovers, and there could be no repairing this relationship. "It was at that point that I felt I didn't owe him anything any more." She moved back in with her parents, and six weeks later went public as a person living with HIV—which was, in 2002 in Nigeria, an extraordinarily brave thing to do. "More than anything else in the world I was tired of the silence." She started giving small public lectures, in churches, schools and workplaces, and soon joined the nascent Nigerian wing of the continent-wide Treatment Action Movement. A journalist asked to write about her, and Rolake agreed, on condition there was no photograph with the article. "Then I asked myself, how long are you going to keep doing this? So I said, 'Okay, use my photograph. But just make sure it's a beautiful one because I don't want to look like 'the AIDS victim.'"

# "Why me? Well, who Would I rather

The day the article was published, her normally frenetic cellphone was silent. "Of course news like that flies." She laughed. "They were all calling each other, but nobody was calling me." Once the phone did start ringing, the reaction from most of her friends and acquaintances was anger. Friends pointed out that her parents could well afford to pay privately for whatever medical care she needed, so there was no reason for her to shame her whole family by taking on this public advocacy.

In 1994, Rolake's younger brother had died of sickle cell anemia, and her community had come together to mourn him. Now, suddenly, friends and relatives were pouring into the house again, holding out their arms and tear-stained cheeks to her mother. Rolake found herself being waked, just like her brother had been. "Watching people come to mourn when you are still alive—it wasn't a very good feeling. My father had to ask, 'Exactly what is the problem now? Have you seen this Rolake you are crying over? She's okay, she's fine, she hasn't changed.'" He dispatched the would-be mourners. But she could understand the shock and dismay: it wasn't just that *she* was infected, it was the implication. "Our kind of people don't get HIV: my cousin, my brother, my sister can't get HIV. People like us don't get HIV—middle-class university graduates. This three million you're talking about"—the number of people then infected in Nigeria—"they're not real."

Rolake figured she might as well make the most of this spokesperson role, and threw herself into the treatment fight. In 2003, she went to South Africa to do a four-month internship with the Treatment Action Campaign, spending time at the pioneering Médecins Sans Frontières clinic in Khayelitsha and with Zackie Achmat, whose pushy activist style caught her imagination. She absorbed TAC's lessons about protest and civil disobedience tactics, a fusion of the in-your-face activism of Western

# should it have been? it was my sister? Hell, no."

AIDS organizations such as ACT UP and strategies honed over years of opposition to apartheid. In South Africa, she marvelled at the noisy protest marches that TAC pulled off, the shouting and the placards—all of it new to a woman who grew up in Nigeria in the repressed years of vicious military dictatorship.

At the Abuja conference where I met her, Rolake was front and centre in a handful of demonstrations where Nigerians and other Africans living with HIV/AIDS interrupted meetings of political leaders, singing, "All we are saying, is free treatment now!" and carrying "dead" comrades in body bags. They were, by the standards of such things, demure demonstrations, but for Rolake they were a breakthrough, the first time Nigerians with HIV had united around their demands in this way.

That day we met at her parents' house, Rolake and I sat outside watching the bustle in the streets, snacking on fried plantain chips she bought from a passing child vendor. I asked her if she ever felt it was unfair, her infection, and the way that HIV had hijacked her life, thrusting her into this role of activist. She shook her head vehemently. "Stephanie, shit happens. Why me? Well, who should it have been? Would I rather it was my sister? Hell, no. At this point HIV is just one of the five hundred things going on in my life." Instead, she was preoccupied by something else. "Being lonely is bigger than HIV in my life. I'm not alone—I live at home with my parents, I have friends—but it's incredibly lonely. Because the things I want to do, the things I really want to say, there's nobody to say them to. What you call beautiful nonsense, you know—I have nobody to do that with and that's incredibly lonely." Her name means "I have found something precious to take care of" in Yoruba. But just then, that was feeling a little hollow.

The prevailing view for people with HIV, she said, is "you can have a relationship with another HIV-positive person. But who says I'm going to like the guy just because he has HIV? I know lots of HIV-positive people who are great but a lot I can't stand." Sex, on the other hand, she has very clear feelings about. "I like sex, I *love* sex—I love orgasmic sex." There were some weirdos who wanted to go to bed with her because they were fascinated by the freak value of HIV, she said: "They want to see if it's different with a positive woman" and if they could somehow sense the virus. "I have HIV, I don't have worms!" she said, rolling her eyes. She had met a few nice men of late, and they were interested, despite her failed marriage and her AIDS-activist profile. But they all wanted a woman who fit the traditional Nigerian wife model, and they bored her. "I want to share my life with someone, not hand it over to any man like my culture and society demand," she said.

"Why aren't I with somebody?" she mused, placing another plantain chip between crimson lips. "Because I still haven't found somebody who deserves me."

MOROLAKE ODETOYINBO

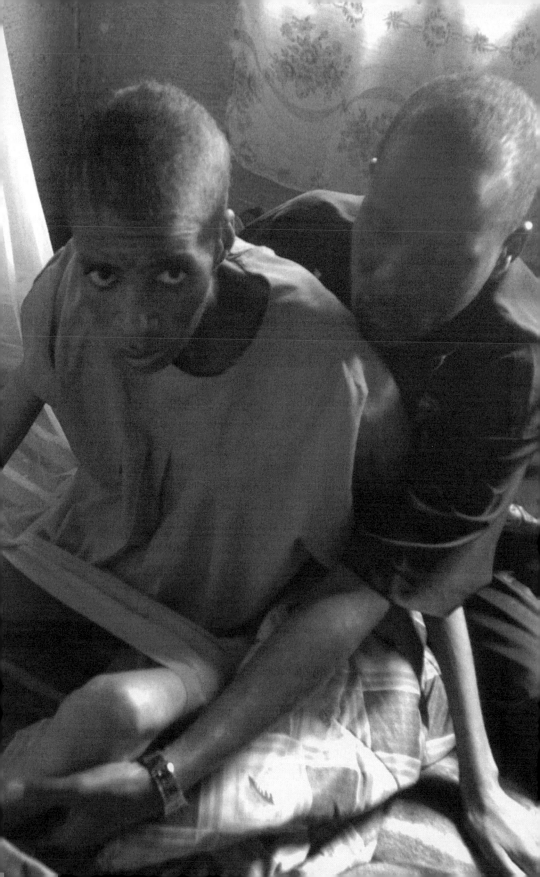

# TWENTY-FIVE

# MoleenMudimu

n seven years of reporting on AIDS in Africa, I had never seen anyone as sick as Moleen. She was so thin that the flesh sank into a crevice between the bones of her forearms. Her hair was gone, her eyes were enormous. She tried to sit up when I came into her room; the effort was clearly agonizing.

"How are you?" I asked, feeling both idiotic for the question and unable to imagine a conversation in polite Zimbabwean society that did not begin this way.

"I'm fine," Moleen said. She couldn't imagine it either.

She wore a bright red cotton nightgown that didn't quite reach her kneecaps—they jutted out of her fleshless legs like golf balls. She lay beneath a garish pink mosquito net in a cramped two-room house in Mabvuku, the low-income neighbourhood outside Harare. South African soap operas played on the tiny black-and-white television beside her, although she couldn't quite focus on the picture. On a hot-plate in the corner of the room, her husband, Benjamin, was boiling a pot of chicken feet. He had spent most of their weekly food budget to buy them: he wanted Moleen to have protein, but the scaly feet were all they could afford.

Moleen was so sick. It made me feel panicked—it was difficult to believe that anyone who looked like this was still alive, let alone still able to talk to me, between gasps for breath, or to joke gently with her husband. He coaxed a laugh out of her, talking about their wedding day, and the bell-like sound that came from her wasted, haunted face was startling.

I met them on a warm Saturday in March 2006. Moleen's pain, and her gentle husband's desperation, were awful, but the worst part was that as we all sat there—me perched on the edge of Moleen's narrow bed, trying not to jostle her, and Benjamin on the low cupboard, in the absence of a chair—we all knew it was totally unnecessary. Moleen, at thirty-two, was dying from AIDS, and the drugs to keep her alive, to make her well again, were for sale at the pharmacy just down the road. Moleen and Benjamin, who was thirty-five, knew about ARVs and they knew how they worked. And, not long ago, they could have bought them—when they were doing okay, by the standards of southern Africa: both are high-school graduates, and Benjamin had a full-time job as a security guard, while Moleen used to make enough to cover their household expenses as a market trader, before she got too sick to stand at the stall. They knew about the drugs, and they should have been able to buy them.

Instead, Moleen lay dying, and Benjamin wondered how long it would be before it was him.

Much of the discussion about the politics of AIDS in Africa focuses, with good reason, on the response, and lack thereof, of the West—on how much funding is provided by rich donor nations, or how international patent laws keep drugs out of reach for African governments. But domestic African politics is just as pivotal. The handful of countries where the governments took early leadership on HIV and drafted comprehensive response plans show the benefit of those actions: declining infection rates and many people on treatment. Then there are countries such as South Africa, where the government's lack of leadership and embrace of AIDS denialism has cost crucial years and thousands of lives.

But it is in Zimbabwe that the effect of domestic politics on AIDS is most starkly visible—and, these days, the effect of AIDS on Zimbabwean domestic politics is fast becoming clear as well.

All over Africa there are people with HIV who, because of cost or logistics, cannot get access to the medicines that would keep them alive.

MOLEEN MUDIMU

Some know what they are missing; many more have never had access to basic information about treatment or have never seen the Lazarus effect of the drugs. But there is a particularly vicious quality to what is happening in Zimbabwe today, where well-educated, gainfully employed people—people well versed in the workings of ARVs thanks to the government's own awareness campaigns—cannot afford to start or to stay on the drugs because their prices have been pushed entirely out of reach by rampant inflation and a crucial foreign exchange shortage.

There was a visceral horror in sitting on Moleen's bed knowing the drugs were there in the corner pharmacy. I knew it and she knew it, and she wasn't a penniless farmer for whom health care has always been an unobtainable luxury: she was a citizen in the country that had, until very recently, one of the best health-care systems in Africa. She knew she was dying because of an entirely artificial crisis, created by a megalomaniac president and perpetuated by the failure of other African leaders and the rest of the world to intervene.

Zimbabwe gained its independence in 1980, after the Rhodesian War ended nearly a century of control by a tiny white minority. When Robert Mugabe, a teacher turned guerrilla, became the new president, the government introduced an ambitious set of social service programs, extending schools and clinics into every corner of the country. Soon Zimbabwe's literacy rates and health indicators were some of the highest in Africa. And Zimbabwe had the economy to support the increased spending: one legacy of white rule was a booming commercial agriculture sector. The country not only fed itself, it supplied grain to most of the region. Cash crops, particularly tobacco, kept Zimbabwe rich in foreign exchange.

But in the late 1990s, it all went off the rails. Mugabe had been president for nearly twenty years by then, and his popularity was waning. But he wasn't willing to hand over power, and he took a series of increasingly drastic steps to hold on to his job. He dealt the country's vibrant economy a first harsh blow, making a massive payment to men who claimed to be veterans of the fight for independence, a buy-off that silenced one sector of burgeoning dissent. Then he undertook a huge land-reform campaign,

# Moleen, at thirty-two, and the drugs to make her well again, pharmacy

supporting violent expropriations of commercial farms and turning them over to new owners—ostensibly, landless black people. There is no question that land ownership in Zimbabwe was terribly skewed: as much as 70 per cent of arable land was then still in the hands of white farmers who had shown little interest in giving up their prosperous holdings or addressing the inequities in land ownership. These farms grew the maize that fed the country, and the tobacco and other cash crops that formed as much as two-thirds of import earnings. But Mugabe's government turned them over not to the skilled black labourers who had worked them for white owners but to cabinet ministers and loyalists of his Zanu-PF party, few of whom had any interest in or aptitude for farming.

The economy crumbled—GDP declined by more than a third from 1997 to 2005, while commercial farm production has declined by 70 per cent since 2000. The Zimbabwe dollar collapsed; soon no foreign bank would take it, and inflation soared to the highest levels in the world. When I met Moleen, it was running at 1,200 per cent per month: that means that a loaf of bread that cost $50,000 Zimbabwe dollars on Monday could be as much as Z$100,000 by the end of the week—bread that was just Z$8 a loaf when Mugabe's land-reform program began.

Meanwhile, in parliamentary and presidential elections, Zanu-PF blatantly manipulated voters, using food aid as well as other more routine tactics of intimidation. While domestic and other international monitors called the elections—which gave Mugabe and his party majorities— patently unfair, observers from Zimbabwe's African neighbours endorsed the vote and his presidency. After national elections in 2005, he targeted

was dying from AIDS,
keep her alive, to
were for sale at the
just down the road.

opposition supporters in a revenge campaign as brutal as it was gratuitous. He sent troops to demolish houses in the slums, where he believed people had voted against him, leaving 700,000 people homeless and hundreds of thousands without jobs. They either returned to the villages they had left years before or moved in with neighbours in the dwellings left standing. Rents quintupled overnight, and, like so many others, the once-prosperous Mudimus and their two children found themselves sharing two rented rooms with six other people.

Zimbabwe's health system collapsed right along with the rest of the country. Clinics that had had 100 per cent coverage in their measles and polio vaccines stopped inoculating children after the vaccines spoiled without the electricity to run the freezers. Grass grew up around the ambulances at rural hospitals because there was no gasoline. And Zimbabwe's nurses and doctors fled the country for vastly better pay in South Africa or England, or went on strike because inflation rendered their chronically late pay packets worthless by the time they arrived.

By regional standards, Zimbabwe had started its response to AIDS early, with public education in the mid-1980s. The country had the money, back then, to launch some wide-ranging programs. Nevertheless, by the late 1990s, one in four adults in the country was infected. But by the end of the century, the payoffs from prevention efforts were beginning to show: young people started waiting to have sex, more people used condoms and everyone cut back on partners. The prevalence rate began, bit by bit, to decline: from 25 per cent in adults in 2001 to 20 per cent in 2004. But that meant there were still 1.6 million people living with HIV/AIDS in a country of

13 million. And by the time antiretrovirals came to Africa, Zimbabwe's political and economic crisis had fatally compromised the country's ability to offer treatment. First, the fractured health system couldn't cope: the nurses fled; legions of people with AIDS choked outpatient departments and medical wards—people with HIV make up 70 per cent of hospital admissions; health officials skimmed off drugs and supplies and sold them on the black market; there was no foreign exchange to buy the supplies to run the national blood bank, so people with HIV were denied transfusions on the grounds this would "waste" precious blood.

The international community isolated Zimbabwe after the disputed parliamentary election of 2000. A belligerent Mugabe responded by piling on laws that made it more and more difficult for international aid agencies to work in the country, and donors began to withdraw, complaining that their grants were being misappropriated to subsidize Mugabe's vicious campaign against his political opposition—or the luxury car collections of cabinet ministers. And so as the AIDS crisis peaked in Zimbabwe, international help went elsewhere. In 2004, Zimbabwe received just $10 per infected person in donor support for AIDS, compared to an average, in southern Africa, of $74. The Global Fund approved a $10-million grant to Zimbabwe in 2002, planning to funnel the money through the United Nations, then rejected subsequent applications when that first grant evaporated in the exchange-rate mirage. Today, the World Bank, which has a major regional AIDS treatment plan, does not fund any projects there at all, while the United States—the main donor for AIDS initiatives in Africa—supports only small local groups. Staff at all these organizations told me they cannot risk "propping up" Mugabe by funding his government's AIDS program: they cannot track where the money goes, and they fear the president may manipulate access to ARVs the same way he has food aid.

When Mugabe's party bullied its way through the 2005 election with only the most muted public protest at home, donors and even the beleaguered opposition began to speculate privately that AIDS might be playing a major role in the country's political drama. So many people were sick, and those who were not themselves ill were nursing relatives or looking after the 1.3 million orphans. Was it any wonder people did not take to the streets in protest—who had the strength?

It is Moleen and Benjamin, of course, who paid the price of the standoff between Mugabe and the donors. They told me they understood why international agencies feel they cannot fund Zimbabwe—they did not want to see any more money in Mugabe's coffers either. But the cost was brutally high: by the time I met them, more than three thousand people in this country were dying of AIDS each week.

I have gone many times to Zimbabwe to report on the political crisis, but as the situation deteriorated still further in 2006, I started to wonder about people with HIV, suspecting that AIDS treatment would not be exempt from the shortages and financial crisis. A call to Prisca Mhlolo and her colleagues at The Centre confirmed that there was an incipient drug shortage, that clinics and hospitals were turning people away. And so I snuck back into Zimbabwe in the preposterous guise of a birdwatcher—because the government bans foreign and most domestic media, and won't let us report there legally—and I relied on Prisca to lead me, as she had before, through the worst-hit parts of Harare, trying not to attract the attention of the ubiquitous agents from the security services. She took me to Moleen and Benjamin's tiny, crowded house.

I knew that Zimbabwe's government had promised to put 145,000 of the 350,000 people needing immediate treatment on ARVs by the end of 2005; in Harare, I soon learned that the drug roll-out didn't manage to reach 15,000. (In contrast, the country's much poorer neighbours, such as Zambia and Malawi, put more than twice as many people on treatment.) Life expectancy for women fell to thirty-four; the WHO said it was the lowest in the world. And in 2006, the situation got even worse: commercial agriculture dried up almost totally, as did all exports, and thus all the hard currency in the country—and so the drug supply began to be erratic. Even the relatively small number of people who had access to the drugs through the national treatment program could suddenly no longer get them reliably; the government clinics stopped enrolling people and tossed out their waiting lists. The army, which had much of its HIV-positive personnel and their families on treatment, turned them away at the clinic door: the cupboard was empty. UNICEF stepped in to bail out Varichem Pharmaceuticals, the company making ARVs in Zimbabwe, to try to maintain supply to some of those already on the medication.

"People are just fighting to get hold of the drugs," the head of one of the few international aid agencies still operating in Zimbabwe told me (although he, like everyone else in Zimbabwe, was afraid to be quoted by name). "And there's not enough. You can't get figures or stats, but we know first-hand that people are off their meds because they can't afford them."

That, of course, not only was a death sentence for the individuals but raised the spectre of a spread of drug-resistant strains of HIV across the region, as thousands of people interrupted their treatment. "If people stop taking them en masse, because supplies run out or they can't afford them, you're going to have resistant strains of HIV all over the country," a senior official with an aid agency told me, his head buried in his hands. His group had scrambled to try to bring in the drugs from other countries; the government held the medication in customs for up to six months, claiming it needed to pass quality tests.

As in any black-market economy, there were still some drugs for people who could afford to pay. A few years ago that would have included urban, working people such as Moleen and Benjamin. They told me that a monthly supply of ARVs would have cost Z$200,000 a year earlier—a fee they could have covered. Even at Z$1 million a month—the cost of ARVs by November 2005, when Moleen realized she would need to start taking them—they might have managed. But not any more.

When I met them, Benjamin was earning Z$4 million a month (then equivalent to $18 on the black-market exchange rate, but dropping all the time) as a security guard in town, spending his nights patrolling office buildings. It wasn't a great job, and he was finding it more and more difficult to stay awake all night because he spent his days nursing Moleen. He walked the two hours to work and the two hours back because he had no money for the bus. The year before, his was a living wage. Hyperinflation, though, meant that by March his pay no longer got the family through the

first four or five days, let alone the month. Before she got too sick to leave the house, Moleen used to buy their food with what she earned cooking and selling *sadza,* the staple cornmeal mush, in a market in town. But now they were trying to cover the rent and food and their two sons' school fees from Benjamin's evaporating salary; meanwhile, the price of ARVs had risen by thousands more dollars every time Benjamin asked at the pharmacy. The test to measure her CD4 count, which Moleen would have had to have in order to get a prescription, cost Z$21 million, up 80 per cent from three months before. The day I came to visit, a four-week course of ARVs cost Z$4 million—Benjamin's monthly wage.

"I need the tablets," Moleen said to me, her voice barely audible from beneath the blankets. "But I can't have them."

Moleen got sick in July 2005, with chest pains and stomach trouble. Her family doctor sent her to the hospital; there the staff professed not to know what was wrong with her. Benjamin and Moleen saw through this polite fiction and went to a public HIV testing centre. Days later, they both had positive results. "We thought it was the end of the day," Moleen said.

And indeed, before long she was unable to get up from their one small bed. "When I look at my kids I feel very weak and unhappy. Maybe I will leave them soon," she said to me. Her sons, Simba, nine, and Terrence, thirteen, were taking care of her at night when Benjamin was at work. The boys had never heard their parents say the word *AIDS.* "But anyway, they are suspicious about the issue," Moleen admitted. With rents so high, all four of them had to share a room, and so there was no hiding the extent of her illness. But Moleen told the children that she was going to live until they finished school. "And I tell them they must not be affected by this sickness in us, because they are building their own lives." So far they had managed to keep the boys in school, but with fees doubling every term, they didn't know how long that would last.

Benjamin and Moleen met back home in Weza, in the west of the country. "Were you childhood sweethearts?" I asked, teasing, and Benjamin laughed. Moleen tried to laugh too, but the sound emerged as a strangled gasp. In fact, they met in high school, and they were married in 1991. "It was a Wednesday—I can even remember the day of the week," Benjamin said. This time, from under the quilt, Moleen managed a giggle.

She had been in bed for several months by that point, and I asked her to tell me what she thought about on those long days. "I miss doing my housework. I used to do it alone and now I can't. I miss doing that—that and selling in the market. I can't walk—I just want to. I'm not worried about being so thin. But I'm worried about not walking."

When Moleen drifted off to sleep, Benjamin and I went out to the little garden behind the house. He was slight and quiet, his face drawn long with worry. He insisted that I take the one stool; he leaned against the rough cement wall. I asked him to tell me what his wife was like before she got sick, and he gave a wistful smile. "She was very lovely. Fit and strong. She was a bit shy." She kept the body of a girl even after their kids were born, he said. She belonged to the Church of Christ, and she went to services every Sunday. "What she liked most was playing with the children. She would sit in the garden and talk to them for hours after school."

These days, Benjamin lifted Moleen and carried her carefully to the latrine; he kept her cold feet in the small cotton socks that perpetually slid off, too loose. When she needed to sit up to eat or drink, Benjamin got behind her and gently cradled the sharp points of her bones against his still-sturdy chest.

His devotion stood in sharp contrast to the attitude of Moleen's own family members, who shunned her after she told them she had AIDS. "When Moleen's parents heard about it, they refused to take care of her or to even come and see her," Benjamin said. "They say I am the one who brought the sickness, and they are blaming me." Not a single member of her family had contacted them since she had been bedridden, and when Moleen's sons tried to visit their grandparents, they were chased away from the home.

Why, I asked her, did she think her family was behaving this way? "I don't know," she said. What are they afraid of? "I don't know."

In a time of serious illness, one's family would normally be closer than ever. In a society that revolves around extended kin ties, it was a strange feeling to be left alone like this. "Now my family is just my wife and kids," Benjamin said. "I feel rejected." His mother is dead, and his sister died a few

years ago, leaving only his father. He, at least, has stood by them. "My father is always on my side," Benjamin said. "He sold his cattle to give us money."

Their only other support comes from The Centre, which sends a home-based care worker, Jocelyn Manieuruki, to see them every three weeks. When Jocelyn's visits had begun a year ago, she brought food parcels and medical supplies, but by March 2006 the food and supplies had run out. "Now she can only talk," said Benjamin.

I asked him what kind of things Jocelyn had to say. "She told me I must not be afraid of her," Benjamin said, his gentle gaze on his wife. "She gave me a paper with a list of certain foods to eat." No doubt the nutrition list was good advice and he would have liked to follow it, but they could not afford most of the foods listed on the page. Jocelyn also taught him how to nurse Moleen without risking new exposure to the virus, and told him which symptoms would require his taking her to hospital—but the few times they went, staff were on "go-slow" and, he said, uninterested in trying to help Moleen. "They say, 'Take her home for home-based care'"—a polite euphemism for palliative.

Jocelyn also told Moleen and Benjamin that the public clinics offering ARVs for free had waiting lists with hundreds of people on them, but that the pharmacy still had the drugs, for a price. "She said it is difficult to get them," Benjamin said quietly. And what, I asked him, did he think about that?

Benjamin opened his mouth to answer, but then the tears came. He turned away. Moleen, watching him, closed her own eyes.

As he nursed Moleen, Benjamin thought about what was coming for him. Would he suffer like her? Who would take care of him?

Sometimes, in the afternoon when Moleen was awake and the house was quiet, they talked about the boys, about what would happen to them. They would go to Benjamin's father, back to the village, most likely. "But it will be very difficult for him—he is old, he's not working at all and he's very poor," Benjamin said.

This was the idea that haunted Moleen. "I'm afraid for them," she said. "I don't want to leave them."

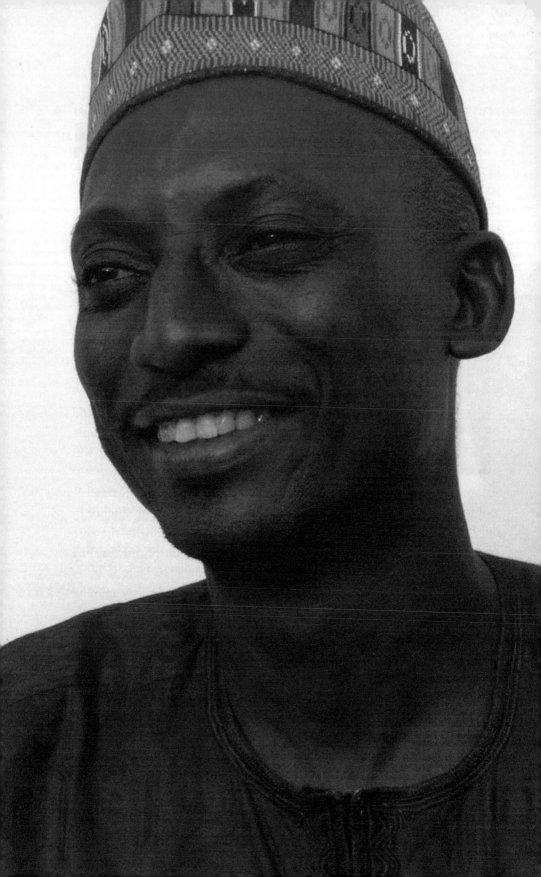

# TWENTY-SIX

# IbrahimUmoru

brahim Umoru looked around one day and realized that he had nothing left to sell. His snazzy white Volkswagen Golf was gone, and so was the land where he had hoped to build a house. He had sold all his electronic gadgets and cut out all household expenditures except for food and school fees. He and his children and the cousins he supported were all living crammed into a couple of rented rooms. He had borrowed what he could, and there was no one left to ask.

And so one day early in October 2003, he woke up, had breakfast—and took no medicine. None before bed either. It left a nagging absence in his day, the disruption of a routine he had followed faithfully for the past two years. He could picture the viruses starting to multiply and spread through his body again. He wondered how much time he had left.

Back in 2000, when Ibrahim was an energetic man of thirty-four, he had come down with a case of pneumonia that resisted treatment and left him spitting blood. He was losing weight off an already spare frame and his feet went numb. His doctor, an old friend, finally despaired of other diagnoses and suggested that he go to the hospital for an HIV test.

It wasn't a totally far-fetched idea, Ibrahim knew—"I have had some funny, funky times," he told me candidly, the first time we met in Lagos. He is a debonair man with a radiant smile and lethal charm. There were lots of girls back in secondary school, and when he played university basketball he was a bit of a star. "I got a little popular and got known around," he said with a grin. "In all honesty I had this unfortunate thing of being liked by older people." Particularly the women who worked in the brothel run by his mother, where Ibrahim spent much of his childhood. Even when he married, in his twenties, he didn't change much.

At the hospital, he tested positive, but staff sang the praises of anti-retrovirals. "The doctors told me with the drugs I had nothing to worry about"—except how to get them. The only ARVs available were imported drugs sold at hefty prices in private clinics. Ibrahim was prescribed Combivir, the cheapest drug on the market, but it cost 21,000 naira a month ($160), while he earned just 16,000 naira a month as the security coordinator for a fisheries company in the Lagos port. He was college educated and better off than most—90 per cent of Nigerians were living on less than $2 a day—but he wondered how he would manage. "I just said, 'God, see me through.'"

He started buying the drugs, and they were a marvel: within months his CD4 count had doubled, and he brimmed with energy. He had a rough time at home—his wife had tested negative for HIV, and then, with the urging of her pastor, left him—but his children were encouraging. Before long, inspired by Rolake Odetoyinbo and other activists he met at a support group, he decided to go public with his status. But at work, his boss insisted he keep the secret. Ibrahim found that diffficult—he started to feel it gnawing away at his health, and he figured that if he told the truth, everyone would adapt. So he told a few colleagues. But they didn't adapt. Soon management made the work environment too hostile for him to stay.

It was harder than he expected to find another job. He burned through his savings, started selling furniture and regretfully parted with his car. A relative gave him enough cash to cover two weeks' worth of drugs. But by October, there was not a naira left. For three months, he took no drugs at all. Each time he coughed, or felt a twinge in an elbow or a knee, he wondered, "Is it starting? And how long will I last?"

Finally, he found work. In the new year, he was hired as a peer educator at the Médecins Sans Frontières AIDS clinic at a Lagos hospital. Ibrahim was a natural counsellor—witty, impossible to shock, comfortable with the frankest discussion. The job paid well, and, even better, the benefits included free treatment for HIV-positive staff. Right away, he resumed his twice-daily dose of Combivir.

A big part of the job was adherence counselling—drilling into people who were starting ARVs that they must take the correct number of pills at the same time of day, every single day, in order to avoid drug resistance. Soon, Ibrahim found he could speak to that issue with a new level of authority. His viral load was creeping up, and he was starting to be plagued by infections. Combivir no longer worked its magic. His virus was drug resistant.

A given cocktail of antiretrovirals can suppress the presence of HIV in a person's body only for a finite amount of time. Slowly—in the West, it generally takes three or four years, although not enough is yet known about poorer African communities—the virus learns to outwit those drugs and its presence begins to grow inexorably in the body again. Eventually people become resistant to Combivir or any other antiretroviral; if they interrupt treatment as Ibrahim did, or take the drugs erratically, then it happens sooner. In North America or Europe, it is relatively easy for a person with HIV to switch to a new, second "line" of drugs at the first sign that an existing regimen is not working. (For a very small percentage of people, the usual "first-line" regimen doesn't work at all, and they must switch immediately.) There are people with HIV in North America on their sixteenth combination of drugs. But in Africa, Ibrahim explained to me, it's not so simple.

Pressure from governments and activist groups such as MSF has driven down the price of first-line AIDS drugs to about $150 per patient per year in low-income countries. But the price of the second-line drugs remains in the thousands of dollars. So much energy and attention has been focused on getting sick people on the initial easiest, cheapest combination of drugs that there has been little pressure on pharmaceutical companies to price second-line medications accessibly. Take, for example, the latest generation of the most effective drugs, called protease inhibitors. "They aren't even sold in Africa!" Ibrahim told me. Pharmaceutical companies don't bother to register them with national drug-approval bodies, knowing that at $5,000 a year they are beyond most every African's budget.

And so when Combivir, the cheapest and most widely used anti-retroviral in Nigeria, ceased to work for Ibrahim, he panicked. "I was staring death in the face," he said. But while Nigeria's public health system still had nothing else to offer, MSF staff had committed to treating patients with whatever it took; they imported second-line drugs from Europe, and Ibrahim switched to a new regimen. Almost immediately, his viral load dropped and his health improved.

His personal crisis was resolved, and anyone he counselled who wound up resistant could also count on getting second-line drugs from MSF. But what about the rest of the country? Nigeria's government remains focused on getting sick people on the first-line drugs; second-line treatment is barely an afterthought in the national plan. Ibrahim can see the problem that looms: through his work with MSF, he knows that having just 2.5 per cent of patients on second-line drugs consumes 30 per cent of the drug budget. Neither his country nor any other in Africa has the cash to put people on to second-line drugs, not when they cost $4,000 a month. What will happen to the hundreds of thousands of people belatedly started on ARVs in Africa, in four or five years when their cheap first-line regimen no longer works? Ibrahim and his colleagues at MSF have tried to sound the alarm, but governments preoccupied with rolling out first-line drugs can hardly spare the time to talk about it.

Ibrahim's body bears the legacy of the treatment interruption. He is still thin, his skin pocked with lesions, and there are stubborn abscesses that won't heal on his feet. But he feels just fine, and he has thrown himself into a lobby campaign for cheaper protease inhibitors. "It can seem a little bit funny—we are talking about dessert when still many people are waiting for a meal," he said, reminding me that 300,000 people a year die of AIDS in Nigeria with no drugs at all.

"I was a lucky man," he said. "But what about everyone else?"

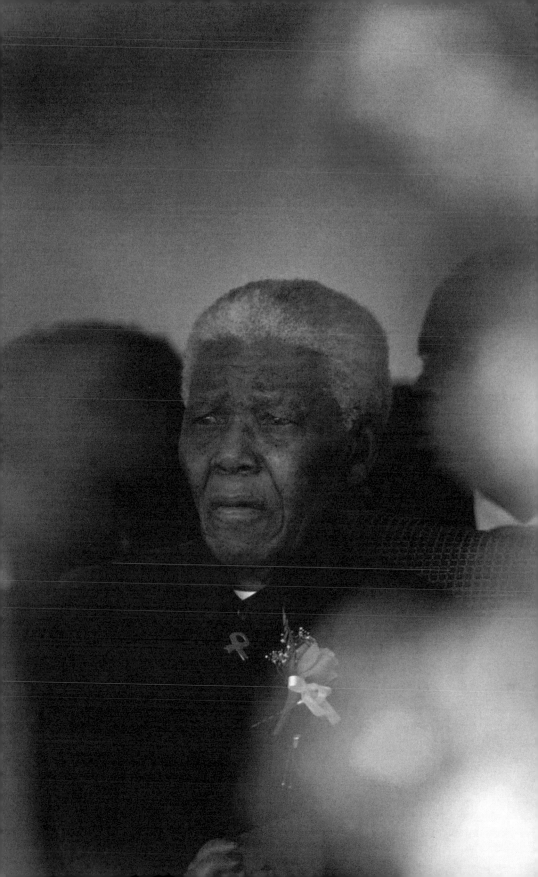

# TWENTY-SEVEN

# NelsonMandela

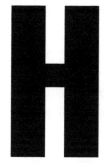

e had never looked more old, more pained, more worn by all that life had asked of him.

On January 6, 2005, Nelson Mandela summoned the Johannesburg media to his home in a leafy city neighbourhood. The reporters lined up in rows on the lawn on a warm summer morning, and Mandela made his way slowly out of the house, stooping to lean on the arm of his elegant wife, Graça Machel. Surrounded by their grandchildren and family friends, he sank heavily into a chair, faced the thicket of cameras and microphones, and began to speak.

"We have called you today to announce that my son has died of AIDS." His famous basso profundo voice was edged in pain, his words, as always, were slow and formal. "Let us give publicity to HIV/AIDS and not hide it, because the only way to make it appear like a normal illness, like TB, like cancer, is always to come out and to say somebody has died because of HIV. And people will stop regarding it as something extraordinary."

And yet it was extraordinary. Makgatho Mandela had died hours earlier in a Johannesburg hospital at the age of fifty-four, after months of illness. He was Mandela's last surviving son. This announcement—this very pointed statement about how he died—shook the country.

It wasn't that nobody knew. In fact, it was an open secret among South Africa's elite that Makgatho had HIV. Had the family said that he had died

# AIDS, Nelson Mandela said.

of pancreatic failure (which was technically what killed him, a problem brought on by immune-system collapse), many people would regardless have quietly assumed that AIDS took his life. His wife Zondi had died young, too, eighteen months before, and the family gave her cause of death as pneumonia, a common ailment in people with AIDS and a common euphemism.

But there was to be no speculating this time: AIDS, Nelson Mandela said. His son had AIDS.

Even in 2005, when eight hundred people a day died of AIDS in South Africa, no one liked to say the word. And that, Mandela said, was why he and the family had decided to go public: to bring dignity to the dying. "Doctors, the nurses and other medical staff in hospital are going to talk about it: 'Did you know that Mandela's son or grandson has died of AIDS?'" he said, mimicking the gossip. "And it gives a very bad reflection indeed to the members of the family that they themselves could not come out and say bravely that a member of the family has died of AIDS."

Nine days later, when the clan gathered in their ancestral village of Qunu for Makgatho's burial, his son Mandla made another announcement: "He is not the first to be killed by AIDS. Our mother died from AIDS. In spite of this, we are not used to death."

The announcement prompted an enormous outpouring of sympathy in South Africa and across the continent. Just as the Mandela family members had hoped, the admission that AIDS had touched them too made it all a bit more normal, a little less shameful.

In some ways, it wasn't surprising that Mandela took this step. Over the previous couple of years, he and Graça Machel had become two of the foremost campaigners on the issue of AIDS in Africa, sponsoring ARV treatment and orphan initiatives through their charitable foundations,

# His son had AIDS.

hosting massive fundraising events, and personally lobbying the leaders of rich nations to provide more funds for research and treatment efforts. But it was not always so. One of the few criticisms made of Nelson Mandela is that he did not do more about AIDS when he served as South Africa's first democratically elected president from 1994 to 1999. While he was in office, South Africa became the most infected nation in the world. Yet Mandela himself rarely spoke the word *AIDS*.

"He, more than anyone else, could have reached into the minds and behaviour of young people," said Edwin Cameron, the High Court judge in South Africa who went public with his HIV infection in 1999 and is now one of the country's most prominent AIDS activists. "A message from this man of saintlike, in some ways almost godlike, stature would have been effective. He didn't do it. In 199 ways, he was our country's saviour. In the 200th way, he was not."

The morning that Makgatho died, the media recorded the spectacle of a very private man sharing his family's most personal moment. There was a sense, that day, that Nelson Mandela himself felt he had much to make up for.

Today, at eighty-eight, Mandela inspires global devotion. I have seen him speak on four continents, and everywhere, people nearly weep with joy at the sight of him, at the high-cheekboned face etched with lines, the tufts of wiry white hair and the trademark African print shirt. He is revered for his leadership of the struggle against white rule in South Africa and the twenty-seven years he spent in prison, including eighteen in the bleak jail on remote Robben Island. While he made a measured choice to use violence against the apartheid state, he was a steadfast advocate of reconciliation and once he was released from prison, he urged black and white South Africans to forge a model of forgiveness for the world—one of his first acts as president was to have tea with the widow of Hendrik Verwoerd, the chief architect of apartheid.

Mandela was elected president by a landslide vote in the country's first multi-racial election on April 27, 1994, and he began to lead South Africa into a new era. The shattered economy started a surge of growth, and millions of poor black South Africans got their first access to clean water, electricity, housing and basic health care. There was almost none of the vicious retaliatory violence that the pessimists had predicted. In 1999, he handed South Africa over to his anointed successor, Thabo Mbeki, as the most prosperous, most stable country on the continent.

Then Mandela announced, with Graça Machel laughing at his side, that he was retiring to do some reading and spend time with his new wife— that they would work on a few causes to which they were committed. But before long, one issue in particular preoccupied them, one that threatened to undermine everything they had built in their long years of fighting for African freedom.

Graça told me about this when we met one sunny winter afternoon in 2006 in the spacious offices of the Nelson Mandela Foundation. The couple had flown back that morning from her big, airy house in Maputo, in Mozambique, where they spend most of their free time these days, and they came in the door holding hands, as they nearly always do. Mandela puttered in the background while his wife sat down with me; a tide of admirers and supplicants came and went, but his most urgent concern was whether the grandchildren were coming for dinner. Graça, brisk and businesslike, plunged into conversation, wringing her gold-ringed hands together while she spoke with the urgency and passion that colours her exuberant English—always with one eye on her husband's slow passage up and down the corridors.

AIDS, Graça said, came before they had so much as a moment to savour what they had won in their long fights for independence. "Naturally you feel this is so unfair, we just did not need this. We deserved to have a good time, in terms of now putting all our energy, all our capacity into building our nations, rebuilding our lives, putting all the troubles of the past really to rest and to be able to say, we have a new beginning, we have a new start."

In the years Mandela was battling apartheid, Graça was fighting for the liberation of Mozambique from colonial rule, alongside her first husband, Samora Machel, the guerrilla leader who became the first post-independence president. She served as minister of education, and later as an international advocate for children's rights, acting as special advisor to the UN on the effect of armed conflict on children. Samora Machel died in a 1986 plane crash for which South Africa's apartheid government is widely viewed as responsible. Mandela, who was godfather to their children, wrote Graça letters of comfort and condolence from his cell on Robben Island. Their long friendship developed into a romance in the 1990s, after Mandela had divorced his second wife, Winnie; he and Graça married in 1998 and began to work together on children's and social justice issues. At sixty, she has the unlined face of a girl, and often wears her hair in long braids or bound in a brilliantly coloured headwrap. She is vivacious, outspoken and feisty, and she too is widely admired across Africa. In recent years, as Mandela's health has declined, he has addressed only the largest gatherings with formal remarks; it is Graça who now articulates the context and the strategy for their work.

"Although the fight for liberation was very hard, this is much more complex, because it's not an enemy where you can say, 'It's there, and I'm here.' There is no demarcation between us and the enemy this time," she said when I asked about AIDS. "This is much deeper than the struggle for liberation—because liberation was ideological, it was political. But this is a terribly human struggle."

Mandela said at that January press conference that he had not known that Makgatho or any other member of his family was infected when he began advocating for support for people with HIV. "I have been saying this for the past years before I even suspected a member of my family has AIDS."

Family friends would say later that although Makgatho had known he had HIV for several years, he kept the news from his father until six months before his death. Makgatho was one of four children Mandela had with his first wife, Evelyn Mase. Only fourteen when his father was sent to Robben

**"This is much deeper than**
**—because liberation was**
**political. But this is a**

Island, he lived far removed from the elite life of political engagement that his siblings embraced. Shy and introspective, he had battled severe alcoholism.

After his death, there was heated debate within the family over whether to make his HIV infection public. "When Madiba decided to pronounce that his son died of AIDS," Graça recalled, using the clan name by which Mandela is universally known in Africa, "most of the family members—yes, of course, they agreed, they understood quite clearly that that was the right attitude, the right decision." Yet some of the siblings and grandchildren were nonetheless resistant. "It was a minority in the family but there were still some people who were thinking, 'Oh my God, what is this?'" They expressed concern that the youngest grandchildren might be shunned at school, she said, although in fact the teachers made sure their classes handled the issue sensitively. "So all those fears, they were not fears because of the children, it was they who had fears: 'How am I going to go out now and say, being a Mandela, that we also, we *also* . . . '"

Graça had been in this situation once before. In November 1999 in Mozambique, her brother-in-law Boaventura Machel died of AIDS. "I told the family, we have to disclose," she said. "Ooh! Some of them—there it was even worse than the Mandelas—they were saying, 'How are we going to go out, and what are people going to think?' I said, 'Exactly because you are the family you are, because you have visibility, you have the responsibility, the sacred responsibility to disclose.'" Graça had her way, and Boaventura Machel's death announcement appeared in the Maputo newspaper *Noticias,* with the stark words "Victim of AIDS" below his name.

It was the first time any prominent family, any public figure, in Mozambique had admitted to HIV infection. But whereas the Mandela family announcement in 2005 won sympathy and admiration, the Machel announcement in 1999 was hotly debated in the country. "Some said, 'She has no right to do that because he did not discuss it, it's his life, how can she?'" Graça recalled. "But other people said, 'The family had the courage to say this thing is happening to us, and to say AIDS doesn't choose and it affects all of us.'"

The Machels weren't the first leaders to admit AIDS had touched them—that was Zambian president Kenneth Kaunda, whose son Masuzyo died in 1986. Kaunda called a press conference to announce that AIDS killed his son and to urge young Zambians to protect themselves. In 1996 Joshua Nkomo, a leader of the independence struggle in Zimbabwe, had announced that his son Ernest died of AIDS. Others would go on to do it— in 2004, Chief Mangosuthu Buthelezi, South Africa's most prominent opposition politician, said at the funerals of a son and a daughter that they both had had AIDS. All these announcements generated headlines and gossip across the continent, for they were every bit as rare in 2004 as they had been nearly twenty years earlier.

In 1986, when Kenneth Kaunda spoke out, it wasn't hard to understand the public's response, because back then Zambians could still deny that AIDS had much presence in the country, although the hospital wards were starting to tell a different story. But by the time Makgatho Mandela died, six million South Africans were living with HIV/AIDS. Yet the stigma endured. There were many reasons for this, but one, as Nelson Mandela would come to say himself, was a failure of leadership: Kaunda, Buthelezi, and Graça Machel were exceptions, as was Uganda's Yoweri Museveni when he began to speak publicly about HIV in the mid-1980s. For the most part, though, Africa's leaders were as reluctant as everyone else to talk about AIDS: they denied it was present in their countries until that fiction could no longer be maintained, they denounced people infected as sinners who got their just reward and they ordered that protesters with HIV be kept well away from any of their public appearances. Graça, in a stinging address to African leaders at a conference in 2000, put it this way: "When historians write about HIV/AIDS, when they write about this period in time, they will ask—'Where were the leaders of Africa?'"

Mandela would not be spared that examination. In the period in which he was president of South Africa, the country's HIV infection rate grew from less than 8 per cent of adults to nearly 25 per cent. Yet he almost never addressed the subject, citing the excuse that it was culturally unthinkable for a Xhosa elder to discuss matters related to sexuality in public. "In our part of the world," Graça told me, "everything related to sex is so private. Only some aunties and some uncles can speak to the younger ones on sexuality, or those who go on the initiation process"—the traditional rites for young men in many tribes, including Mandela's Xhosa. The spread of a sexually transmitted infection was not viewed as a presidential matter in newly-free South Africa.

In 1997, with AIDS in mind, Mandela oversaw the passage of a law that overrode patents, allowing South African pharmaceutical companies to produce cheaper generic versions of essential medicines. Beyond this, however, AIDS was rarely on Mandela's agenda. He delegated the file to his brilliant and influential deputy, Thabo Mbeki. Day-to-day management of the issue was handled by the Health Ministry, where AIDS was one of a dozen competing disease priorities. Few people then believed that the impact of HIV could possibly be as bad as a handful of public health experts were warning.

In recent years, Mandela has suggested that he regrets not having handled the issue differently. As we spoke that day over tea in a cozy meeting room, Graça told me that, with the benefit of hindsight, she and Mandela see things they should have done—but without being an apologist, she added, it is important to remember what it was like in South Africa as apartheid ended. "In the first years of freedom in this country, the leadership concentrated on building the relationships to make sure the transition would work—and not to allow anything to jeopardize what was being built so carefully, to make sure above all that we prevent bloodshed in this country," she said. "So quickly we take freedom for granted, and we forget how difficult it was, and how many times many of us could not sleep because we did not know the following day what was going to be happening in this country. But now, because things are much better, they say, 'Oh, why he didn't he do this, why didn't he do that.' That's human nature."

It is also true that although HIV infection rates shot up while Mandela was in office, that didn't necessarily make the extent of the problem evident: subtype C, the strain of the virus most common in southern Africa, typically progresses slowly from infection to illness, and the first large wave of deaths in the region did not begin until about 1997. Because no country in the world had any experience of the astronomical infection rates that would soon be commonplace in the region, it was difficult for anyone to imagine what AIDS would soon do to South Africa.

Only as she and Mandela began to contemplate their post-political life did they realize how this disease dwarfed other issues. "We saw that this is the biggest challenge any—at the beginning we would say, that any nation can face—and then we came to realize that it's not only national, it's not only global, it's even family, it's at the most personal level," she said. "We knew that even young people are being wiped out by this. We both knew that there is no cure and they will die—that is the critical element—they will die soon. And you don't allow this to happen, you cannot be indifferent."

When he left office, Mandela turned to work with his Children's Fund, which focused on children's rights, and he also started an eponymous foundation to support education, particularly in rural areas. Bridgette Prince, the foundation's first program director, told me that within weeks Mandela felt a growing need to focus on AIDS as well. "He had never done health things—he had always done education-based things—but if you have a developmental mind you can see what issues will be with us for a while. And Madiba was certainly visionary."

Now he sought a way to take action on AIDS without competing with the government. First he met with traditional leaders—because, Prince said, Mandela felt that while South Africans in cities had access to information and other role models, people in rural areas were still very much in the sway of traditional authority figures. "So he embarked on sessions with them where he was open and honest with them on their behaviour about sex and sexuality and their role in communities, and what their role should be in terms of providing for orphans and making sure that abuse of women doesn't take place—and about becoming advocates for AIDS." Over time, Mandela's initial discomfort with talking about sexual matters began to ease, although he would always do so in a formal manner; friends credit Graça for some of this change, because she has long argued that frank talk about sex and personal relationships, among and across generations, is a key step in fighting HIV.

Troubled by the lack of hard data on the presence of AIDS in the country, the Mandelas next had the foundation put up the money for a sweeping national door-to-door survey of HIV infection rates—something other governments in the region were scrambling to do, but which the Ministry of Health in South Africa had yet to show interest in. When the survey's alarming results (nearly 30 per cent of adults in poor urban areas tested positive) were in, the foundation turned them over to the national government.

Then the issue got somewhat more complicated. Mandela had become convinced that it was possible to treat AIDS with antiretrovirals in Africa. Yet Thabo Mbeki, his successor as president, was lost in the world of AIDS dissident science. While Mandela was growing more and more engaged with AIDS, the elite of his African National Congress was divided on the issue— they saw what HIV was doing to their own families, but Mbeki demanded loyalty. The lack of engagement of the Mandela era was now compounded by Mbeki's radical views and unwillingness to listen to his critics.

After Mbeki infamously opened the International AIDS Conference in Durban in 2000 by saying that AIDS was a disease of poverty, questioning whether it was caused by HIV and doubting the efficacy of ARVs—to the horror of the thousands of delegates—it fell to Mandela five days later to close the conference, and he addressed the issue head on:

> The president of this country is a man of great intellect
> who takes scientific thinking very seriously and he leads a
> government that I know to be committed to those princi-

ples of science and reason. The scientific community of this country, I also know, holds dearly to the principle of freedom of scientific enquiry, unencumbered by undue political interference in and direction of science. Now, however, the ordinary people of the continent and the world—and particularly the poor who on our continent will again carry a disproportionate burden of this scourge—would, if anybody cared to ask their opinions, wish that the dispute about the primacy of politics or science be put on the backburner and that we proceed to address the needs and concerns of those suffering and dying . . . In the face of the grave threat posed by HIV/AIDS, we have to rise above our differences and combine our efforts to save our people. History will judge us harshly if we fail to do so now, and right now.

Mandela had been at pains to stay clear of matters political, knowing his very presence could easily eclipse Mbeki. But now he was widely perceived as the only person with the moral authority to make the president listen.

And so in February 2002, Mandela made his first overt foray into politics since leaving office: he told the media that he was seeking to meet with the ANC leadership to try to spur action in the response to AIDS and end the bickering. "This is a war," he said. "It has killed more people than has been the case in all previous wars and in all previous natural disasters. We must not continue to be debating, to be arguing, when people are dying."

When he met with the ANC national executive, Mandela chose the supremely uncontroversial issue of babies; he pleaded with the council to provide ARVs to pregnant women to block transmission of HIV. The government had said it planned to appeal the court decision, won by Zackie Achmat's Treatment Action Campaign, that ordered that nevirapine be made publicly available to pregnant women. Mandela urged the senior party members to reconsider. "My view is that a perception has been created that we [the government and the ANC] don't care for lives, we don't care that babies are being born almost every day to women with HIV," he said.

"This is a war," he said.
than has been the case
in all previous

It would prove to be a seminal moment in Mandela's political life: instead of the respectful hearing the elder statesman no doubt anticipated, he was openly heckled. People called from the audience, "Sit down, old man." Their primary source of pique was that he was showing up the president— but they made clear what they thought of Mandela's efforts on HIV.

A few weeks later, he travelled to the International AIDS Conference, held that year in Barcelona. His keynote address contained what many people saw as a veiled shot at Mbeki. "There is no doubt that strong leadership is the key to any effective response in the war against HIV," he said. "When the top person is committed, the response is much more effective."

Next he paid that seminal visit to Zackie, who was at the height of his drug strike. In front of a horde of television cameras in Cape Town, Mandela hugged the activist and called him a role model. "What I've come here to do is to find out under what conditions he will be able to take treatment," he said. "I have a case to take to the president to acquaint him with his position."

Zackie believes this gesture was the most courageous of Nelson Mandela's whole political career. "I think for Mandela this is a much more important stand to take than his stand at [the treason trial for which he went to prison for twenty-seven years] . . . Why? Because when he did it in the ANC under apartheid, he had everyone's support. He stood on the shoulders of giants—and morally the whole world was completely onside—not immediately, but they came onside," Zackie said. But when Mandela publicly aligned himself with the Treatment Action Campaign, he "stood alone against his own party. And that party, for all of us, was our parents, it was our home."

Mandela was walking an uncomfortable line, making clear he disagreed with the government and yet refusing to criticize outright. The same

# "It has killed more people in all previous wars and natural disasters."

week he visited Zackie, he endorsed the Mbeki argument that further research was necessary on the effects of antiretroviral drugs. Bridgette Prince recalled the whole issue of AIDS, and treatment in particular, as a "minefield" into which Mandela felt obliged to walk. After a series of briefings from experts on antiretroviral therapy, she said, Mandela decided to go a step further and provide ARVs: his foundation would fund two pilot sites, one in a rural area in the Eastern Cape and another in Cape Town.

"We made ARVs available even before the government did, and that was quite a serious dilemma," she said. "But in his mind, we needed to make sure people could get ARVs." Mandela was careful to involve the provincial government, which had none of the national leadership's hesitancy about treatment. It was a source of wide relief when the foundation acted, she said; many people had been wanting to do something similar, but only Mandela had the "moral clout" to do it without the move being perceived as outright insurrection.

Mandela tried to bring that moral authority to bear on governments outside his own country as well. By the time he left office he was an icon, and countries that had once scorned him clamoured to give him honorary citizenship and other awards. Increasingly, Mandela used those occasions to appeal to rich nations to fund the fight against AIDS. He spoke about the impact of poverty on the spread of the disease and of the developed world's inadequate response to that poverty. He made the links between multinational debt, trade regulations and paltry foreign aid spending. And he decried the cost of treatment.

"We need to remind ourselves why so many of these children are orphans today: because their parents were not able to get access to treatment for AIDS, most likely because they could not afford it," he said in Barçelona.

"Or because they lived in a country which was too poor to provide their basic health care." Why was life-saving treatment solely the prerogative of the rich? he demanded. "I ask all leaders in the world: Is this acceptable? We know that there are treatments available which restore the immune system, which stop the opportunistic infections, especially TB, and which return AIDS sufferers to good health, for several years, at least. Is it acceptable that these dying parents have no hope of access to treatment? The simple answer is no . . . Regardless of whether they can pay for it, or where they live, or for any other reason, why should treatment be denied?"

Graça, meanwhile, was using her own considerable influence to push for action on the aspects of the pandemic that most alarmed her: she became a patron of the campaign for microbicide research; she met with groups of youth and urged that they be given information and tools to protect themselves from the virus; she tackled the delicate issues of culture and gender inequality, saying that traditional ideas of manhood that valued multiple sexual partners would have to change. And she repeatedly targeted African leaders, urging them to do more. "What is the point or use of a government if it cannot or will not lead its people?" she demanded of a room full of dignitaries at the African Development Forum. "Our governments in Africa must stop looking at all the obstacles holding them back from action . . . Lack of resources is not a sufficient excuse. When governments lead their countries to war they can spend [much of] the countries' resources on that war. What percentages of national budgets are currently being spent to vanquish HIV/AIDS?"

Together, she and Mandela drew on their celebrity and their unparalleled access to people of influence to try to spur public action. They brought Oprah Winfrey to Africa to meet AIDS orphans, and they strategized with former U.S. president Bill Clinton about how to force drug companies to lower their prices. Mandela formed an organization called 46664 (his prison number on Robben Island) that staged a series of giant rock concerts aimed at AIDS awareness, and the world was treated to the spectacle of Mandela, his hand clasped in Graça's, nodding his grizzled head to the beat of songs by rapper Will Smith and R&B diva Beyoncé Knowles. During the Live8 concerts of 2005, Graça helped him onto a stage in Johannesburg where he made an appeal televised to more than a billion people. "We live in a world where the AIDS pandemic threatens the very fabric of our life," he said, "yet we spend more money on weapons than for the support for the millions infected by HIV. It is a world of great promise and hope. It is also a world of despair, disease and hunger. Overcoming poverty is not a gesture of charity; it is an act of justice."

Their presence charmed the crowd—Mandela's appearance at Live8 drew more hysterical applause than any rock star or actor—but then the throngs in London and Philadelphia and Tokyo went home and AIDS in Africa slipped off the agenda again. The political leaders who lined up for photo-ops with Mandela dodged new funding commitments. The Global Fund could not meet its pledges; the UN talked of a global AIDS funding shortfall of more than $8 billion.

Mandela's public words showed signs of increasing frustration. At least twenty-six million people have already died of AIDS, he said, 95 percent of them in the developing world, and forty million have HIV: "These numbers are staggering, in fact incomprehensible. By all accounts we are dealing with the greatest health crisis in human history." And even though science had found some solutions to the problem, these were out of reach of the poor. "This is a global injustice. It is a travesty of human rights on a global scale."

Graça said they found the lack of response bewildering. "The terrible thing with this pandemic is you have to reach a certain peak to get people to wake up," she said. "We shouldn't have to pay that price—it's terribly high—before people wake up and get involved." The necessary course of action was so clear: fully finance the Global Fund. Cancel unpayable debts. Give realistic amounts of foreign aid. "I find it very difficult to understand how those who have the power to make resources available to save the lives of people can hesitate—they can't afford to hesitate," she said.

While their lobbying efforts on funding were met with disinterest, the Mandelas took on an equally obdurate aspect of the African pandemic: the stigma around the disease. They used the simple approach (as they eventually would with Makgatho's death) of showing that they personally cared. They embraced HIV-positive activists at conferences, visited clinics, addressed words in every speech to people with the virus, telling them "the world cares about you." Stigma itself kills, Mandela reminded audiences, when people deny their illness and don't seek treatment, or are afraid to tell. "It is inexcusable to subject any person infected or affected by HIV/AIDS to such abuse and rejection," he scolded in Barcelona.

Graça said they often discussed the shame, wondering how people could turn against even their own children. "This thing brings up the ugliest part of us as human beings." She worried that it will take at least another generation to end the shame associated with sexually transmitted illness. "It's more than shame, it's taboo. And taboos take a long time to unravel, to become a normal thing. They take generations. It's not a question of knowing, because we know—it's simply that that taboo is so deeply entrenched in our psyche that we don't manage to overcome it." The taboo warps the response that might have been made, she added, had HIV been spread by mosquitoes, or sneezing, rather than sex. "It was not meant to be brought to an open and daily discussion—not meant to be intergenerational with parents talking to their children—not meant to have church leaders talking about it. It's all those things that take so long to change in our attitudes."

For Graça and her husband, the most troubling aspect of the African pandemic is the fate of orphans. There is still no comprehensive strategy for Africa's orphans; funding for prevention, care and treatment remains inadequate. As devoted grandparents who head a sprawling clan, they have a heightened awareness of how the disease is radically reshaping demographics—and a profound sense that none of the interventions to date can replace what's being lost. They get some small sense of that burden when

# ugliest part of us as human beings."

they try to supervise the homework and plan the birthdays of their own orphaned grandchildren.

"To be honest, I don't think I comprehend the dimensions of the havoc, disruption, discontinuity," Graça said. "You have young couples dying in their late twenties, early thirties, and the grandparents have to fill the void, have to try to connect the chain of knowledge, experience, values, that goes from one generation to another—when you jump a generation, there is a void and you can't fill it. Even when the grandparents fill the basic needs, the food and clothing and a shoulder to lean on so you feel someone is there, you don't fill it. And this will be for many generations. I have no idea how it is going to impact, what kind of citizens these children are going to be, how they will cope. We say it disrupts the social fabric but we don't go deep enough to say what this means. It will be a different society. Especially in rural areas, where it's not like it's hundreds of families, it's thousands of families gone—we can't fill all the spaces that are left."

It is this that drives them, Graça said—this that keeps them from simply settling down in her hilltop house in Maputo and savouring time with their grandchildren. There are still things that they can do, influence that perhaps only they can have, and they fought for too much for too long to pass up any occasion to try to preserve those achievements.

And these days, it isn't just about their countries, or their continent, it's about their family. "People know that this is something very, very close to his heart," she said, her eyes on her husband as he moved slowly across the foundation office, leaning heavily on his cane. "It is not only solidarity with millions of South Africans. It has touched him in a very personal manner."

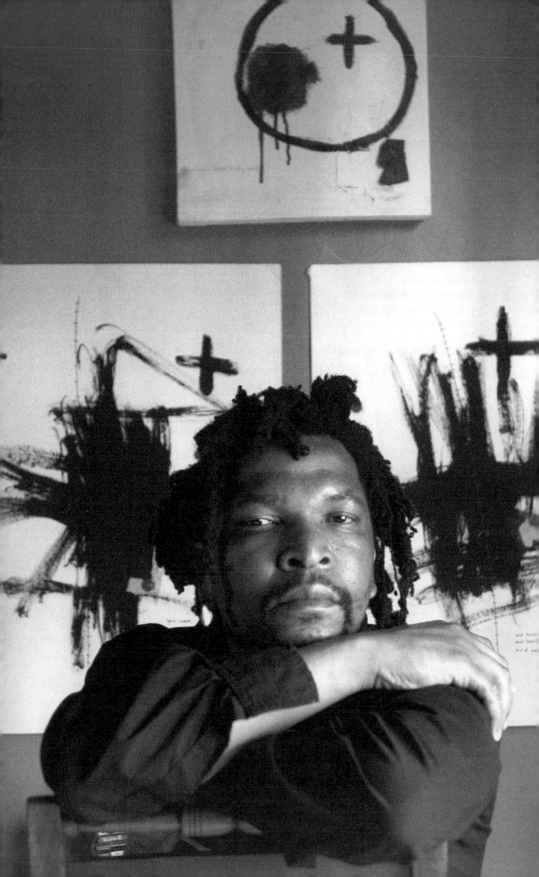

# TWENTY-EIGHT

# Thokozani Mthiyane

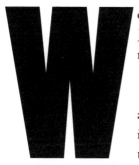

e sat at my kitchen table in the coppery light of a Jo'burg late afternoon, and Thokozani patiently repeated the word for me.

"*Ushayabhuqe,*" he said.

"Oo-shy-a-boo-kay," I recited, struggling, as always, with the sharp click sound represented by Q in isiZulu. He repeated the word, made me say it three more times.

Thokozani has taught me all the euphemisms: *amagama amathathu*—"the three words," for H-I-V. *Iqqhok'si*—high heels—for the wanton women who are blamed for bringing the virus. And *ushayabhuqe*—the catastrophe—the word people use instead of *AIDS.*

I met Thokozani, a soft-spoken poet and artist with leonine features and heavy dreadlocks studded with cowrie shells, not long after I moved to Johannesburg. Early on, TK, as his friends call him, agreed to try to teach my partner, Meril, and me to speak isiZulu. We have never progressed very far with the language, but our long-suffering teacher grew in the course of our lessons to be a better friend.

TK and I both make a living from words, and we share an interest in how language works. I need the vocabulary of AIDS to do my job, and I am also fascinated with the secrecy and the fear that underlie the euphemisms, with the ways in which people choose words that will shield them from having to name what is happening here.

Often, after a lesson, TK and I sit at the wooden table in my airy house near the park, and I talk about my latest trip to another AIDS-ravaged patch of Africa, and TK talks about here, about the bookstore where he works, how another employee is mysteriously sick, how people whisper about what might be wrong. He talks about home, too. He grew up in Clermont, a township outside Durban in the South African province of KwaZulu-Natal, which is now the absolute heart of the global AIDS pandemic. Positive HIV tests of pregnant women in KwaZulu clinics run as high as 60 per cent. Clermont was a violent place when Thokozani was growing up, a hotbed of resistance to apartheid—and not long after freedom came, the young people started dying again, killed not by soldiers or vigilantes but by the illness no one likes to name. Over the past decade, TK has seen cousins and friends, boys with whom he used to play soccer and run in the streets, all die by age thirty. Every couple of weeks, he slouches into my kitchen, slings his coat over a chair and says, "There's a funeral this weekend" or "I heard about a cousin." And playing dumb, I say, "Oh, sorry. How'd he die?" TK grimaces and says, "You know, they say he was sick." And we roll our eyes at each other in a grim and shared recognition.

I rely on TK to translate more than isiZulu for me. He talks me through the mysteries of this place, the layers of tension between black and white, the crazy violence. And he helps me understand AIDS. I tell him about the people I meet on my travels, and we talk about our friends, too—people we know right here in Jo'burg, where one in three people has HIV, guys who we know are having unsafe sex, because their girlfriends keep getting pregnant.

At first I used to marvel at it—at why people have gone on making such choices in defiance of what might seem like the most basic survival instinct. But in talking to TK, I realized that it's not, in the end, so hard to understand. Infection rates are much higher here than in, say, Canada or France, but the variables that go into decisions about love and sex and intimacy, those are no different here. People have sex without condoms because it feels good to say you trust someone that much—or because there is a particular pleasure that comes in taking risks. Or, my friend points out, just because it feels nice. We all do things we know we know we shouldn't—especially when we're in love, or filled with lust, or lonely.

TK helped me see the other reasons, too, the ones that have more to do with this place. There is the fatalism of the guys he grew up with. They don't worry too much about this mysterious, invisible virus because there are so many other things that could kill them tomorrow—political violence, car-jacking, malaria, an accident in the mine shaft. For young men in parts of KwaZulu, there is a 70 per cent lifetime chance they will contract HIV. If that's the case, some say, why not get it over with? And these days, as access to treatment spreads, poor understanding of ARVs also leads people to believe that if they do get the virus, they can "fix it" with a pill.

TK talks, too, about the politics of race in all of this. He reminds me that those who live in communities where people have suffered or died for years from entirely treatable illnesses have a justifiable suspicion of health advice from rich outsiders. On his travels in Europe, he has learned how many people view the African pandemic as some sort of aberration that has its roots in uniquely African behaviour, even though a pile of research shows they have no more sexual partners than people in any other part of the world, but simply have them concurrently rather than serially. And while TK and I agree that Thabo Mbeki's stance on AIDS is bizarre, he has helped me come to see that the president has a point when he rails against Western stereotypes of licentious black men. His words ring true for TK, as they do for many Africans irritated by the one-dimensional portrayals of sexually predatory men and silent, long-suffering women that continue to characterize discussion of the pandemic by experts in the West. And then there is the potent, seductive force of denial: nobody likes to think too long or too hard about what's happening here. So they make choices that are, in the end, risky. But none of that is irrational, he points out—it's simply human.

Thokozani speaks to these questions of trust and risk with some authority. His urban hipster look disguises the fact that he is a gifted athlete who could have played professional soccer. He cultivates his township-boy demeanour, but he has won international recognition for his art—harsh, richly coloured abstract paintings that evoke Mark Rothko and Jean-Michel Basquiat. He can analyze the politics of race and class with sharp insight; he can also, as I often end up snapping at him, be a shocking sexist. The contradictions combine into a compelling and charismatic presence, and he rarely lacks for female company.

As TK and I grew to be closer friends, there was something I worried about, something I couldn't bring myself to ask. It was none of my business, but when you live in the middle of *ushayabhuqe,* you get paranoid. I tried to think of ways of poking into TK's private life—wondering if I could casually ask, while we chopped onions for dinner, if he was having safer sex, if he had been tested for HIV.

Then one afternoon, Thokozani started talking about how many of his friends in the township had messed up their lives by having kids so young—and how, growing up, he resented the way each of his parents had children with other partners, siblings he barely knew. He was determined to avoid that, he said, and he never had unprotected sex: at first from fear of pregnancy, then AIDS came and made him extra cautious. I had heard this "it won't happen to me" avowal from dozens of men, and usually regarded it with some skepticism, but TK spoke with such harsh conviction that I believed him. And I felt a flood of relief.

In the middle of 2005, Meril and I went home to Canada on holiday. The day we came back, my good friend Ngaire and I went for a walk in the park, and she said, after a lull in conversation, "I have some bad news. It's about TK."

I thought, Oh God, it's HIV. Because that's what you think, in southern Africa, when you hear those words.

# I said to him, "they're going to figure it out."

But then I thought, No, not TK. He's too careful. Too smart.

Ngaire said, "He's got HIV."

He came by to see me a few days later; we simply sat, for a long time, and looked at each other. I've talked a hundred times with people who have recently learned they are HIV-positive, but this was something different. Just like always, we made tea and we chatted about the latest political scandal—but everything was utterly changed. I understood with a new and visceral clarity how bizarre HIV is, how people look the same and know they're dying, how the presence of minute strands of RNA in tiny cells can become the biggest thing in a room. Suddenly I was revisiting, in an urgent and intimate way, all the things I believe about AIDS—that it can be a chronic illness, that it doesn't have to change everything, most of all that a cure will be found. "There will be a cure," I said to him. "A few more years, they're going to figure it out." The words sounded feeble; TK gave me a smile that said, I appreciate what you're trying to do.

He was still coming to grips with the idea of this germ festering inside him, killing him slowly; with the fear and distaste he sensed from his friends, many of whom had stopped calling; with how to break the news to his frail mother. He showed me poems he was working on, heavy with images of bleached bones and blood-soaked earth. TK, with his dark, dark sense of humour, was trying to cope with an irony so black that it defied even his ability to laugh at the nastiness of fate. All those years of condoms and fastidiousness—*ushayabhuqe* had him anyway.

Another year went by before he could bring himself to tell me how it happened.

One evening in May 2003, TK went out to dinner with his girlfriend, Samantha, and afterwards she dropped him off at home, a row house in

Yeoville—a somewhat sketchy Johannesburg neighbourhood popular with young artists. His housemate was out clubbing; the housemate's brother was asleep in the small room he rented in the yard at the back of the house. TK went to bed.

"In the middle of the night my housemate arrives and wakes me up and says, 'There's a burglary at the neighbour's—the burglars saw the taxi dropping me and ran away—but all her things are outside and they need to be brought in.'" In Jo'burg, which has one of the highest crime rates in the world, the only thing unusual about this was that the burglars had run off. Together they woke up their neighbour, an older woman who lived alone. She had slept through the pilfering of her home, and was grateful to the men for toting her television back inside. When they were finished, TK went back to bed.

Not long after, he woke again, to the sound of screaming. It was his neighbour, yelling that there were men in her house. TK, his housemate and his brother all ran next door again. There they found a wild-eyed young stranger, who cried, "I'm going to shoot you! My brother is here under the bed and he's going to shoot you!" TK remembers his housemate calmly confronting the burglar, telling him to go.

"There was commotion. I had a hammer in my hand, and the next thing I know I was bleeding profusely—I did use the hammer. I just have a recollection of a silhouetted movement on my head but I can't recall it correctly. I kind of blacked out and when I regained composure I thought, 'We should have just locked the door and called the police.'" But by now his housemates were involved in a brawl and the lights were smashed. TK ran back to his own flat and called the police, an ambulance and Samantha. Then he tried to go back next door, but found he couldn't stand. His housemate's brother was at his door and he was bleeding everywhere. TK made a painful effort to hand him something to hold over his wounds, and realized that he was streaming with blood himself. "I sat on the floor. I was just bleeding, just bleeding. I felt like I was—I thought that was the end."

Samantha arrived, then the police, but no ambulance, and Sam decided to take the injured men to the hospital herself. "I remember holding my housemate's brother—because he was really, really stabbed—worse than me, and I had a huge gash on my head, twenty-eight stitches worth, and cuts on my hands," TK said. "But he was bleeding more, he was stabbed under the armpit and stabbed in the back. He was crying, he thought he was dying. The wound was like a living thing." Thokozani remembers reaching over to try to comfort him, to try again to stanch the blood.

At the hospital, a medical student stitched his head. He went home that night; it would be ten days before the brother was released. TK soon moved out of the house and he went for trauma counselling. The therapist suggested he have an HIV test. "She said she believes it's one in three people here who are infected, and she said, 'The way you're describing the situation you were in, it's likely that you contracted HIV. This thing may go deeper than you see. The stitches will heal and you will cope, but you need to know that there was a lot of blood, a lot of people injured and bleeding.'"

So he had a test. And it was negative. In post-test counselling they told him about the window period (it can take a couple of months for a newly infected person's body to produce enough antibodies that he or she tests HIV-positive) and suggested he come back in eight weeks. "But I didn't go. I went to Amsterdam to be part of a theatre production and I was gone for three months. While I was there, I got sick—the glands under my armpits swelled and I was cold. I thought maybe it was the cold weather—then miraculously I was fine, and I continued to do the production." He would later learn that this is a classic story of what's called seroconversion: at the point at which the body develops detectable antibodies to HIV, usually a few weeks after infection, a person often suffers flu-like symptoms. These pass after a couple of days, and then it can be years before any other symptoms are noticeable. Nevertheless, when TK returned to Jo'burg, he went to the doctor, who poked at his glands. "She said I should have an HIV test. I said, 'I'll have to go home and think about it.'"

Much later, I asked him why he'd been reluctant to test again. "Since I had the last test I had been with one person," he said, "and she's had a test and she's negative and I had a test and I'm negative, so where could I have got this thing?" It was, he said after a long pause, fear, and old-fashioned denial.

And then one night he was chilling with a couple of friends, watching soccer, idle gossip flowing back and forth, and they mentioned that the guy stabbed with him in the housebreak six months earlier was ill. With AIDS.

"I had this amazing fright—my body just went cold from the bottom of my feet to the top of my head."

But again, he quashed the panic: he had had a test, and it was negative, and he felt fine. What could be wrong? He was leaving for an artists' residency in France, a wonderful opportunity that he had been looking forward to for months. He didn't tell me, or anyone else; he put the whole thing out of his mind.

But by the beginning of 2005, he was back in Johannesburg and feeling tired and sick once more. With the news about his housemate's brother on his mind, he decided it was time to go for another HIV test—although he never seriously entertained the idea that it might be positive. When the counsellor said that word, he thought almost immediately about suicide. Then he had another thought: What about his lovers? Could he have infected anyone else? If the women were at risk, he felt he had to tell them before he did anything.

His most pressing concern was for his close friend Samantha, whom he'd dated for a couple of years. They had had condoms break a couple of times, and he was consumed with the fear that he might have infected her with HIV. So he went to see her that night, told her the news. She was, as always, staunchly supportive, much more concerned for him than for her own health. She tested the next day, and again a few weeks later, and was negative both times.

"Then I made this odyssey to look for everybody I thought I could have infected or been infected by. And to this day, that is if they're telling me the truth, they are free from the virus—and I'm the only one." Those years of protected sex had done just what he intended.

The counsellor who saw him after the housebreak was prescient. The man who stabbed him may have bled on him—TK thinks he was wounded. And of course, there was his housemate's brother, the guy they said had AIDS: TK remembers pressing his own wounded hands against the man's serrated flesh.

THOKOZANI MTHIYANE

# "This has nothing to do with justice."

Stories like TK's are a phenomenon almost unknown in the West. In countries where the HIV infection rate is below one per cent, there is only the most infinitesimal risk of ever encountering the virus this way. But in a country such as South Africa, and so many other African nations where there is a generalized epidemic, every fender bender, every broken glass at a crowded party, every child with a scraped knee in a sandbox full of friends takes on a new and terrible dimension. HIV in Africa is almost always discussed, and researched, in terms of sexual transmission of the disease, and it is true that these cases make up the vast majority of infections, but it also true that unsafe blood supplies, reuse of unsterilized medical equipment, sharing of razors for traditional scarring or circumcision or prison tattoos, car accidents and violent crime all spread the disease, and there is little solid data on how much these kinds of transmission are accelerating the epidemic.

TK tells himself that, ultimately, it doesn't matter how he got the virus. "The fact is that I'm infected." And yet it's ironic: "All my sexual partners are free from it because I protected them like I protected myself." More than ironic, it's patently unjust. But then, as he reminds me, "This has nothing to do with justice."

Thokozani manages to be both a tremendous cynic and a person preoccupied with questions of justice. He grew up in the worst, bloodiest days of the fight against apartheid and became an adult just as his country gained its freedom. His life—travelling to Europe for artists' residencies, going to poetry readings in bookstores, heading downtown late at night to join friends at a bar in the heart of the city—is more than a world away from the life his parents lived or could have imagined.

His name means "be joyful, people" in isiZulu. He had an English first name once, too—black children had to, to go to school—but he left it behind long ago; he refuses to tell me what it was. When he was born in February 1969, his father was a labourer and his mother worked as a maid for white families, one of the few jobs open to black women. TK's parents split up when he was young, and he was raised by his grandmother.

He quit school for the first time when he was seven, because the teachers whipped disobedient students and he thought the rules were dumb. He quit again a few years later, when the teacher made him sit in the back row because his granny couldn't afford shoes and a uniform for him. He got a job as a "garden boy," helping to tend white people's yards, and used his wages to buy himself clothes on the long-term payment plan at the shops. "Then when I was thirteen or fourteen, shit started hitting the fan—the riots started. The apartheid government would send soldiers to monitor the schools. We would throw stones, they would return with tear gas and we would all leave." A school day never lasted more than a couple of hours. So Thokozani started a program of self-education, saving up pennies for taxi fare to a white neighbourhood with a public library. Township boys weren't allowed to borrow books, but he could sit there and read. He discovered Oscar Wilde, James Joyce, Bernard Shaw, Franz Kafka—his habit of quoting at length from these dead Europeans makes me laugh. "So you're in this black power struggle but you're sneaking off to read James Joyce?" I asked him once.

He shook his head in disappointment at my narrow mind. "In spite of all that," he said about the black-consciousness rhetoric then emerging, "you had in the back of your head that literature, wherever it comes from, is the great liberator. It offered a different way of thinking—someone like Oscar Wilde would say things that were applicable even though he was talking about another environment." In any case, it was difficult then to get hold of African literature. "In 1992 we discovered Ngugi wa Thiong'o, *Decolonizing the Mind*—he said African writers should cease to write in English and explore their own languages. But for him to be heard he had to write in English."

TK got a job in a record store and added a music habit to his book addiction. He became a Rastafarian, drawn to the politics of the movement: "*Songs of Freedom* by Bob Marley or *African* by Peter Tosh, they were about black consciousness, African identity under siege by apartheid." And he started painting, after rudimentary lessons from other black artists. "I thought I could develop it as a skill and make a living—but also I was trying to find another way of articulating my society, my woes and aspirations. It gives you another way of thinking. And there was nothing else to look forward to living in a township in the early '90s—just work in a factory and watching soccer on Sundays."

Thokozani is so much of my world, when we argue about books and eat pizza and gossip about friends, that it is hard for me to believe that just a few years ago, he felt his life so circumscribed. He talks of how it was both normal—the way it had always been—and constantly galling. How the white schools had books and playing fields, how he and his friends were chased off the whites-only beach. "You start to develop a real admiration and a hate for white people—you see them in town and think they're nice—but at the same time you are in this prison and they are enjoying apartheid."

And then came 1994. After years of protracted negotiations, and the deaths of thousands of people—the majority in the townships around Durban—South Africa held its first democratic election and Nelson Mandela became president and everything looked different. Except that just as one enemy was vanquished, the other was emerging.

"The first time I heard about HIV was 1987—the biology teacher mentioned it: human immunodeficiency something—the word was so long. The teacher said it was an incurable new disease, sexually transmitted but mostly found among homosexuals. It was never seen as a thing that would spread in such magnitude. There were no details. It remained a mystery for many years. Then in the mid-1990s I heard about it in the community—it was just a rumour, 'So-and-so died, they were sick, it might be AIDS.' I remember thinking about this song by Prince, 'Sign of the Times,' remember it? *A skinny man died of a big disease with a little name.* The big disease with the little name—I wondered about that."

# "You wake up one day it's a black flood

By 1999, a lot of people were dying, and TK decided to get tested for the virus; he had a serious girlfriend and they were talking about having children. Knowing he was being needlessly overcautious, given his history of protected sex, he tested again six months later; still negative. He moved to Jo'burg to be near his girlfriend, and got a job at South Africa's main bookstore chain. Friends got sick, and cousins died, and that was frustrating and sad, but he felt personally safe from AIDS. "When something is 'over there,' you think its going to remain over there. And then you wake up one day and it's right here—it's a black flood flowing in your veins."

The first person TK told he was positive, after Samantha, was his manager at the bookstore. "Because I worked for her and also because I needed someone that I trusted—she was really calm, and told me I would be fine. She knew a lot of people infected who had been living with it for years. She got a friend to call me—he said, 'I'm also like that and it's been years and there is a lot to fear but that fear can be overcome and I know what you're going through.'" The friend went to see TK, brought him information on HIV. More than the pamphlets, though, it was the sight of him, calm and normal looking after six years of living with the virus, which was immensely reassuring.

Thokozani saw no reason to keep the news a secret, and started to tell his friends. Some said it couldn't be true, because he didn't *look* sick. Others didn't say anything at all, and just stopped calling.

After his positive test, he had gone to the clinic at a big Jo'burg hospital, one of the main sites for the South African government's public treatment program. "I found it pathetic. The guy tells me that this isn't the end of world, I'm still going to live—they're going to maintain

# and it's right here— flowing in your veins."

me on multivitamins and exercise. I was despairing. I needed something more concrete than 'this is not a death sentence' when I do know that people eventually die. I lasted less than ten minutes there." Although his bookstore salary barely extended to small luxuries like CDs and paperbacks, he decided he would pay for the care of a private specialist.

A year and a half after he learned he was infected, his CD4 count was hovering just above 300, and we began to talk about antiretrovirals. Thokozani is an Africanist, a man with a healthy skepticism about imports from the developed world; I had a secret fear that this would extend to AIDS treatment, that I would find South Africa's treatment-denialism drama playing out in our friendship. I told him about all the people I knew who had been so desperately, terribly ill and suddenly got their lives back when they started taking the drugs. I told him that the side effects of ARVs are unpleasant, but most pass after a couple of weeks. I told him about the men I knew back in Canada who had been living well on ARVs for more than a decade. He only cocked an eyebrow at me.

He went back to the specialist, who found a CD4 count of 281 and sent him to get a viral load count done. TK called me right after the appointment. "He says it's over 100,000." My stomach knotted: that wasn't good. That, in fact, was potentially really quite bad: more than 100,000 copies of the virus in a millilitre of blood. "That's not the best news," I said carefully. "You probably want to talk to him about treatment." In fact, the doctor was already pushing Thokozani to start ARVs.

He came by that night. I made a pot of his favourite rooibos tea and we talked through the pros and cons. On the one hand, beginning the drugs now meant he was starting something he would never be able to stop. The sooner one begins, inevitably, the sooner one moves towards eventual drug resistance. There would likely be side effects; the drugs would be expensive. On the other hand, I told him, he was at risk now: if someone coughed on him in a shared taxi, and he caught tuberculosis, it was going to take his body much more effort to heal. While the treatment guideline used everywhere in Africa is to start people when their CD4 drops below 200, in the developed world, people start at 350 or 400. The less the immune system is damaged, the easier it is to recover.

He called a few days later to say he'd started taking the drugs. And within a couple of months, he felt very changed. "I'm more productive and stronger—my mind has moved away from fear of facing imminent mortality to a possible prolonged life. Now I'm much, much, much better—my eyes are clear, I run further and faster than I did before I took them."

Because he was doing well on the drugs, he felt more comfortable talking about the fact that he was infected, less like a freak who might waste away and die at any moment. At a bookstore staff meeting, he read a poem he was working on about living with HIV. A couple of young women wept; he encouraged them all to ask questions, but no one did. But after that, if he took a day off, everyone scrutinized him for signs of illness when he went back to work. He was frustrated about the silence—especially when a couple of his co-workers got visibly sick, took more and more days off, and no one talked, except in whispers, about what might be wrong. He also tried to get his friends to engage in honest conversations about HIV, but they hurriedly changed the topic. "When your friends tell you, 'If I get infected I'll just eat properly,' and you're like, Yo—just because Thabo Mbeki told you it's a disease of poverty and Manto"—the health minister—"is telling you to eat garlic and beet root. Really, it makes me feel bitter about my government." He finally told his sisters he was infected; his mother passed away in late 2006, before he had found a way to tell her.

For all that Thokozani feels physically well, he is at the same time irrevocably changed, and through him I have come to a new understanding of what life with *ushayabhuqe* means. There is no longer any immediate risk that TK will die, or even be ill. "There are days when I don't even think of it," he said. "Until I have to take my pill, then I remember." And yet the virus has reshaped his life on every level. He can't indulge his fashion-junkie streak in a new jacket, and has had to cut back on his other weaknesses, books and CDs. "I can't travel and spend money as I used to because I have to spend it on medication." His drugs cost 600 rand a month, about $100, from his 5,000 rand monthly salary. He has to think about nutrition. "I can't go through the day just having bread and chips, I have to think about what I eat." He starts to talk about events far in the future—when the soccer World Cup comes to South Africa in 2010, for example—and then catches himself, gives a small sardonic laugh.

And what about the future? "When I see someone that I really like or feel there's a mutual attraction—I can't go out. I have to go home and take my medication. And the conversation—you have a glass of wine, 'Are you coming home with me?' and you say, 'No.'" Thokozani, the dedicated flirt, laughed at this, a little darkly—at the idea of the possibilities he has walked away from. He feels compelled to tell women, within hours of meeting, that he is living with HIV. Sometimes one he really likes will, either immediately or after talking to her friends, break it off. And if she doesn't, TK feels guilty—"knowing that she has the potential for a much happier life than with a person who might fall sick."

The drugs gave Thokozani his energy back, and a certain calm, but there are many things they can't restore. He does not think he will simply get used to all of this. A person doesn't get used to living with the clock ticking.

"Sometimes I don't know who I am, Stephanie.

"I miss myself."

# Epilogue

have not been able to follow all of the people whose stories are told in this book—their homes are beyond the reach of communications networks, or the political or economic instability in which they live makes it difficult to trace them. Many, however, I have kept in touch with over the years since we met.

SIPHIWE HLOPHE continues to lead Swapol, which has grown into one of the most powerful social forces in Swaziland. She fears her health is declining, but the country's public ARV program provides drugs only for people with CD4 counts below 200—that is, late-stage AIDS—and so she does not yet qualify for treatment. TIGIST HAILE MICHAEL and her brother, Yohannes, are doing well in school in Addis Ababa, and the local burial society has managed to continue renting their small house for them. In 2004, PRISCA MHLOLO began taking ARVs smuggled into Zimbabwe, the only way drugs were available at the time. The next year, she was able to switch to ARVs provided by The Centre; she was in good health for some time but lost her job in 2006 after allegedly misappropriating funds to buy herself drugs to treat a severe case of tuberculosis. She remains in poor health. REGINE MAMBA is raising her grandchildren, and now five great-grandchildren, for a total of 18 children. She is still a key part of the granny support group in Malala, Zambia, which is caring for 478 orphans. LYDIA MUNGHERERA continues her energetic politicking on the global stage and has thrown herself into a project that she calls the Mamas' Club, supporting young HIV-positive women with children through TASO, which remains one of the most powerful AIDS support organizations in Africa. NOÉ SEBISABA struggles to build up the activities of Stop SIDA in Burundi. After living for five perilous years with a CD4 count teetering at or below 200, Noé managed at last to get into the public ARV program in Bujumbura, which is able to provide drugs to fewer than seven thousand of the fifty thousand people who needed them by late 2006. His country remains peaceful but badly short of funds for reconstruction. CHRISTINE AMISI has 750 patients on ARVs in her clinic on the hill in Bukavu, where a fragile peace is holding. Tina gave birth to a fourth son in April 2006; three months later, Congo held its first democratic elections since 1960, a cause for tentative optimism. CYNTHIA LESHOMO fell critically ill with tuberculosis near the end of 2006; it appeared that her immune system was so damaged that even her faithful adherence to ARVs could no longer defeat the virus. MFANIMPELA THLABATSE died a month after I met him again. He had made several trips to the ARV clinic in the city but was always told to come back a few weeks later; he couldn't afford the transport and he never made it to the top of the waiting list. Siphiwe paid for his coffin. ANDUALEM AYALEW is out of work after years of activism; as the Ethiopian military geared up its official response to AIDS in 2006, it declined to use his one-man educational service any longer. He and his wife, Tigist, moved to an even smaller room outside Addis Ababa, and he resumed his hunt for paid employment. They are both in good health. ALICE KADZANJA's first-line ARVs began to fail her in early 2006, but she was able to switch to a new regimen through Dignitas International. The Dignitas project in Zomba, Malawi, of which she remains a key part, had two thousand people on treatment by the end of 2006 and was adding 150 more each month, a remarkable pace for a clinic anywhere. ZACKIE ACHMAT stepped down from the national leadership of the Treatment Action Campaign to work on documentary films and his own writing. He has a new boyfriend and a new dog and has taken up going to the gym. TAC is working with South Africa's government to expedite the expansion of treatment across the country. Young LEFA KHOELE is thriving on ARVs: he gained 8 kilograms in his first six months on the drugs and in September 2006 he began Grade 4. His grandmother Julia says he is unrecognizable as the child she first took to see Dr. Prinitha Pillay. The MSF project in his area enrolled 1,300 people into HIV care in its initial six months of operation. PONTIANO KALEEBU continues to run HIV vaccine trials in Entebbe. WINSTONE ZULU left Kara Counselling in mid-2006, after fifteen years with the group. He and a few friends from his earliest days of activism bought a farm outside Kabwe, Zambia, where they plan to teach new techniques to local subsistence farmers— because, he says, after all his years of lobbying for access to treatment, he realizes that many people don't have the food to eat with the drugs. Winstone is on second-line ARVs; his wife, Vivian, remains healthy without treatment. AGNES MUNYIVA is still HIV-negative, and still selling sex in Majengo. MPHO SEGOMELA'S grandmother Magdeline died three weeks after Mpho did. Her aunt Ellen remains ill but alive on ARVs, to which she gained eleventh-hour access with the help of nurse Rosina Letwaba. ANNE MUMBI'S Children in Distress centre adds a half-dozen new orphans to its rolls each week; she says that while neither the debt relief nor aid increases pledged by the G8 have yet had much discernible impact on Zambia, she remains optimistic. GIDEON BYAMUGISHA'S organization, ANERELA, is expanding its ranks of HIV-positive religious leaders; Gideon, in good heath, runs his parish outside Kampala and focuses on care for orphans. IDA MUKUKA remains the backbone of HIV counselling and support services in Zambia, and has now toured North America talking about her life with HIV. She is also well. MOROLAKE ODETOYINBO fulfilled a long-time dream in late 2006 when she gave birth to a healthy son, whose name, Eyilayomi, means "I have found my joy." She had access to the full range of HIV-prevention techniques in her pregnancy through the Nigerian public health system. She continues to direct the Nigerian branch of the Pan-African Treatment Access Movement in Lagos. She has yet to find a man of suitable calibre to consider as a husband. MOLEEN MUDIMU died of AIDS two weeks after I met her, in April 2006. Her husband, Benjamin, is in poor health and cannot afford ARVs. He is raising their sons alone. Zimbabwe continues its economic and political decline under Robert Mugabe; the UN is attempting to establish a multi-donor fund to procure ARVs directly for the public health service while withholding funds from the Mugabe government. IBRAHIM UMORU is thriving on protease inhibitors and continues both his counselling and lobbying activity with MSF. He is engaged to a woman he met at the AIDS clinic. NELSON MANDELA and Graça Machel remain, despite their retirement, committed advocates for people living with HIV/AIDS. THOKOZANI MTHIYANE is in good health in Johannesburg. He continues to write and paint, but has given up on the largely futile task of trying to teach me isiZulu.

I have not been able to find out what happened to MOHAMMED ALI, MANUEL COSSA or ANITA MANHIÇA.

In many vital ways, AIDS in Africa today looks very different than it did when I first began to report on the pandemic nine years ago.

First, on an epidemiological level, the disease appears to have peaked: the rate of new infections has hit its highest level, and has stabilized or even begun to decline in a few of the hardest-hit countries, such as Kenya and Zimbabwe. Of course, because of the way HIV works, that doesn't mean the worst of the impact is over—it will be years yet until the rate of deaths begins to decline, and in some countries, such as South Africa, it is still climbing. Epidemiologists extrapolate from the peak in the incidence rate in Africa, and a similar one in South Asia, that global HIV incidence has also hit its highest point. Part of the decline in the rate of new infections is likely the result of behaviour change—but ultimately it had to drop, because of, as an article in the medical journal The Lancet put it, "the diminishing number of those at most risk of acquisition of the virus as the epidemic matures." In other words, death.

While the rate of death has not declined, there is hope on this front as well. In late 2006 just over a million people in Africa were taking antiretrovirals—a tenfold increase since I began reporting on the pandemic (although still less than a quarter of those who need the drugs). The spread of treatment reflects the influence of the powerful international actors who have engaged with AIDS in the past few years. PEPFAR, the U.S. AIDS response, continues to be dogged by controversy over its emphasis on abstinence programs and reliance on brand-name drugs, but this debate has begun to fall away as African countries themselves choose to emphasize abstinence and the U.S. government purchases increasing amounts of generic medicines. PEPFAR had paid for or supported ARV treatment for nearly 900,000 people across the developing world by the end of 2006.

The Global Fund to Fight AIDS, Tuberculosis and Malaria has not proved to be the early success that AIDS activists had hoped. Its funding for AIDS programs moves through tortuous bureaucracy (although many of those layers of bureaucracy were, in a grim irony, instituted at the insistence of the U.S. government, which now criticizes the fund for being too slow). Many African AIDS organizations say the fund is a disappointment because it moves so slowly and its partnerships with national governments—rather than local groups—mean there are many opportunities for corruption. A handful of countries that receive Global Fund grants, including Kenya and Nigeria, have had those reviewed or suspended because of misuse of funds by staff at national AIDS programs. However, African groups retain the hope that these problems can be remedied, because the fund—with its global reach—remains the best hope for sustainable assistance in fighting AIDS. Some 500,000 people are receiving ARVS through the Global Fund.

There was a breakthrough in pediatric treatment in December 2006, when Bill Clinton negotiated a deal with the two main Indian generic-drug makers to produce a three-in-one dispersible first-line ARV tablet for kids for 16 cents a day; the former U.S. president said it would allow poor countries to treat hundreds of thousands more children, whose access to ARVs continues to lag far behind that of adults. The Clinton HIV/AIDS Initiative continues to be a powerful player in making treatment more accessible.

However, little progress has been made in lowering the prices of second-line drugs; they remain priced beyond the reach of most African programs, although the need for them is growing quickly. Equally grim, the tightening of patent laws under the World Trade Organization increasingly restricts access to the generic drugs on which most African treatment programs depend. Treatment-access groups say that at the current rate of expansion, the G8 will not meet its goal of universal access to treatment by 2010—rather than treating the ten million people in poor countries who need the drugs, AIDS programs will reach only half that number.

In the field of HIV prevention, there is new excitement about methods such as male circumcision. In December 2006, two trials, in Kenya and Uganda, found that circumcised men contracted HIV only half as often as men who had not been circumcised. But other important prevention methods—especially for women, who still struggle for sexual autonomy—remain elusive: a half-dozen microbicides are in phase III human trials for efficacy, but the first results will not be available until late 2007. And while trials of the most urgently needed product, an HIV vaccine, are expanding, a successful vaccine remains at least a decade away.

The funding gap continues to plague efforts to respond to the African pandemic. The United Nations says that while $20 billion is needed to fight AIDS in 2007, less than half of that will be available.

Each day in Africa, 5,500 people die of HIV/AIDS—a treatable, preventable illness. We have twenty-eight million reasons to act.

# GLOSSARY

ABC
The acronym given to a package of strategies to prevent HIV infection, first used in Uganda in the 1980s and today championed by UNAIDS and international donors, particularly the United States. It stands for Abstain (from sexual intercourse, and also implies delay of sexual debut); Be faithful (have sexual relations with only your regular partner or partners); and use Condoms (consistently and correctly).

ACT UP
The popular name for the AIDS Coalition To Unleash Power, a radical activist organization founded in Manhattan in 1987, which pioneered dramatic civil disobedience such as the "die-in" (where hundreds of activists lay on the ground feigning death outside government offices and pharmaceutical companies) to draw attention to government inaction and funding inequities.

ADHERENCE
Adherence refers to how closely one follows a treatment regimen—taking the correct dose of a drug at the correct time, exactly as prescribed. Failure to adhere to an anti-HIV treatment regimen can lead quickly to drug resistance and to illness, because the virus has the opportunity to reproduce during the gaps when doses are skipped. To suppress HIV effectively,

a person must be at least 90 per cent adherent, or take the drugs correctly 90 per cent of the time.

AIDS
The *A* stands for acquired. This means that the virus is not spread through casual or inadvertent contact, the way a germ like flu is. In order to be infected, people have to do something (or have something done to them) that exposes them to the virus. *I* and *D* stand for immunodeficiency. The virus attacks a person's immune system and makes it deficient, that is, less capable of fighting infections. *S* is for syndrome: AIDS is not one disease but rather presents itself as a number of diseases that attack as the immune system fails.

ARVs
Antiretroviral therapy (ART) uses antiretroviral (ARV) drugs to treat people living with HIV. These drugs inhibit the ability of the virus to reproduce in the body. They are most effective when used in combinations, which is called highly active antiretroviral therapy, or HAART.

AZT
The first antiretroviral drug to be approved by the U.S. Food and Drug Administration, in 1987. It had some success in suppressing HIV, although patients eventually grew resistant; combined with other ARVs, it is much more effective. It was first manufactured by GlaxoSmithKline, as Retrovir; the patent expired in 2005, and AZT is now widely marketed in generic form as zidovudine.

CD4 CELL
A white blood cell, or lymphocyte, that leads the body's attack against infections, named for the proteins called CD4 studded on its surface. HIV invades the cell by attaching to the CD4 receptor. During the incubation period, when a person is infected with HIV but still healthy, up to 5 per cent of the body's CD4 cells may be destroyed each day by the virus. In a

healthy person there are 1,200 CD4 cells per microlitre of blood. A person is said to have AIDS when his or her CD4 count is less than 200. Clinicians in Africa may diagnose AIDS based on a CD4 count, measuring the number of these cells; anyone with a CD4 count below 200 is at serious risk for opportunistic infections and should have ART.

## DISCORDANT
Not having the same HIV status. A discordant couple is a pair of long-term sexual partners in which one person is HIV-positive and the other is not.

## EPIDEMIC
A disease that has spread rapidly through a segment of the population in a given geographic area. Epidemic is a relative concept: a small absolute number of cases of a disease is considered an epidemic if the disease incidence is usually very low. In contrast, a disease (such as malaria) is considered endemic if it is continuously present in a population but at low or moderate levels.

## G8
The Group of Eight major industrial democracies, whose heads of state meet annually to discuss major global economic and political issues. The G6 was founded in 1975 by France, the United States, Britain, Germany, Japan and Italy. They were joined by Canada in 1976 to form the G7, and from 1991 by the USSR/Russia to form the G8.

## GENERIC DRUGS
Drugs come in two basic forms: proprietary (or brand-named) drugs that are developed and produced by large multinational pharmaceutical companies, and generic drugs that are either copies of or use the basic formula of a proprietary drug. Brand-name drugs are typically protected by patent for twenty years, after which other companies can produce the generic version. In countries without patent protection, companies can re-engineer (essentially, figure out the ingredients) of the brand-named drugs and produce them at any time. Generic drugs typically cost a fraction of the

price of the brand-named version. Generic ARVs, most from India, made ARV treatment in Africa possible.

## GLOBAL FUND

The Global Fund to Fight AIDS, Tuberculosis and Malaria was established in 2001 by the United Nations General Assembly Special Session on AIDS, after Secretary-General Kofi Annan and African heads of state called for a massive scale-up in resources to fight the three disease, which together kill more than six million people each year. The fund is an independent public–private partnership, primarily financed by rich-country governments. Countries with epidemics of any of the three diseases submit proposals to the fund for new mitigation programs, and the fund awards grants over the period of two to five years. By August 2006 the fund had committed $5.5 billion in 132 countries, but is chronically short of cash, as donors fail to deliver on promised pledges or to renew their funding.

## HIPC

The Heavily Indebted Poor Countries initiative was created in 1996 by the World Bank, out of a recognition that many developing nations had unsustainable and unpayable loads of debt to rich nations and international financial institutions. Under HIPC, the debtor nation could apply to have its debts suspended and eventually cancelled if it undertook a World Bank–approved program of economic reform and channelled the funds released into poverty reduction.

## HIV (HUMAN IMMUNODEFICIENCY VIRUS)

The virus that weakens the immune system, ultimately leading to AIDS. It is found in two types: HIV-1 is responsible for most HIV infections throughout the world; the more rare and less virulent HIV-2 is found primarily in West Africa.

## NEVIRAPINE

Approved in the U.S. in 1996, nevirapine is an ARV drug patented by Boehringer-Ingelheim (marketed as Viramune). It is used in combination with other drugs as part of an ARV regimen. Delivered in a single dose on its own to a woman in labour, and to a newborn, it can significantly lower the risk that a mother with HIV will infect her child.

## OPPORTUNISTIC INFECTIONS

Conditions not typically seen in people with healthy immune systems but which can cause serious disease when the immune system is weakened. Persons living with advanced HIV infection may suffer opportunistic infections of the lungs, brain, eyes and other organs. Opportunistic illnesses common in Africans with AIDS include *Pneumocystis carinii* pneumonia (PCP), the skin cancer Kaposi's sarcoma, candidiasis and tuberculosis.

## PANDEMIC

A pandemic refers to an epidemic of worldwide proportions—outbreaks of infectious disease that affect people all over the world, such as influenza in 1918 or AIDS today.

## PEPFAR

The U.S. President's Emergency Plan for AIDS Relief. Announced by President George W. Bush in 2003, the plan is a five-year, $15-billion initiative to provide AIDS prevention, care and treatment in some of the worst-hit countries, the bulk of which are in Africa. While dogged by criticism for politically driven programming such as funding abstinence education and using brand-name drugs rather than generics, PEPFAR has nonetheless been successful at rapidly disbursing funds and helping to scale-up programs in Africa. In its first three and a half years, it paid for or supported ARV treatment for 822,000 people; HIV testing and counselling for 18.7 million people; care for three million AIDS orphans; and interventions to prevent an estimated 101,500 transmissions of HIV between pregnant women and their babies.

## PMTCT

Stands for prevention of mother-to-child transmission, also referred to as parent-to-child transmission. A pregnant woman with HIV has odds as high as 50 per cent of transmitting the virus to her baby. Roughly a third of the infections are passed in utero; a third from the exchange of blood and fluids during delivery; and a third in breastfeeding. By using a combination of interventions (ideally, ARV therapy for the mother from 28 weeks gestation, a Caesarean delivery and substituting formula feeding for breastfeeding), the risk of infecting the child can be lowered to about 2 per cent. PMTCT+ refers to programs that include ARV treatment for mothers afterwards so that they can stay healthy and care for their children.

## PREVALENCE

HIV prevalence refers to the total number of infections at a particular point in time. Prevalence is usually presented as a percentage of adult population—so, for example, a 20 per cent HIV prevalence means that one in five adults are infected. HIV incidence refers to the number of people who have become infected with HIV during a specified period.

## RESISTANCE

Some micro-organisms, such as bacteria, viruses and parasites, can adapt so that they can multiply even in the presence of drugs that would normally kill them. As HIV replicates in the body, it mutates, and the new forms it takes can be impervious to drugs that previously succeeded in suppressing it.

## RETROVIRUS

HIV is a type of pathogen known as a retrovirus, the first of which was identified in the 1970s. A retrovirus consists of two strands of RNA, and once inside a host cell, they make DNA copies of their own RNA, preventing the cell from carrying out its natural function and instead turning it into a factory to make new viruses. This, plus the ability of the virus to mutate rapidly, makes it difficult to treat with drugs.

### SEROCONVERSION

The point at which the body begins to produce antibodies to a pathogen. With HIV, this occurs a few weeks to a few months after infection and is often marked by flu-like symptoms. (The most commonly used and inexpensive HIV test looks for antibodies and is ineffective before sero-conversion occurs; an infected person tested this way before seroconversion will test negative.)

### SIDA

The French, Spanish and Portuguese acronym for AIDS.

### TRIPs AGREEMENT

The Trade-Related Aspects of Intellectual Property Rights is an agreement drawn up by the World Trade Organization to ensure intellectual property rights are respected within international trade. It came into force on January 1, 1995. The agreement means that WTO member nations cannot produce generic versions of AIDS drugs—although eventually an agreement was reached that a country with a public health emergency could issue a "compulsory licence" and override some drug patents.

### VCT

Abbreviation for voluntary counselling and testing. This is widely viewed as the most appropriate way to do HIV testing in Africa—with pre- and post-test counselling, with a guarantee of confidentiality and with informed consent. The approach originated in the North American and European epidemics, where the first infected groups were gay men and drug users who, it was thought, would not otherwise seek testing.

### VECTOR

The Latin word for "bearer"; in epidemiology it refers to a person who carries a disease. In vaccinology, it refers to a harmless virus or bacteria used to deliver pieces of a disease-causing organism (such as HIV) into the body's cells in order to stimulate a protective immune response.

## Viral load

The amount of HIV in a blood sample. A viral load count measures the amount of HIV in an infected person's system. A person on successful ART will have a viral load that shows as "undetectable." U.S. treatment guidelines suggest that anyone with a viral load over 100,000 should be offered treatment.

# HOW YOU CAN HELP

The most valuable thing that you can do to fight the AIDS pandemic in Africa is talk about it. There has, in the past year or two, been a swell of interest at a grassroots level, and international stars and philanthropists have taken up the cause. But the crisis continues to fail to draw the political and financial response it merits because too few people in the West yet understand or care about what is happening.

That said, many people who do know what's happening in Africa want to help. I hear from a couple of dozen of them every week, and most of them ask me one of three questions.

First, people want to go to Africa to help in a hands-on way, and they ask me to suggest a community or organization they can assist. It's a commendable idea, but not always the best solution. I have seen how volunteering in Africa can be a fantastic experience for volunteers, but often a less than terrific one for the project or community they join, which may pay a high price for the skills the volunteers bring. However well-intentioned, Western volunteers can be a drain on the communities they go to help: if they don't speak the language, they cannot assist with education or AIDS awareness, and usually they don't have the particular skills that are needed (for the perfectly good reason that most of us rarely need such skills in our home countries: when was the last time you dug a borehole?). All too often, the already overburdened and under-resourced community that the volunteers want to help ends up translating for them, figuring out their housing and food needs, and taking them to the expensive clinic in the city when they get malaria or jiggers or dysentery.

If you are a physician, nurse, midwife or pharmacist with expertise in AIDS care, then many African governments may be glad to have you. But otherwise, it may be that the most useful thing you can do is education and advocacy work at home. The Doctors Without Borders Access to Essential Medicines Campaign, for example, or Debt, AIDS, Trade Africa (DATA) have good suggestions on how you can raise awareness on important issues such as access to AIDS treatment and the impact of unfair trade laws. Is talking about trade barriers as interesting as going to live in a Kenyan village? No. But trade law is tremendously important, and letters to your Member of Parliament or Congress do make a difference. If your real desire is to be of help, rather than to see the world, then that's the place to start.

Second, there is the question of donations. Many people want to know how to send *stuff* to Africa: medical supplies, soccer balls, textbooks. I tell them that instead they should send money: the shipping costs and customs duties on anything sent from North America or Europe typically far exceed the value of the actual goods. A Tanzanian AIDS group can't afford to pay the import tax. And often, the items people propose to send are in any case available right there in Tanzania—the issue is that people can't afford to buy them. It is much more effective to send money and let the group buy the school books or latex gloves themselves. They can make the decisions about what they most urgently need, and the local economy gets a boost, too.

The third question I hear is from people who want to know how to send money directly to one grandmother, or to one community group. I certainly understand that: we've all heard stories about waste, mismanagement and corruption within big charities, UN agencies and governments. It is much more appealing to think of helping one granny pay school fees than to put your donation into a giant UNICEF pot. Unfortunately, this idea is rarely practical. In many of the places worst hit by AIDS, there are no banks and there is no postal system. How are the Zambian grandmothers going to receive your donation—and what will they do with a cheque in euros or Canadian dollars?

Following is a list of international charities whose work in Africa I have personally been impressed by, and groups—founded by or working with the people in this book—that are able to receive international funds through bank transfers or a service such as Western Union. Money, of course, is desperately needed. These are great places to send it.

## AIDS CARE AND TREATMENT ORGANIZATIONS IN AFRICA

### CHILDREN IN DISTRESS

www.cindi.org.zm
PO Box 21663
Kitwe, Zambia
tel. +260.2.229.369

### DIGNITAS INTERNATIONAL

www.dignitasinternational.org
P.O. Box 145
40 Dundas St. West, Suite 323
Toronto, Ontario M5G 2C2
Canada
tel. +1.416.260.3100

### GRANDMOTHERS TO GRANDMOTHERS CAMPAIGN

c/o The Stephen Lewis Foundation
www.stephenlewisfoundation.org
260 Spadina Ave., Suite 501
Toronto, Ontario M5T 2E4
Canada
tel. +1.416.533.9292

KARA COUNSELLING
   www.kara.org.zm
   P.O Box 37559
   Lusaka, Zambia
   tel. +260.1.229.847/222.776

NELSON MANDELA FOUNDATION
   www.nelsonmandela.org
   Private Bag X 70 000
   Houghton 2041
   South Africa
   tel. +27.11.728.1000

PAN-AFRICAN TREATMENT ACCESS MOVEMENT
   www.patam.org

STOP-SIDA (BURUNDI)
   www.stop-sida.org

SWAZILAND POSITIVE LIVING
   www.swapol.net
   P.O. Box 2030
   Manzini, Swaziland
   tel. +268.505.7088

THE AIDS SUPPORT ORGANIZATION OF UGANDA (TASO)
   www.tasouganda.org
   Old Mulago Complex
   P.O. Box 10443
   Kampala, Uganda
   tel. +256.41.532.580/1

TREATMENT ACTION CAMPAIGN (TAC)
www.tac.org.za
34 Main Road
Muizenberg 7945
South Africa
tel. +27.21.788.3507

# INTERNATIONAL AGENCIES

CARE (UK)
http://www.care.org.uk
CARE
53 Romney Street
London SW1P 3RF
UK
tel. +44 (0)20 7233 0455

CLINTON HIV/AIDS INITIATIVE
www.clintonfoundation.org
The William Jefferson Clinton Foundation
55 West 125th St.
New York, NY 10027
USA

THE GLOBAL FUND TO FIGHT AIDS, TUBERCULOSIS
AND MALARIA
www.theglobalfund.org
Chemin de Blandonnet 8
1214 Vernier
Geneva, Switzerland
tel. +41.22.791.17.00

MÉDECINS SANS FRONTIÈRES (UK)
    http://www.msf.org/unitedkingdom
    67–74 Saffron Hill
    London EC1N 8QX
    UK
    tel. +44 (0)20 7404 6600

OXFAM (UK)
    http://www.oxfam.org.uk
    Oxfam (Head Office)
    Oxham House
    John Smith Drive
    Cowley
    Oxford OX4 2JY
    tel. +44 (0)870 333 2700

# ADVOCACY FOR AIDS IN AFRICA

ACCESS TO ESSENTIAL MEDICINES
    www.accessmed-msf.org

AIDS VACCINE ADVOCACY COALITION
    www.avac.org
    101 West 23rd St., #2227
    New York, NY 10011
    USA
    tel. +1.212.367.1279

DATA: DEBT, AIDS, TRADE IN AFRICA
    www.data.org
    1400 Eye St. NW, Suite 1125
    Washington, DC 20005
    USA
    tel. +1.202.639.8010

FRIENDS OF THE GLOBAL FIGHT
    www.theglobalfight.org
    901 15th St. NW, Suite 410
    Washington, DC 20005
    USA
    tel. +1.202.789.0801

GLOBAL CAMPAIGN FOR MICROBICIDES
    www.global-campaign.org
    c/o PATH
    1800 K Street NW
    Washington, DC 20006
    USA
    tel. +1.202.822.0033

MAKE POVERTY HISTORY
    www.makepovertyhistory.org

MAKE TRADE FAIR
    www.maketradefair.org

AVERT
www.avert.org
4 Brighton Rd.
Horsham, West Sussex
RH13 5BA UK

INTERNATIONAL AIDS
VACCINE INITIATIVE (IAVI)
www.iavi.org
110 William Street, Floor 27
New York, NY 10038–3901
USA
tel. +1.212.847.1111

INTERNATIONAL PARTNERSHIP
FOR MICROBICIDES
www.ipm-microbicides.org
1010 Wayne Ave., Suite 1450
Silver Spring, MD 20910
USA
tel. +1.301.608.2221

RESULTS UK
http://www.results-uk.org
25 Clemens Street
Leamington Spa CV31 2DP
UK
tel. +44 (0)1926 435 430

STOP TB PARTNERSHIP
www.stoptb.org
tel. +41.22.791.4650

UNAIDS
www.unaids.org
20, avenue Appia
CH-1211 Geneva 27
Switzerland
tel. +41.22.791.3666

UNITED NATIONS
VOLUNTEERS
www.unv.org
Postfach 260 111
D-53153 Bonn
Germany
tel. +49.228.815.2000

WORLD HEALTH
ORGANIZATION
www.who.int/hiv/en/
Department of HIV/AIDS
20, Avenue Appia
CH-1211 Geneva 27
Switzerland

# BIBLIOGRAPHY

Abdool Karim, S. S., and Q. Abdool Karim. *HIV/AIDS in South Africa.* Cambridge: Cambridge University Press, 2005.

Amnesty International. *Marked for Death: Rape Survivors Living with HIV/AIDS in Rwanda.* London: April 6, 2004.

Barnett, Tony, and Alan Whiteside. *AIDS in the Twenty-First Century: Disease and Globalization.* New York: Palgrave Macmillan, 2002.

Behrman, Greg. *The Invisible People: How the U.S. Has Slept Through the Global AIDS Pandemic, the Greatest Humanitarian Catastrophe of Our Time.* New York: Free Press, 2004.

Bergstrom, Ida. "A Second Life." *African Woman* (Kampala), April 2006.

Cameron, Edwin. *Witness to AIDS.* Cape Town: NB Tafelberg, 2005.

Chen, Lincoln, and Helen Epstein. "Can AIDS Be Stopped?" *The New York Review of Books,* March 14, 2002.

Chirwa, Wiseman Chijere. "Malawian Migrant Labour and the Politics of HIV/AIDS, 1985 to 1993." In Jonathan Crush and Wilmot James, *Crossing Boundaries: Mine Migrancy in a Democratic South Africa.* Cape Town: Institute for Democracy in South Africa, 1995.

Conover, Ted. "Trucking through the AIDS Belt." *The New Yorker,* August 16, 1993.

Crush, Jonathan. "Contract Migration to South Africa: Past, Present and Future." Briefing for the Green Paper Task Team on International Migration, Pretoria, 1997.

D'Adesky, Anne-Christine. *Moving Mountains: The Race to Treat Global AIDS.* London: Verso, 2004.

De Cock, Kevin, et al. "Shadow on the Continent: Public Health and HIV/AIDS in Africa in the 21st Century." *The Lancet,* July 6, 2002.

Debt, AIDS, Trade Africa. *The DATA Report 2006.* Washington, June 2006.

Epstein, Helen. "The Hidden Cause of AIDS." *The New York Review of Books,* May 9, 2002.

——"The Mystery of AIDS in South Africa." *The New York Review of Books,* July 20, 2000.

Epstein, Helen, and Daniel Halperin. "Concurrent Sexual Partnerships Help to Explain HIV Prevalence: Implications for Prevention." *The Lancet,* July 3, 2004.

Farmer, Paul. *Infections and Inequalities: The Modern Plagues.* Berkeley: University of California Press, 1999.

Feldbaum, Harley, et al. "The National Security Implications of HIV-AIDS." *PLoS Medicine,* June 2006.

Garrett, Laurie. *Betrayal of Trust: The Collapse of Global Public Health.* New York: Hyperion, 2000.

—— *The Coming Plague: Newly Emerging Diseases in a World Out of Balance.* New York: Penguin Books, 1994.

Gill, Peter. *Body Count: How They Turned AIDS into a Catastrophe.* Johannesburg: Jonathan Ball Publishers, 2006.

Global Movement for Children. *Saving Lives: Children's Right to HIV and AIDS Treatment.* London, 2006.

Greene, Melissa Fay. *There Is No Me Without You.* New York: Bloomsbury, 2006.

Gumede, William Mervin. *Thabo Mbeki and the Battle for the Soul of the ANC.* Cape Town: Zebra Press, 2005.

Hallett, T. B., and G. P. Garnett. "Has Global HIV Incidence Peaked?" *The Lancet,* August 7, 2006.

HelpAge International. *AIDS: The Frontline.* London, November 2005.

Hooper, Edward. *The River: A Journey Back to the Source of HIV and AIDS.* London: Penguin Books, 1999.

Hunter, Susan. *Black Death: AIDS in Africa.* New York: Palgrave Macmillan, 2003.

Iliffe, John. *A History of the African AIDS Epidemic.* Cape Town: Double Storey Books, 2006.

Kahn, Patricia, ed. *AIDS Vaccine Handbook: Global Perspectives.* New York: AIDS Vaccine Advocacy Coalition, 2005.

Kalipeni, Ezekiel, et al., eds. *HIV and AIDS in Africa: Beyond Epidemiology.* Malden: Blackwell Publishing, 2004.

Kidder, Tracy. *Mountains Beyond Mountains.* New York: Random House, 2004.

Kasambala, Tiseke, and Joseph Amon. *No Bright Future: Government Failures, Human Rights Abuses and Squandered Progress in the Fight against AIDS in Zimbabwe.* London: Human Rights Watch, 2006.

Lewis, Stephen. *Race Against Time.* Toronto: House of Anansi Press, 2005.

Lurie, Mark, et al. "The Impact of Migration on HIV-1 Transmission in South Africa." *Sexually Transmitted Diseases,* vol. 30, no. 2 (2003).

Lurie, Mark, et al. "Who Infects Whom? HIV-1 Concordance and Discordance among Migrant and Non-migrant Couples in South Africa." *AIDS 2003,* vol. 17, no. 15.

McGregor, Liz. *Khabzela.* Johannesburg: Jacana Media, 2005.

Mishra, Vinod. "Patterns of HIV Seroprevalence and Associated Risk Factors (Evidence from the Demographic and Health Surveys and AIDS Indicator Surveys)." Presentation to PEPFAR annual meeting, Durban, 2006.

Oxfam. "The View from the Summit—Gleneagles G8 One Year On." Oxford, June 2006.

Peterson, Susan, and Stephen Shellman. "AIDS and Violent Conflict: The Indirect Effects of Disease on National Security." 2006. http://mjtier.people.wm.edu/intlpolitics/security/papers.php.

Poku, Nana, and Alan Whiteside. *The Political Economy of AIDS in Africa.* London: Ashgate Publishing, 2004.

Power, Samantha. "The AIDS Rebel." *The New Yorker,* May 19, 2003.

Sachs, Jeffrey. *The End of Poverty.* New York: Penguin, 2005.

Schoofs, Mark. "All That Glitters: How HIV Caught Fire in South Africa: Sex and the Migrant Worker." *The Village Voice,* April 28, 1999.

—— "Debating the Obvious: Inside the South African Government's Controversial AIDS Panel." *The Village Voice,* July 5, 2000.

—— "Proof Positive: How African Science Has Demonstrated That HIV Causes AIDS." *The Village Voice,* July 5, 2000.

—— "Lost Opportunity: South African President Hedges on Cause of AIDS, Ignores Access to Medicine." *The Village Voice,* July 12, 2000.

Shelton, James D., et al. "Is Poverty or Wealth at the Root of HIV?" *The Lancet,* September 24, 2005.

Singh, Amarnath. "Zackie Achmat: Light on the Meaning of Life." Johannesburg *Financial Mail,* May 7, 2004.

Spector, Michael. "The Vaccine: Has the Race to Save Africa from AIDS Put Western Science at Odds with Western Ethics?" *The New Yorker,* February 3, 2003.

Treatment Action Campaign. "Equal Treatment: The Science of HIV/AIDS." Cape Town, March 2006.

United Nations Development Program. "The Impact of HIV/AIDS on Human Resources in the Malawi Public Sector." Lilongwe, February 2002.

# ACKNOWLEDGMENTS

There are no words for my gratitude to the twenty-eight people who trusted me to tell their stories in this book. I am the very fortunate beneficiary of their wisdom, their courage and their generosity.

Hundreds of other people, in my nine years of reporting in Africa, have helped with translation and logistics and understanding the stories, and I am grateful for their assistance and their patience.

Many of the stories and ideas in this book began as articles for *The Globe and Mail,* and I have been graced with editors who took the unlikely step of sending me to Africa to report on AIDS at a time when the issue barely registered on the North American news agenda. My thanks and admiration to Philip Crawley, Edward Greenspon, John Stackhouse and Stephen Northfield.

My brilliant agent, Jackie Kaiser, helped me figure out how to tell this story, and I am grateful for her guidance. I have an extraordinary team of publishers: George Gibson at Walker Books in the United States, Laura Barber at Portobello Books in the United Kingdom, Britta Egetemeier at Piper in Germany, Haye Koningsveld at Ambo Anthos in Holland, Michael Heyward at Text Publishing in Australia, Oyvind Arneberg at Arneberg in Norway, Martina Wachendorff at Actes Sud in France and Lise Bergevin at Leméac in Quebec have all been unwavering in their enthusiasm, while my heartfelt thanks go to the incomparable Louise Dennys at Knopf Canada, who has championed *28* and whose graceful and insightful editing made it a much better book. I am immensely fortunate to be published by Louise and her crack team at Knopf, including Adrienne Phillips, Deirdre Molina, Scott Sellers and Scott Richardson.

David Tu, Brian Brink, Alan Ronald, Paul Spiegel, Andrew Chadwick and Pontiano Kaleebu all read parts of this book and helped me to avoid the worst errors. Paula Donovan, Stephen Lewis, James Fraser, James Lorenz and Lucy Matthew, all of whom are passionately engaged in the fight against AIDS, have also been generous with their assistance in my travels. John Morstad, whose portraits grace this book, has shared many of my most enlightening African adventures.

Anurita Bains, Ngaire Blankenberg and Lynn Heinisch were insightful early readers. Sisonke Msimang has talked me through many aspects of the pandemic and the book is better for her friendship. David and Tamara Rasmussen provided shelter for writing; Jen McDonald and Aran Rasmussen, great support. Marney McDiarmid was a source of wisdom, inspiration and faith; she makes many things possible. My family—Barbara, Brad and Amy Nolen—offered great encouragement.

My son, Darragh, thoughtfully delayed his entry into the world until a few days after I wrote these final words. And my partner, Meril Rasmussen, has lived these stories alongside me; he helps me write better, makes my life better, in infinite ways.

Johannesburg, 2007

# INDEX

chlamydia, 245–46
Christianity, history of in Africa, 278–79
CINDI. *See* Children in Distress
(CINDI)
Cipla Ltd., 109–10
circumcision (male), 378
Clermont, South Africa, 358
Clinton, William J., 15, 186, 219, 352, 377
coal mining, 123
colonialism, AIDS and, 12
Como, Italy, 231
concurrent sexual networks, 14, 172, 359
condoms, 379
forbidden use of, 98, 280, 283
ignorance about, 23, 157–58
made easily available, 38, 49, 102, 130,
161, 217, 241, 246, 252, 283
their role in delaying microbicides, 304
unavailability of, 52, 112, 210, 261
unwillingness to use, 14, 50, 52–53, 65,
95, 139, 142, 171, 174, 205, 247, 253,
296, 300, 358–59
Congo. *See* Democratic Republic of the
Congo (D. R. C.)
Coping Centre for People Living with
HIV/AIDS, 142
copper mining, 123
Corridors of Hope (project), 49
corruption among social and civil servants,
13–14, 31, 51, 185, 259, 261, 265–68,
377
Cossa, Manuel, 121–32, 376
cotrimoxizole, 131, 203
cryptococcal meningitis, 77, 83, 114

Dakar, 47
Dar es Salaam, 47
DATA (Debt, AIDS, Trade Africa), 388,
393
debt (national)
pernicious effects due to, 13, 262–63,
268–70, 292, 351
promised cancellations of, 269–70, 353
dementia, 81, 77
Democratic Republic of the Congo
(D.R.C.), 8, 12, 105–6, 111–18, 267, 374

denial of HIV infection/prevalence/risks,
61, 168, 186–87, 196, 293, 322, 359,
363, 369. *See also* AIDS: "dissidents"/
deniers of
diamond mining, 123, 137
diarrhea, 1, 7, 58, 62–63, 65, 129, 140, 154,
191, 200, 203, 230, 290
dictators (African), 12, 39, 151, 173, 269,
317
Diflucan (drug), 182, 189
Dignitas International, 173, 176–77, 374,
389
divorce, cultural unacceptability of, 40,
176, 313–14
Dlamini, Gugu, 182
Dlamini, Siphiwe, 22
Dlamini-Zuma, Nkosazana, 184
Doctors Without Borders (MSF), 105,
107–18, 175, 190, 205, 316, 334–35,
375–76, 388, 392
Driefontein gold mine, 129
drug companies. *See individual organizational*
*names, e.g.* Pfizer Inc.
marketing practices of, 17–18, 184, 352
*See also* AIDS: drug therapy for; patent
law
drug regimes, adherence to, 110. *See also*
HIV: drug resistance of
Duesberg, Peter, 232–33
Durban, South Africa, 47

East London, South Africa, 81
Ebola (virus), 5
efavirenz, 207
Eritrea, 152, 161
Erwin, Alec, 190
Ethiopia, 36–39, 151–53, 161
culture of, 39–40

Family Health Trust (Zambia), 228
Fowke, Keith, 247–50
Front for the Liberation of Mozambique
(FRELIMO), 122, 128

Gaborone, Botswana, 135
Gachit, Ethiopia, 151–52